HEALTH
in the
later years

HEALTH
in the
later years

Armeda F. Ferrini
California State University–Chico
with
Rebecca L. Ferrini

Copyright © 1989 by Wm. C. Brown Publishers. All rights reserved

Library of Congress Catalog Card Number: 87–070668

ISBN 0–697–00311–6

Printed in the United States of America by Wm. C. Brown Publishers
2460 Kerper Boulevard, Dubuque, IA 52001

10 9 8 7 6 5 4 3 2 1

Contents

Preface

The projected increase in the number and proportion of older people in the United States makes the study of aging relevant to everyone. Courses on aging are now commonly taught on college campuses as more students desire to learn about elders. Courses on aging and health are particularly in demand, as health is a paramount concern to those growing old, those who work with them, and society as a whole.

This text is designed for use in courses on health and aging for upper-division college students. Students enrolled in these courses usually come from diverse backgrounds, including biology, medicine, dietetics, social work, psychology, sociology, and recreation, among others. Some students are preparing to work with older people, others are primarily wishing to learn how to age successfully. The text is intended to meet the needs of both populations. The text is also appropriate for graduate students and professionals who desire continuing education in health and aging.

The health topics addressed in this text provide a broad overview of health and aging. Chapters discuss the major topics relevant to personal health, health-related issues of concern to those working with elders, and psychosocial and political factors which affect elders' health. To meet the needs of students with little health background, basic health principles are included as well as their application to older people. Facts are amply referenced to enable advanced students to study health issues in more depth. The text also includes boxed inserts and exercises to personalize the learning process.

The authors wish to acknowledge the following persons who have played a part in development of the final manuscript: Marilynn E. Koerber, Lowman Home; Ruth Ann Althaus, Illinois Benedictine College; Richard W. Wilson, Western Kentucky University; Sherman K. Sowby, California State University, Fresno; Susan J. Eklund, Indiana University; Carolyn Plonsky, St. Francis College; Susan Radius, Towson State University; and Linda C. Campanelli, The National Council on the Aging, Inc.

Studying the Health of Elders

Old and young, we are all on our last cruise.

Robert Louis Stevenson

Introduction

Before initiating the study of the many issues of health in the later years, it is important that students become familiar with the terminology and research methods used by those who study aging. This chapter will present common methods that researchers use to collect information about elders and the aging process. The importance of the study of aging and health on both a personal and professional level will also be addressed.

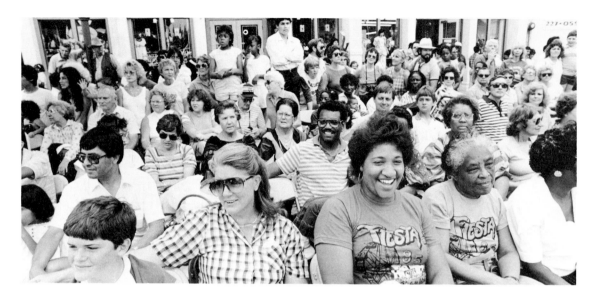

How Old Is Old?

Although death and taxes are said to be inevitable, living to be old is not. It is only in the last century that a significant number of people have lived long enough to become "old."

The definition of *old* varies over time. Today, we consider age sixty-five or so to be old, whereas two hundred years ago, age fifty might have been considered old. Further, the definition of *old* varies according to the age of the person being asked. A child may consider someone over twenty old, a teenager may think forty is over the hill, and a sixty year old may consider seventy as elderly. In essence, old is often thought of as an age beyond one's own. Most elders do not consider themselves old until they become sick or dependent upon others.

The process of aging is a complex, continuous process that begins at maturity and continues until death. It is difficult to define the ages of childhood, middle age, or older adulthood. For consistency, *chronological age* is typically used. Age sixty-five has traditionally been used to define the beginning of old age because this is the age of full retirement benefits from Social Security in

the United States. However, some gerontologists make distinctions between the young-old (sixty-five–seventy-four) and the old-old (seventy-five and above) because there are often significant differences between these groups. Generally, the young-old are more vigorous, have higher incomes, are more likely to be married, and have fewer health problems than the old-old. However, even these divisions are not absolute. Some elders are in extremely good health well into old age while some individuals in mid-life exhibit many disabilities and illnesses. For this reason, many gerontologists distinguish chronological or numerical age, from *functional age,* the physiological capacity of the body. Thus, a marathon runner may have a chronological age of eighty, but physiologically function as well as a forty-year-old. Further, we all know individuals who psychologically and socially grow old before their time; for example, individuals who use their age as an excuse for inactivity, dependence, and disengagement from society. In a sense, these individuals have died before their bodies. Without a doubt, *sociological* or *psychological* age is also an important part of aging.

Definition of an Elder

 An Elder is a person who is still growing, still a learner, still with potential and whose life continues to have within it promise for, and connection to the future. An Elder is still in pursuit of happiness, joy and pleasure, and her or his birthright to these remains intact. Moreover, an Elder is a person who deserves respect and honor and whose work it is to synthesize wisdom from long life experience and formulate this into a legacy for future generations.

The Live Oak Project

Despite these caveats, the definition of old used in this text is the chronological age of sixty-five and older because most data are available in this form. When available, information on age sub-groups will be included.

Many and varied terms have been used to describe older people: senior citizens, golden agers, retired persons, mature adults, elderly, aged, old people. There is no clear preference among older people for any of these terms. For instance, some people grimace at being called a senior citizen while others like the term. Many gerontologists have chosen to adopt the term *elder* to describe those age sixty-five and older. This term is an attempt to redefine aging in a more positive way that connotes wisdom, respect, leadership, and accumulated knowledge. This text will use *elder* to reflect that attitude. The term *older people* will also be utilized to describe those sixty-five and older. This term makes it clear that aging is a continuum with older people at one end and younger people at the other.

The Study of Aging

Gerontology is the term used to describe the study of aging. The word gerontology comes from the Greek terms *geron* and *-ontus,* which means "old man." Gerontology is a multidisciplinary field with a major focus on the biological, behavioral, and social sciences. However, gerontology may be applied to such diverse areas as anthropology, history, literature, and economics.

The term *geriatrics* refers to the medical care of older people. In contrast to gerontology, geriatrics is primarily concerned with changes that occur with age as a result of disease. Geriatricians, physicians who specialize in the medical care of elders, and geriatric nurses are the more common medical professionals with specialties in meeting the medical needs of elders.

Because the number and proportion of elders are expanding rapidly in the United States, both gerontology and geriatrics will become increasingly important as society looks to these experts for guidance regarding social and public policy changes, medical care innovations, and future direction of health services to meet this increasing consumer pool.

Methods to Collect Information

In order to learn more about older people, gerontologists must gather unbiased information. This section will discuss the four most common methods used to collect data on aging: laboratory experiments, field experiments, field studies, and survey research.

In a laboratory experiment, the researcher can isolate what is to be studied by limiting the effect of extraneous variables. For instance, if a researcher wants to isolate the effects of low light on reading ability, other factors that might affect reading ability (e.g., background noise, size of print) could be controlled except the level of light intensity. However, these studies are conducted in an artificial environment and the results may not be applicable to real life. The subjects' knowledge that they are in a laboratory situation can cause alterations in behavior, especially among elders. For instance, an older person may perform more poorly on an intelligence test in the laboratory than at home because of the anxiety induced by the artificial environment.

Laboratory experiments may also be conducted on animals. These experiments allow the investigator to perform experiments that may be unethical or impractical with human subjects. Because laboratory animals have short life spans, studies can be concluded more quickly. For instance, researchers can manipulate weight, lifetime diet, body temperature, or genetics to see the effect on aging in one to two years, rather than seventy or so. Animals can be injected with drugs, deprived of sleep, have organ implants, or be sacrificed to examine organs—techniques that are impossible to use on humans. However, the biggest drawback to animal studies is that the results may not be generalized to humans.

Field experiments are similar to laboratory experiments except that these experiments are conducted in a natural environment. The field experiment manipulates a selected variable, while keeping others constant, to determine the effect of one particular variable. For instance, researchers might offer weekly lectures on accident prevention at a senior center to a select group of participants and offer no such service to another group (the control). After a certain number of weeks of educational seminars, the researchers may determine the frequency of accidents in both groups and conclude that the educational presentations were or were not effective in reducing accidents. This type of study may be more effective than laboratory studies because they are conducted in more natural situations; however, many variables cannot be controlled in the field. For instance, in the study described above, the researchers cannot be sure that the accident risk decreased because of the information presented in the seminars, or because the participants' interest in accident prevention stimulated them to read more material on accident prevention and discuss the topic with friends and family.

In field studies, no variables are manipulated. Researchers seek to uncover the relationship (or correlation) between variables in the natural setting by observing, questioning, and interviewing subjects to find correlations between certain variables. For instance, a researcher may interview elders in a senior center who do not visit their physicians regularly. Asking them questions about their health, financial situation, and view of physicians, the researchers would try to determine if any of these variables are correlated with the tendency to underutilize medical care. These experiments are helpful because they use natural settings. However, they are limited by the types of questions asked. Further, these studies are often misinterpreted. Just because two factors are correlated, does not mean that one causes the other. For instance, because older people with low incomes often underutilize medical care does not mean that poverty causes underutilization of services. Other variables, such as self-reliance, physician attitudes, motivation, availability of transportation, or knowledge of available health services may be more closely related than income.

Survey research commonly uses personal interviews, written questionnaires, or phone interviews to collect data on the incidence, distribution, and interrelationships of psychological and social variables. Survey research utilizes large or small population groups by selecting random samples that ideally represent the population as a whole. A good example of survey research is the National Health Interview Survey in which a large

Introduction

sample of elders were asked to report on several of their health habits. This type of study is advantageous because a great number of people can be surveyed. However, like all methods that use interviewing, the respondents may not remember or may adapt answers to please the interviewer. Another disadvantage is that the sample that responds to the survey may not be generalizeable to all older people but may only represent a subgroup, such as those who are motivated or literate. For instance, those who responded to the Starr-Weiner study on elder sexuality may have been more open, sexually active, or willing to discuss sexuality than the rest of the elder population.

Another type of survey research involves the reanalysis of existing records. In these types of studies, researchers utilize data from public documents and previously collected statistics, such as the United States Census Bureau, to uncover new connections.

Cross-Sectional and Longitudinal Approaches

One of the most salient issues in the study of aging is ascertaining which proportion of changes are due to age and which are due to other factors. For instance, gerontologists who want to determine the effect of age upon function of a particular body system need to distinguish the effects of aging itself from other variables (e.g., poor nutrition, physical inactivity, chronic illness, cigarette smoking). All research attempting to distinguish the effect of age on particular variables utilizes either cross-sectional or longitudinal methodology.

In a cross-sectional approach, the researcher draws a sample of individuals from different age groups and collects data on the presence of a certain trait. After the data are collected, the various groups can be compared to ascertain differences and similarities among the groups. For example, a cross-sectional study might measure attitudes about death across age groups by examining three age groups: twenty to thirty-nine year olds, forty to fifty-nine year olds, and those age sixty to eighty. The researchers then compare the data obtained for each group. In another example, to determine whether height is lost with advanced age researchers may collect height data on various age groups and compare the averages to determine if elders lose inches in stature.

Cross-sectional analyses have many advantages and disadvantages. They can be accomplished over relatively short time periods and are less expensive than longitudinal analyses. The limitations of cross-sectional research can be illustrated using the two examples outlined above. In the first, an alternative conclusion from the data would be that elders are more apt to talk about death because they have more recent experience with the deaths of those close to them than younger persons. Thus, it may not be age that causes a preoccupation with death, but recent experiences with the death of loved ones. In the second example, the conclusion that older people lose stature with age may be erroneous because the researchers did not take into account the fact that average heights have increased with every decade in the United States. Thus, older people may not have significantly shrunk in stature with advancing age, but may have been shorter to begin with. Further, cross-sectional studies do not take into account that older people may react differently to tests or laboratory situations than younger people, affecting test results. Finally, they are ineffective in distinguishing changes due to age and those due to generational differences or other factors.

A research methodology to better discern changes that occur among individuals with age is the longitudinal study in which a series of measurements are conducted on the same individuals over an extended period, generally for at least seven years. For instance, cognitive function may be tested in a group of fifty-year-olds, then these same individuals may be similarly retested at age sixty, seventy, and eighty. Because the same individuals are tested over an extended period of time, it is more likely that any changes uncovered are due to age, rather than generational differences. However, even longitudinal studies are not foolproof because physical condition, motivation, attitude, and other variables may affect the results and unless accounted for, may be mistaken for age changes. Since longitudinal studies take a long time it may be difficult to keep track of study participants and such studies are often quite costly. Further, individuals may become more familiar with the testing situation or interviewer with time, affecting the results.

A problem inherent in any research methodology is sampling. It is obvious that all older people cannot participate in every study, so researchers attempt to choose a sample that is representative of the entire population (in terms of income, education, living situation, and other variables) so the results of the sample can be generalized to the general population. Many experiments use a random sample of individuals; however, since studies generally rely on voluntary participation, the results may be biased. Those who volunteer for experiments may be more healthy, outgoing, intelligent, and independent than those who do not. On the other hand, many studies obtain their volunteers from clinic outpatients or those who are institutionalized. Obviously these populations do not represent the healthy elder population and the presence of drug effects, chronic illness, and inactivity may affect the results.

Why Study Health and Aging?

One of the most powerful incentives to study health as it relates to aging is a personal one. Information about the many variables affecting health status in the later years can help people make better-informed health choices to increase the quality of their later life.

Whether old age is to be endured in an unhealthy, debilitated state, or with energy and vigor is largely up to individual responsibility and the value placed on healthy behavior. One common response of an individual who is practicing an unhealthy behavior (e.g., smoking cigarettes, overeating) is, "I'm going to die anyway, might as well be from this." However, there is a large flaw in this reasoning. The chance of growing old with disabilities due to poor health behaviors is much greater than the chance of dying quickly from them. It is ironic that many of the diseases and disabilities formerly believed to be inevitable are now thought to be brought about by our own thoughtless behaviors. Thus, the short-term enjoyment of unhealthful activities exacts a long-term cost on health. Whereas health may not seem a large concern when young, when one becomes old, health becomes a crucial concern. Perhaps the most important reason to discuss health in later years is to get a perspective on the direction our own health behaviors may be leading us.

Aside from the impact on our personal lives, the study of health and aging will assist us to better manage the aging process of those close to us—our friends and families. It is much more likely now than it was fifty years ago that our parents, grandparents, and other kin will live to old age. Concurrent with this, it is more likely that family members will spend some of their lives dealing with impaired spouses or relatives. Accurate knowledge about health and disease, appropriate measures to minimize health problems, available medical and social services and means to finance them will be valuable in meeting that challenge.

The study of aging and health may enhance our professional careers. With the demographic shifts in the next few decades, the number of careers for those who choose to work directly with elders will increase dramatically. Researchers, teachers, social workers, physicians, nurses, nutritionists, counselors, psychologists, pharmacists, physical therapists, and many others with special knowledge of the needs of elders will be in demand. Those entering other careers, such as advertising, fashion designing, tourism, and mass media will do well to understand the needs and desires of elders as older people become an increased proportion of our total population.

Finally, knowledge of health and aging and its impact upon health care provision is a critical economic and political issue. Health care expenditures currently account for 11 percent of the Gross National Product, and cost the nation over a billion dollars a day. About one-third of that cost pays for the medical care of elders. With the expected population shifts, important issues will have to be faced: Who should pay for health care? How can health care policy be modified to better meet the needs of elders? Barring early death, sooner or later we will all join the ranks of elders, and will be either helped or harmed by these policy decisions. Questions such as these are crucial to answer for our nation and our future.

1 Elder Americans: Myths and Facts

Wisdom would suggest that the most foolish and least affordable of prejudice is that directed against a group which we must all join.

Alex Comfort

Introduction

One of the first tasks in the study of aging and health is to dispel some of the half-truths about the aging process and the experience of being old as these lead to prejudice and discrimination against elders. One way to counteract such misconceptions is to present current information about characteristics of elders in the United States. Although the elder population is tremendously heterogeneous, it is helpful to study the income, living situation, health status, education, life expectancy, and geographic distribution of elders since these impact directly or indirectly on the health of elders. Finally, special concerns of minority elders will be addressed, especially those that influence health status.

We need to rid ourselves of the mistaken notion that after a particular age, people become different, even impaired. We must stop imposing this notion on others—and ourselves.

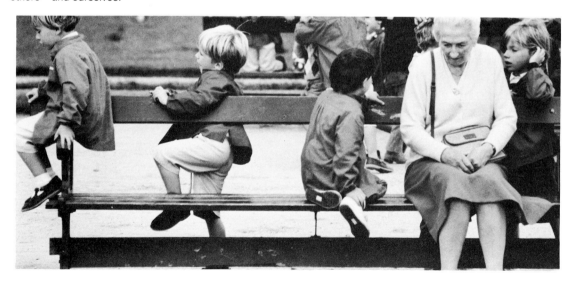

Ageism

Robert Butler coined the term "ageism" to describe prejudice and discrimination against the old because of ignorance, misconceptions, and half-truths. Ageism is the assumption that personal traits of older individuals and their situation are due to age, not other factors. These perceptions, whether negative or positive, are usually over-simplified generalizations about elders, based on limited experience with members of that group. Although some myths of aging may be true for some older people, ageism is the blanket application of these stereotypic characteristics to all elders. Ageism may come about because elders are viewed as separate or different, and they no longer experience the same thoughts and feelings as the rest of the population. Comfort asserts that like racism, ageism needs to be met by information, contradiction, and when necessary, confrontation. We need to reject ageism for ourselves and to refuse to impose it upon others. He puts it bluntly when he says, "By ignoring an oppressed minority, which we are inevitably going to join, we do not realize that we are slashing our own tires." (1976)

Myths and stereotypes about elders affect how others act towards older people. A study by the National Council on Aging (1981) revealed that those under age sixty-five attributed a

---

Stereotypes of the Ideal Aged American

Let us look at the stereotype of the ideal aged American as past folklore presents it. He or she is a white-haired, inactive, unemployed person, making no demands on anyone, least of all the family, docile in putting up with loneliness, rip-offs of every kind and boredom, and able to live on a pittance. He or she, although not demented, which would be a nuisance to other people, is slightly deficient in intellect and tiresome to talk to, because folklore says that old people are weak in the head, asexual, because old people are incapable of sexual activity, and it is unseemly if they are not. He or she is unemployable, because old age is second childhood and everyone knows that the old make a mess of simple work. Some credit points can be gained by visiting or by being nice to a few of these subhuman individuals, but most of them prefer their own company and the company of other aged unfortunates. Their main occupations are religion, grumbling, reminiscing and attending the funerals of friends. If sick, they need not, and should not, be actively treated, and are best stored in unsupervised institutions run by racketeers who fleece them and hasten their demise. A few, who are amusing or active, are kept by society as pets. The rest are displaying unpardonable bad manners by continuing to live, and even on occasion by complaining of their treatment, when society has declared them unpeople and their patriotic duty is to lie down and die.

If this picture of aging offends you, visit a few of the places where old people are kept. If you dislike what you see, recognize that you have a few years to change it before the stereotype hits you. If it has hit you already, you will know it better than anyone and you will want any help available to fight back.

Reprinted from *A good age* by Alex Comfort. Copyright © by Mitchell Beazley Publisher, Ltd., 1976. Used by permission of Crown Pub., Inc.

number of problems to older people that elders did not find true in their daily life. For instance, the young thought elders had significantly more problems with income, poor health, loneliness, and crime than elders actually experienced (table 1.1). These misconceptions may promote a fear of growing old among the young as well as further alienation from older people. Comfort's quote is well-taken, we are foolhardy to perpetuate prejudices against older people since we will all become the eventual victims.

Myths and stereotypes about elders also affect how elders view themselves. In the same study, older people themselves had exaggerated views about the problems facing the elder population as a whole, even though they did not personally experience them. In essence, many elders also exhibit ageism, but see themselves as the exceptions (table 1.1).

The following are only a few of the many ageist attitudes perpetuated in American society.

"After age sixty-five, life goes steadily downhill."

Sixty-five is not a magic age that defines the boundary between healthy middle age and total decrepitude. Aging is a dynamic process that begins from the moment we are born. As a group, the health status of elders is generally poorer than

---

Table 1.1 Differences between personal experience of Americans sixty-five and over and expectations of other adults about those experiences

Rank As Actual very Serious Problem for 65 and Over		Personal Experience	Public Expectation	
		"Very Serious" Problems Felt Personally	"Very Serious" Problems Attributed to Most People Over 65	
		By Public 65 and Over	By Public 18–64	By Public 65 and Over
(No.)		(%)	(%)	(%)
4	Not having enough money to live on	17	68	50
3	Poor health	21	47	40
6	Loneliness	13	65	45
9	Poor housing	5	43	30
2	Fear of crime	25	74	58
8	Not enough education	6	21	17
9	Not enough job opportunities	6	51	24
7	Not enough medical care	9	45	34
1	High cost of energy such as heating oil, gas, and electricity	42	81	72
5	Getting transportation to stores, to doctors, to places of recreation, and so forth	14	58	43

Source: NCOA. *Aging in the Eighties: America In Transition.* Washington, D.C.: The National Council on the Aging, Inc., 1981. Reprinted by permission.

the health of younger groups. However, changes are extremely variable among individuals and are influenced by both psychological and environmental factors. In general, changes associated with age and chronic disease onset are minor and most individuals adapt well with little alteration in daily routine. Although some physical decrements are associated with advanced age, many changes are positive. The later years can be a time to continue old roles and interests or develop new ones. Aging may bring more free time, independence from raising children, and lack of job-related stress. Nevertheless, life does go steadily downhill for a few who lose social roles and good health and become increasingly debilitated.

"Old people are all alike."

There is more variability among elders than any other segment of the population. Individuals become more unique with age as their collection of experiences and attitudes exert a tremendous influence on development. Elders experience drastically differing rates of physiological and psychological aging and decline of health. The characteristics of an immobilized elder in a nursing home are very different from an elder marathon runner or statesperson. Further, the age of old people varies from sixty-five to over one hundred, a span of thirty-five years. Using that same age range in another group, we can see the variability; what does a fifteen year old have in common with a fifty year old? Although statistics used will necessarily focus on generalizations, it is important to be aware that there are a myriad of differences among elder sub-groups.

"Old people are lonely and ignored by their families."

The common belief that elders are more likely to be lonely than other age groups is not substantiated by research. In fact, one study reported that elders are the least lonely and the most satisfied with social relationships of all age groups. The same study found that neither gender nor living alone was correlated with loneliness among elders

(Revenson and Johnson 1984). When given a choice between living alone or with their children, elders overwhelmingly prefer to live alone if personal finances can support it (Johnson and Bursk 1977). Presumably, the isolation created by living alone is counteracted by social relationships outside the home. The desolation following the loss of an intimate attachment correlates more highly with loneliness in the later years, not isolation itself (Revenson and Johnson 1984).

The majority of old people who live alone are in close contact with their children, either in person or by telephone. Further, it is estimated that 80 percent of those who are frail in our country are cared for by family members. When spouses are not available, adult children, especially daughters, act as caregivers. It is estimated that children provide care to one-fourth of the disabled men and one-third of the disabled women in our country. Most of those in nursing homes have no living children to care for them.

"Old people are senile."

The term *senility* has often been used loosely to describe any memory loss or confusion in older people. However, memory loss or confusion are symptoms of a disease that affects a small proportion of elders and is called dementia. Severe cognitive impairment is present in only about 5 percent of elders living in the community. Contrary to popular belief, intelligence, learning, and memory do not decline in old age. Significant impairment is due to disease processes, not old age. It is interesting that the young, or those around them, do not worry when they forget, but when an older person forgets something, both the older person and those around see it as significant.

"Old people have the good life."

Along with the many negative myths about old age, many people believe that elders have it easy and that life after retirement is paradise with time to travel and rest. Although elders on the whole enjoy their older years, it is fallacious to think that old age is easy for all. In fact, old age

Self-Test for Age Discrimination

For each of the following situations, two persons are listed as having asked you for your advice and opinion. How would you respond to each person? Notice your feelings about each circumstance. What would you do if:

1. She came to you and said she was contemplating marriage?

    Your twenty-one-year-old niece: _____

    Your seventy-one-year-old grandmother: _____

2. He told you he wanted to become a nurse?

    Your twenty-one-year-old nephew: _____

    Your sixty-year-old uncle: _____

3. He said he wanted to learn how to bowl?

    Your eighteen-year-old cousin: _____

    Your eighty-year-old father: _____

4. He said he was joining an art class?

    Your sixteen-year-old brother: _____

    Your seventy-three-year-old grandfather: _____

5. She was planning to campaign actively for a presidential candidate?

    Your twenty-two-year-old niece: _____

    Your seventy-five-year-old friend: _____

6. She was going to start college after being out of school for years?

    Your thirty-year-old aunt: _____

    Your sixty-year-old aunt: _____

7. She wanted to learn a trade?

    Your twenty-year-old sister: _____

    Your sixty-five-year-old mother: _____

8. She started coming home at 2:00 or 3:00 in the morning?

    Your twenty-one-year-old sister: _____

    Your seventy-year-old grandmother: _____

9. He became an old-movie buff and started to travel around to see old movies wherever they were shown?

   Your sixteen-year-old brother: _____

   Your sixty-five-year-old grandfather: _____

10. All he did for recreation was play cards?

   Your twenty-five-year-old cousin: _____

   Your seventy-five-year-cousin: _____

In which of the situations did your answers vary most? Why do you believe the variance occurred?
Did your answer vary by whether the person was related to you or not?
What criteria (besides age) did you use in responding to the individual's requests?
If you were the older person in each situation, what response would you prefer?

Reprinted with permission from Epstein: *Learning to Care for the Aged*, Reston Publishing Co., Reston, Md. 1977.

is a time of great losses for many elders—the loss of loved ones, the loss of health, the loss of physical appearance, and the loss of value in society. Further, retirement reduces income significantly. Many minority elders may never retire because their life expectancy is shorter or they must continue to work because they have insufficient money to survive otherwise. Although aging is not a negative experience for most elders, there are negative aspects of growing old that must be addressed. These include coping with negative stereotypes, chronic illness of self or spouse, limitations in mobility, death of loved ones, increasing dependency, and reduced income.

"Most old people are sickly."

Most elders experience at least one chronic condition and some have several. However, the majority of elders do not have health problems that limit their ability to manage their own households. Although concerns of those with severe health problems and the institutionalized should be addressed, the majority of older people cope well with only minor activity limitation. A household survey of community-dwelling elders revealed that only about 18 percent of elders in the community report that they are limited in carrying out daily living activities (U.S. Senate Special Committee on Aging 1985). Despite the multiple physical decrements associated with later life, the majority of elders rank themselves in better health than others their age. About 70 percent of elders reported their health to be good or excellent in comparison with others their own age and only 9 percent reported themselves to be in poor health.

"Old people no longer have any sexual interest or ability."

Although there is a slight alteration in sexual response with age, older people in reasonably good health have active and satisfying sex lives. Sexual interest does not decline with age. Rather, sexual interest and activity in the later years is correlated with interest and activity in the younger years. However, sexual activity may decrease in the later years for elder widows, not because of a lack of interest, but because of a lack of a partner. The myths of aging sexuality will be discussed further in Chapter 11.

"Most old people end up in nursing homes."

At any point in time, only 5 percent of those sixty-five and older are in a nursing home. The likelihood of living out one's final years in a nursing home increases with advancing age. Only 1 percent of those age sixty-five to seventy-four are in nursing homes in any given day. In the seventy-five to eighty-four age group, 7 percent are in nursing homes and this number increases to more than 20 percent of those eighty-five and older. The chances of being institutionalized also increase with lack of spouse or family. Nevertheless, the majority of older people will not reside in a nursing home, even for a short time.

Demographic Profile of Elders

Physiological state is an important component in determining overall health status. However, a number of other social and economic considerations, such as marital status, living arrangements, education, income, degree of social support, and cultural background exert a strong influence upon health status and behavior. The following cases exemplify the complex interactions among physiological, socioeconomic, and other environmental factors upon health.

Case 1: The seventy-five-year-old woman has slight visual impairment and has to walk with a cane because of osteoarthritis. She is unable to drive, but relies on public transportation to go to church and functions at the historical society of which she is the chairperson. She is mentally alert, reads well with glasses, and has a positive attitude about life. She has some college education and lives alone.

Case 2: The sixty-five-year-old black man with a history of congestive heart failure lives in a three-story walk-up because he does not have enough money to move. His children live nearby and help him with housecleaning and meal preparation. However, he has refused their offer to stay with them. He has been prescribed medication for his heart trouble, but takes it only when he experiences pain because of cultural beliefs that medicine should only be taken when one is sick.

Case 3: The eighty-year-old woman has recently returned from the hospital after hip surgery and is temporarily disabled. She needs physical therapy, but cannot get there because she fears she will be attacked in the city neighborhood. She has neighbors to help her fix meals, but is very hesitant to ask for any other type of help because she is unable to pay for it.

Case 4: The sixty-five-year-old woman is a retired dancer and continues to dance daily in a local studio. She is fully mobile and drives well. She is highly educated about the importance of diet and exercise in maintaining health. She lives with her husband in a house behind her adult daughter's family and helps with babysitting and light housework.

This section provides an overview of the demographic factors that impact directly or indirectly upon the health of older people. Demography is the study of the size, geographical distribution, and composition of a particular group.

Most of the demographic data available define elders as those sixty-five and older, however, it is important to remember the tremendous variation among elders. Further, the information is generally presented in terms of average values and does not address the variation among individual elders. Thus, it is important not to use these general data to make predictions about the situation of a particular older person. For instance, the average income for an older woman in 1985 was $6,313/year. However, some older women may be penniless, while a very few had incomes of over $20,000/year. Unless noted otherwise, the facts and figures cited were culled from the U.S. Bureau of the Census and the diverse material gathered in a report by the U.S. Senate Special Committee on Aging (1985).

Figure 1.1 Number of persons 65+: 1900 to 2030. Note: Increments in years on horizontal scale are uneven. (Based on data from U.S. Bureau of the Census).

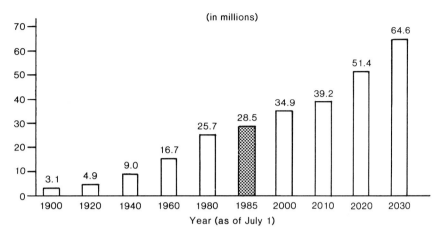

(in millions)

Year (as of July 1)

Number and Growth of the Elder Population

The number and proportion of those over sixty-five have grown faster during most of this century than any other segment of the population. This growth is especially evident in technologically advanced societies, such as the United States, where the rates of infectious diseases and maternal and infant mortality are low. In 1985, there were 28.5 million people age sixty-five and older in the United States. At the beginning of the century, less than one in twenty-five people (40 percent) was sixty-five or over. By 1985, one person in nine (or 12 percent) fell into this category.

Within the last two decades, the elder population has grown twice as fast as the rest of the population. The number and proportion of elders in the population continues to increase rapidly. According to U.S. Bureau of Census projections, the nation's total population is expected to increase by one-third between 1984 and 2050, and the fifty-five-and-over population is expected to more than double. By 2050 one in three persons is expected to be at least fifty; one in four will be sixty-five or over. The population over seventy-five

is experiencing especially rapid growth; by 2000, half of all elders will be seventy-five and older (figure 1.1).

In 1985, white elder Americans accounted for over 90 percent of the total elder population, black Americans comprised 8 percent, and Hispanics (who may be of any ethnicity) made up 4 percent. According to 1980 census figures, Asian Americans and native Americans made up about 1 percent of the population. Ethnic minorities comprise reduced proportions of those over sixty-five mainly because of their shorter life expectancies and higher birth rates. For instance, white elders are almost 12 percent of the white population, but black elders are only about 8 percent of the total black population, native Americans sixty-five and older comprise 6 percent of their total population, and Hispanic elders comprise only about four percent of the total Hispanic population.

The nonwhite elder population comprises 10 percent of all elders in the country. However, the number of nonwhite elders in the United States has grown faster than the number of white elders in the last decade and this trend is expected to

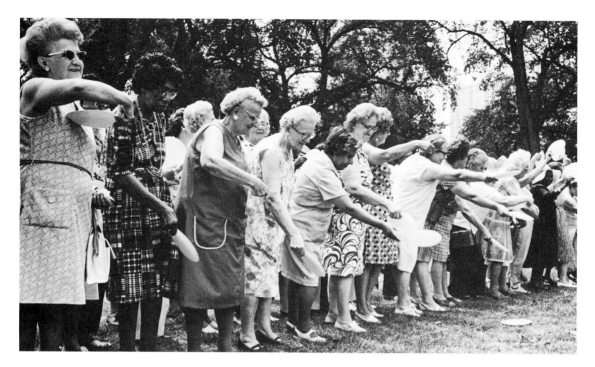

continue. Between 1980 and 1984, the black population grew by 6.7 percent while the number of whites grew 3.2 percent. When all elder ethnic minorities were combined, their numbers increased almost 30 percent in four years. This is due to immigration, increased fertility, and decreased mortality among nonwhites.

The increased numbers and proportion of elders in the United States will have profound consequences on our society, especially upon the provision of medical care. A higher number of elders increases the need for hospitals, long-term care facilities, and home health services, and will place a heavier burden on publicly funded insurance such as Medicare and Medicaid. Additionally, the eighty-five and over age group is growing the fastest and is expected to increase seven-fold between 1980 and 2050. Since those who are very old are more likely to live alone, have multiple illnesses, or be institutionalized, this increase will significantly influence the future demand for health and social services in our country.

Life Expectancy

Life expectancy for both men and women has been increasing in our country. Those born today can expect to live more than twenty-five years longer than those born in 1900 (table 1.2). The life expectancy for women born in 1985 was 78.2 years; for men, 71.2. Life expectancy has increased rapidly in the last century largely because of reduced infant and maternal death during childbirth and the control of infectious diseases. In the last two decades, an increasing proportion of the population has survived to old age because of reduced mortality in middle-aged and elder populations. Life expectancy is highly dependent on ethnicity, income level, and gender.

Gender has the largest influence on life expectancy. In the United States, both white and nonwhite women live longer than men and the gap has been widening through the years. In 1984, elder women outnumbered elder men three to two and the difference increased with advancing age.

Table 1.2 Life expectancy at birth and age 65 by sex and calendar year 1900–2050				
	Male		Female	
	At Birth	At Age 65	At Birth	At Age 65
1900	46.4	11.3	49.0	12.0
1910	50.1	12.1	53.6	12.1
1920	54.5	12.3	56.3	12.3
1930	58.0	12.9	61.3	12.9
1940	61.4	11.9	65.7	13.4
1950	65.6	12.8	71.1	15.1
1960	66.7	12.9	73.2	15.9
1970	67.1	13.0	74.9	17.0
1980	69.9	14.0	77.5	18.4
1990	71.4	14.5	78.9	19.2
2000	72.1	14.8	79.5	19.5
2010	72.4	15.0	79.8	19.8
2020	72.7	15.2	72.7	20.1
2030	73.0	15.4	73.0	20.3
2040	73.3	15.6	73.3	20.6
2050	73.6	15.8	73.6	30.8

Source: Social Security Administration, Social Security Area Population Properties, 1984; Advanced Study No. 92.

A woman has a one in three chance of reaching age eighty-five, but a man's chance of reaching that age is only one in six.

Ethnicity also affects life expectancy. In the United States, whites live longer than blacks and both live longer than Hispanics. Some Asian groups have even longer life expectancies than whites. Native Americans have the shortest life expectancies. In 1985, the life expectancy was 65.3 years for black men and 73.5 years for black women. The life expectancies of native Americans is estimated to be eight years less than the average for the general population.

Marital Status, Living Arrangements, and Social Supports

It is clear that gender is one of the most important determinants of marital status and living arrangements in later years. Older men are twice as likely to be married than older women. In the United States, half of the older women are widows, five times more than the number of widowers. In 1984, two-thirds of women seventy-five and older were widowed, while two-thirds of men that age were married. Women are more likely to be widows not only because they generally outlive their spouses, but also because they often marry men older than themselves. More than one-third of men sixty-five and older are married to women younger than sixty-five. In addition, elderly widowed men have remarriage rates about seven times those of elder women. The average widow who does not remarry is sixty-five, has been widowed for six years, and can expect to live over nineteen years as a widow.

Two-thirds of the older people in the United States live in a family setting. Living arrangements generally reflect marital status. Older women are less likely to live with a spouse than older men. In 1984, over four-fifths of the men

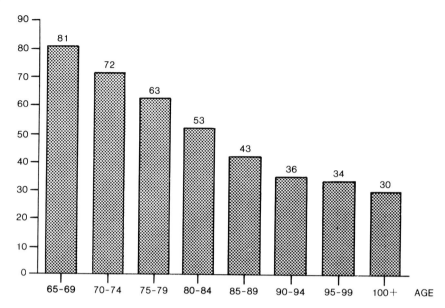

Figure 1.2 Number of men per 100 women by elderly age group, 1984. (Source: U.S. Bureau of the Census, Current Population Reports, Series p.–25, No. 952 estimates).

sixty-five and older lived with a family while three-fifths of the women that age lived in a family setting. About 30 percent of older people live alone; 41 percent of older women and 15 percent of older men. Most elders choose to live alone and prefer that lifestyle to living with adult children (Johnson and Bursk 1977). However, living alone can be a liability because those who live alone are more likely to have lower incomes and are at greater risk of institutionalization than those who live with families (Siegal and Hoover 1982).

Most older people receive social support from their children. According to one national study, of the elders who lived alone, 70 percent had at least one surviving child and had frequent contact with offspring. Most elders lived near their children and either saw their children or talked with them frequently on the telephone. About three-fourths of those with children said at least one of their children was minutes away from them. Sixty-three percent had seen at least one child within the week prior to the survey, another 16 percent saw a child once a month and most of

the remainder saw a child several times during the year. Less than three percent of those living alone who had a child saw them less than once a year (Kovar 1986).

Neighbors and other relatives also provide important social supports to the aged. In the survey mentioned above, 70 percent of the elders living alone had met with family or neighbors within the past two weeks and 81 percent had talked with them on the telephone. Half of them had been to church within the past two weeks. Only 11 percent of the respondents had not visited with children, siblings, friends, or relatives in the last two weeks (Kovar 1986).

Marital status, living arrangements, and the availability of social support play a major role in determining whether an older person is in need of formal care. Family members supply 80 percent of the care of disabled elders, often at significant physical, psychological, and financial cost. Spouses provide the majority of care and children provide care to one-fourth of disabled elder men and more than one-third of disabled elder women. When a spouse or child is not present, elders are more likely to be institutionalized. Only 25 percent of institutionalized men and women are married as compared to about 40 percent of those not institutionalized. In addition, over 80 percent of elders in the community have at least one child as opposed to fewer than half of the nursing home residents (who generally have just one) (U.S. Department of Health, Education, and Welfare 1977).

Current trends, such as the increasing divorce rate, tendency to have fewer children, more women in the work force, and the expanding gap in life expectancy between men and women will exacerbate the problem of familial support for elders. Currently about one-tenth of elderly persons have been divorced, but this figure is expected to rise to 50 percent by 2020.

Education

As a group, older people have completed less schooling than younger adults. However, this gap continues to narrow. In 1985, elders had completed a median 11.7 years of school, compared to 12.5 median years for the entire population. Nearly half of the elder population were high school graduates and about 9 percent had four or more years of college. The median years of school completed vary considerably by ethnicity. Hispanic elders are the most educationally disadvantaged with an average of 7.1 years of schooling. Blacks completed an average of 8.1 years of schooling. Elder whites and Asian Americans completed about twelve years of schooling. Blacks, native Americans, and Hispanics fell far behind whites in the number of high school and college degrees received.

Although elders may have fewer years of education than other adults, they do not stop learning when they reach age sixty-five. Half a million elders are enrolled in educational classes and this trend is expected to continue as educational institutions cater more to elder learners (Hendricks 1983). Since many workers have not been prepared for the free time that comes with retirement, they return to education to enhance

quality of life, develop their interests, and refine new skills (Sterns and Sanders 1980). Elderhostel programs where older people meet in the summer for short-term coursework on special topics are increasing by over 20 percent a year (Elderhostel 1985).

Economic Status

As a group, elders in the United States have a lower income than other adults, mostly due to retirement from the workforce. Families with heads of household sixty-five or older averaged $19,162/year in 1985 ($19,815 for whites; $11,937 for blacks), about 60 percent of the median income of those age twenty-five–sixty-four. In 1985, about one of six families with an elderly head of the household had incomes below $10,000. On the other end of the scale, 35 percent of families with an older adult as head of the household had incomes of $25,000 a year or more.

A significant amount of elders live in poverty. In 1985, 12.6 percent of elders lived in poverty; for those eighteen to sixty-four, the rate was 14.1 percent. The official 1985 definition of poverty for elders is an income of $6,503 (a weekly income of $125 or less) or $5,156 (a weekly income of $99 or less) for individuals living alone.

It needs to be mentioned, that the federal government applies a different poverty base to elders than to other groups, creating a discriminatory standard based solely on age. Historically, this occurred because it was thought that older people needed less food per month than younger people. This amounts to $437 for persons living alone and $928 for couples. If the same standards were used for elders as the rest of the population, elders would be considered the poorest adult group (Villers Foundation 1987).

The poverty rate among elders is an improvement from 1970 when 25 percent of elders had incomes below the poverty level or 1959 when 33 percent of elders were poor. Even though fewer elders are subsisting below the poverty line, a disproportionately high number are still living on marginal incomes. Elders have higher rates of near poor (incomes of 25 percent above the pov-

Figure 1.3 Median income of persons aged 65 and older by marital status, 1983. (Source: U.S. Bureau of the Census, March 1984 Current Population Survey.)

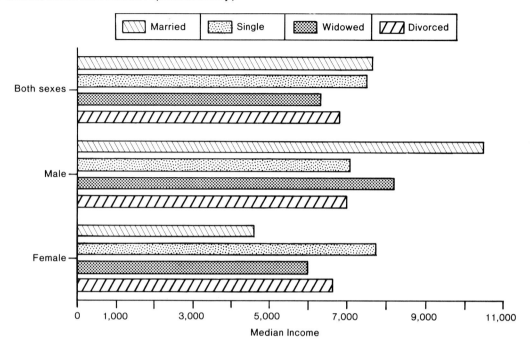

erty level) than other adults. Over one-fifth of those sixty-five or older were either poor or near poor in 1985.

Low income among elders is associated with age, gender, ethnicity, absence of a spouse, and living arrangements (figure 1.3). Those over eighty-five have a significantly lower income than younger elders and are more likely to be poor or near poor. Poverty is also disproportionately high among women; elderly women are significantly poorer than elderly men (16 percent vs. 8 percent). Nearly three-fourths of elderly poor are women; at all ages, women have lower incomes than men. In 1985, white men sixty-five and older had a median income of $10,900; white women $6,313. Elders of both sexes who live alone are more likely to be poor than those who live in families (26 percent vs. 6 percent). In 1985, the median income for elders living alone was $7,568, only half that of younger adults living alone. Half the elders living alone reported incomes of $7,000

or less; one-fourth reported incomes below $5,000. On the other end, one-fifth of elders living alone had incomes of $15,000 or more.

Minority status increases the likelihood of poverty in the later years. Data from 1985 reveal that almost 11 percent of elderly whites were below the poverty line while blacks had almost three times that figure (32 percent). The percentage of elder Hispanics falls between the black and white figures: twice as many Hispanics were below the poverty level (22 percent). Further, the median income of white men over sixty-five is significantly higher than that of black or Hispanic men. For women, income differences were not as great among ethnic groups. However, minority elder women, especially those living alone, are still the hardest hit by poverty. In 1985, about 55 percent of black women living alone had incomes below the poverty level.

Chapter 1

Elders depend on a number of sources of income including social security, supplemental security income, veteran's benefits, savings, pensions, and income properties. The single largest source of income for those over sixty-five is Social Security benefits with about 90 percent of elders receiving them. In 1985, about 35 percent of the average older person's income came from Social Security. However, not all elders depend on Social Security payments to the same extent. Only 15 percent of elders rely on Social Security as their sole source of income, but over one-third depend on Social Security for more than 80 percent of their income.

The second most important source of income for elders is personal assets such as annuities, income properties, and savings. In 1985, personal assets comprised about one-fourth of elders' income. However, there is wide variability among elders in number of assets. While some elders have many assets, most have little to none. For instance, in 1985, one-third of elders had no personal assets while another third had less than $500/year.

Earnings are an important source of income for younger elders, but their importance decreases with age. Those age sixty-five–sixty-seven received 35 percent of their income from earnings, but only 4 percent of the income of those eighty and older was from earnings.

Although national figures show that elders have accumulated significantly more assets than younger adults, their major asset is a home, which cannot be easily liquidated. Further, most elders have only a modest amount of other assets. The average assets figure for elders is inflated, mainly due to a few individuals (7 percent) with assets over $250,000.

Geographic Distribution

About 70 percent of older people in the United States live in metropolitan areas—either in the city or in the suburbs. Almost half of these live in the inner city. Elders are more likely to live in suburban areas than nonelders. White elders are more concentrated in the suburbs, while ethnic minority elders are more predominant in the central cities.

About one in five elders live in rural areas, primarily small towns. About half the nation's rural elders live in the South. Many rural counties in the agricultural heartland of the United States have a high proportion of elders because elders have remained while younger people have moved to urban areas. Other communities in Florida, Arizona, and Texas have high elder populations because of a move later in life to a more suitable climate. The states with the highest number of older people are California, New York, and Florida, each having over two million residents. Other states having over one million elder residents are Illinois, Michigan, Ohio, Pennsylvania, and Texas.

Mortality and Morbidity

Death rate, or mortality, is defined as the number of individuals per 1,000 who die per year. Females have lower death rates (about 34 per 1,000 per year) than males (almost 60 per 1,000 per year). Death rates for both sexes have declined significantly in the last forty years.

In the United States, heart disease, cancer, or stroke kills four of five elders. Heart disease, the number one killer in all age groups, is responsible for over 40 percent of all deaths among those aged sixty-five and older. Cancer follows with 20 percent, and strokes, 9 percent. Deaths due to cardiovascular disease and stroke have decreased over the last ten years while those due to cancer continue to rise. Although suicide ranks low as a cause of death among the elderly, the rate for those sixty-five and older (especially men) is higher than for other age groups.

Mortality rates provide much information about the health and longevity of a population. However, mortality statistics must be examined with care; decreased mortality rates do not necessarily mean more years of good health, rather they often translate into a longer period of illness (morbidity) and increased need for medical services to limit the progression of chronic illness.

Morbidity rates provide information about the incidence of disease in a population. Elders have the highest morbidity of all age groups; in the later years, the majority of morbidity is chronic illness. Chronic illnesses are progressive, mainly incurable conditions that vary in their degree of severity. Common chronic disorders among older people include arthritis, hearing and vision disorders, hypertension (high blood pressure), heart conditions, osteoporosis, and digestive conditions. Elders are less likely to suffer from most mental impairments than younger groups, but rates of depression and cognitive impairment increase slightly with age. Alzheimer's disease is the leading cause of cognitive impairment.

More than four of five elders have at least one chronic condition and many manifest more than one. Although most cause only minor alterations in daily routine, chronic illnesses account for the majority of disabilities for the middle-aged and elderly. On the average, one in five individuals age sixty-five or older needs help from another to perform one or more personal care or home management activity because of chronic conditions. However, only 3.5 percent of elders are so severely limited that they cannot complete their daily routine.

Disabilities due to chronic illness increase with advanced age. Fourteen percent of those between sixty-five and seventy-four need help with at least one activity. Among those age eighty-five and older, almost 50 percent have some limitation because of chronic conditions; about one-fourth of them are severely disabled.

Although indices measuring the extent of chronic illness in the population are one way to measure health, personal perception of health is another measure of health status. Contrary to the popular belief that most elders are sick, one survey reported that two-thirds of elders living in the community describe their health as excellent or good compared to others their age. One-third percent report their health as fair or poor (Kovar 1986).

Health Care Utilization and Expenditures

Because elders have a higher prevalence of chronic illness than the rest of the population, they use health services more often. Elders are hospitalized twice as often, use one-third of all acute hospital beds, use twice as many prescription drugs, and visit physicians slightly more often than younger populations. Elders are also the primary users of nursing homes.

Although those sixty-five and older account for 12 percent of the nation's population, they are responsible for almost one-third of the total personal health care expenditures. In 1984, those sixty-five and older spent $4,202/year on medical and related services. Hospital expenses accounted for the largest share of health expenditures for elders (45 percent), followed by physicians and nursing home care (21 percent each).

While the younger population is more likely to finance their health care through private insurance, those over sixty-five often rely on public funds including Medicare (a federal health insurance for those over sixty-five) and Medicaid (a shared state-federal public welfare program for the poor of all ages). Even with the contribution of public funds, on the average elders still pay about one-fourth of their total medical care bill. In 1984, elders paid an average of $1,059 from their own resources, approximately 15 percent of their total income.

Despite the high average expenditures for medical care, many elders spend little for medical care. Sixty percent of elders in 1980 had total medical expenditures of less than $500/year. On the other hand, elders approaching death or institutionalization face extremely high health care expenditures. Chapters 12 and 13 will discuss these issues further.

Minority Elders

Ethnic minority elders comprise only 12 percent of the total elder population, but their numbers are increasing due to higher fertility rates and gains in life expectancy. It is estimated that by 2050, about one-fifth of America's elders will belong to a minority group. Although the groups are diverse, minority elders have many commonalities—age, high poverty level, and racial discrimination. Not only do they occupy an inferior status because of their ethnicity, they also must cope with the problems of poverty and ageism. Differences in language, education, appearance, and customs have kept minorities out of well-paying jobs, positions of authority, and consequent financial security. Many minority elders are becoming more isolated from younger members of their culture because their lifestyle and background are no longer valued by a more Americanized younger generation and vice versa. In general, ethnic aged are less educated, poorer, have more health problems, and die sooner than their white counterparts.

Despite many negative aspects, the minority aged do have some unique resources. Identification with an ethnic group and cultural traditions are a source of support in the later years. In addition, ethnic groups tend to maintain stronger extended social networks, within both the family and the local community.

Even though ethnic groups share a number of commonalities, each group is more dissimilar than similar. Even within an ethnic group, there is much variation in education level, financial status, cultural background, length of time in the United States, family structure, geographical distribution, and degree of adherance to cultural practices. Statistics necessarily focus on generalities, but the reader should be aware of their diversity as it affects health status and behavior. Ethnic minority elders generally have poorer health status, more activity limitations due to chronic illness, and less access to medical care than their white cohorts. Further, Hispanics and blacks are more likely to view their health as fair or poor than whites (National Center for Health Statistics 1984). Income, traditional health beliefs and practices, and attitude toward standard medical practices are only a few of the critical determinants of their health status.

Black Americans

The black population is the largest group of minority elders in the United States. In 1984, they comprised about 8 percent of the total elder population (U.S. Bureau of the Census 1985a). The Census Bureau estimates that by the year 2000, the rate of growth of the black population will exceed that of whites by over 25 percent. As in other population groups, there are more elder black women than men. The life expectancy of blacks is increasing rapidly. In 1940, black Americans lived about eleven years less than whites. By 1980, this disparity was reduced to five years. Once blacks and whites reach age sixty-five, differences in life expectancy are small and death rates after age seventy-five are higher for whites than for blacks.

As a group, elder blacks are more apt to suffer from chronic health problems than their white counterparts: about half have chronic conditions as compared with just over a third of whites. Although the three major causes of death—heart disease, cancer, and stroke—are the same in both blacks and whites, hypertension is more prevalent in the black population. It is assumed that blacks are more likely to suffer from untreated illnesses as a result of poverty, malnutrition, and inadequate medical care. When compared with whites their age, elder blacks have more restricted activity, disability, and lost work days per year. They visit physicians less often and stay longer in the hospital, supporting the belief that they postpone seeking medical attention until health problems become severe (National Center for Health Statistics 1984).

Black elders are less likely to utilize public services because they have come to expect little from such agencies. Racism is still prevalent in the health care system and many blacks are suspicious of health care facilities. Their low income

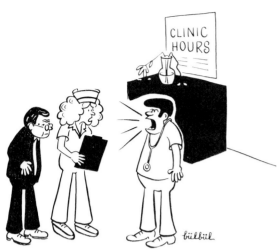

"Stop yelling, doctor. He's not deaf or senile. He just doesn't speak English."

may prevent them from seeking medical care until the problem is severe. They commonly rely heavily on extended kinship networks for social support (Dancy 1979).

Hispanic Americans

Hispanics are the second largest minority in our country. They are highly diverse: they may originate from Mexico (60 percent), Puerto Rico (14 percent), other Central and South American countries (8 percent), Cuba (6 percent) and others (12 percent). Hispanic elders (of various ethnicities) comprise about 4 percent of the total elder population (U.S. Bureau of the Census 1985b). The Hispanic population is considerably younger than the white population. This is due to higher fertility rates, shorter life expectancies, and historical patterns of immigration and deportation. For instance, many middle-aged and elder Mexican Americans return voluntarily to their homeland.

Demographic data on the Hispanic population is very inaccurate. The Bureau of Census has been inconsistent in categorizing those of Spanish descent and members of this group have been placed under both white and nonwhite categories. In addition, the number of Hispanics is difficult to estimate because many are here illegally, are illiterate, unable to speak English, and suspicious of census takers.

Traditionally, Hispanic elders are highly respected by their children and are the core of the extended family network. They act as repositories of cultural traditions, values, and history. More than the young, they have retained their native language and culture. Mexican Americans have more kin in town, more frequent interactions with relatives, and more exchange of aid with kin than whites (Keefe 1979). However, in the United States, some believe the extended family network of the Spanish-speaking population is being replaced by the nuclear family, threatening the emotional and financial support of Hispanic elders (Maldonado 1975).

Hispanic elders are poorer and less likely to receive Social Security benefits than whites primarily because they were not employed consistently (especially farm, household, and service workers) or because their wages were paid under the table (Lacayo 1980). Little information is available regarding the health status of elder Hispanics. It is reasonable to believe that those with lower incomes have the same health problems as other ethnic groups (Bell, et al. 1976).

Native Americans

Native Americans (American Indians, Eskimos, and Aleutians) comprise less than 1 percent of the United States population (U.S. House of Representatives 1984). Less is known about native American elders than any other sub-group. Although estimates vary, their life expectancy is about eight years less than that of the general population. About 6 percent of their total population is over sixty-five. Because most native Americans never reach age sixty-five, some believe they should be eligible for full Social Security retirement benefits earlier. As of 1980, elder native Americans comprised less than 2 percent of the native American population and numbered about 75,000 (U.S. Bureau of Census 1981). Although the majority of native Americans have moved from reservations to urban areas, for the most part, their elders still live on reservations or in rural areas (Leukoff, et al. 1979).

Native Americans are the poorest minority group in the United States. According to the 1980 census, 50 percent of native American families survive on incomes of less than $4,000/year and almost half live below the poverty level. Because of the high unemployment rate among native Americans (80 percent), most elders are ineligible for Social Security benefits and must depend on government support as their sole source of income.

The extended family kinship network is utilized by many native Americans and families have a commitment to their elders. Because of the high unemployment rate, elders may provide over half the income for their extended families through governmental subsidies (Williams 1980). This provision of support may indirectly preserve the status of elders within the family. However, traditional family support is ineffective in families with no resources and many native American elders are left impoverished on the reservation when their children leave to seek a better life. The plight of native Americans is exacerbated by their low educational level, shorter life expectancy, serious health problems, poor housing and lack of access to and stringent governmental controls on health and social service programs for native Americans (Applewhite 1983).

As a group, elder native Americans have a high incidence of chronic illness. Death rates from tuberculosis are six times that of the general population. Alcohol-related deaths occur five times more frequently among native Americans. Diabetes deaths are twice as frequent and the presence of diabetes on some reservations is six times the national rate (U.S. House of Representatives 1984). Almost three-fourths of native Americans have health impairments severe enough to affect their ability to complete tasks of daily living. In fact, fewer native Americans age fifty-five and older are free of disability than the rest of the population age sixty-five and older. Despite the consistent increase in per capita health care expenditures for the rest of the population, expenditures for health care for native Americans are significantly less. Since the chronic impairments are many, the decreased expenditure is likely due to lack of access to care.

Asian Americans

Asian American elderly come from a variety of countries: Japan, Phillipines, Korea, Samoa, Malasia, Vietnam, and Cambodia. Asian American elders comprise less than 2 percent of the total United States population. Information on Asian American elders is very sparse and is mostly limited to the two largest Asian groups, Japanese and Chinese. The vast majority of Asian Americans live in urban areas (almost 70 percent live in San Francisco); most live in California and Hawaii. Although a sub-group of younger Asian Americans have a higher median income and a lower unemployment and poverty rate than the national average, elder Asian Americans still suffer the same poverty, discrimination, and language difficulties as other ethnic minorities (Lum 1983). Many receive no Social Security because they were employed farmworkers or self-employed. Many elder Asians, especially men, live alone because strict immigration policies of the past prohibited the immigration of women. Many have little formal education and speak English poorly. In general, their health status is similar to white elders. However, as a group, elder Asian Americans have a higher incidence of suicide—three times that of their white counterparts. Like other minorities, elder Asians are less likely to utilize medical care services, instead relying on traditional medical practices.

Special Considerations in Working with Minority Elders

- These individuals often lack full knowledge or understanding of the services and benefits to which they are entitled.

- They are likely not to understand and to be bewildered by bureaucratic jargon, yet may appear to agree with authorities so as to avoid embarrassment and frustration.

- They are likely to seek emotional support primarily from their kinship network, and secondarily from friends, neighbors, co-workers, and other groups.

- They may see more than one health care specialist (i.e., herbalist, traditional healer, medical doctor, chiropractor) for an illness, and may be taking herbs and other combinations of medication.

- They may have traditional food preferences and be more comfortable with a native language.

- They may be accustomed to relying on one dose of a medication for a cure and may not understand the need for a number of pills over an extended period of time.

- They may be accustomed to taking traditional medications at various times and for numerous ailments, tending to borrow and lend them at will. They may attempt to do the same thing with medications recommended by the physician.

- They often say little, comply with most requests, rarely complain, and in general exhibit exemplary behavior which may mask communication problems and cultural barriers.

- They need not follow all the traditional practices of their culture and may not reveal the extent of their commitment to traditional ways from external appearances.

- They are likely not to fully understand "patients' rights" and the current encouragement of inclusion and self-determination in health matters.

- They may be under pressure from family members who are in conflict with each other regarding the use of Western medical practices or traditional folk remedies.

From Evaneshko, V., 1984. Ethnic and Culture Considerations. In B. Steffel, ed., *Handbook of Gerontological Nursing*. Reprinted with permission of Van Nostrand-Reinhold Publishing Co.

Traditional Asian culture dictated that children care for their elder parents and elders were venerated for their wisdom and experience. For Asian Americans, however, filial piety has begun to take a back seat to such traditional American values as independence, self-reliance, and future potential. Still, aged Chinese and Japanese Americans have a tendency to retain the old ways—to live in small, close-knit groups with others who share their language and culture. Although this serves as a needed social support, it tends to isolate these populations from the dominant society.

Summary

To study elders and their health status, it is important to debunk widely held myths of aging with demographic facts. These myths arise from ageism—the negative stereotyping and discrimination against older people because of half-truths, ignorance, or misconceptions. An understanding of demographic data is crucial to understand elders and the multiple factors that impact on their health status. Such factors as living situation, financial status, health care utilization, morbidity, and geographical distribution provide a glimpse of the characteristics and needs of American elders. Statistical data may lead one to the erroneous conclusion that elders are a homogeneous population, rather than a widely varied group. Nevertheless, statistical information is invaluable in dispelling stereotypes about elders and planning to meet the future demands of that group. Finally, since the elder group is one we eventually will all join, the information can assist us to be more realistic about our later life.

Activities

1. Visit the document section of your library and find out the demographic characteristics of elders in your community. Find the proportion of older people, proportion of ethnic group elders, income, and other pertinent material. Compare with national figures.
2. Using the material you gathered for question 1, what health needs can you predict for your community? Interview a public health official, social worker, or planner of the local Area Agency of Aging to get other perspectives on the status and needs of elders in your community.
3. Collect materials from print media that reflect myths and stereotypes about elders. Pay particular attention to advertisements.
4. Analyze current television programming, newscasts, and television advertisements to determine whether the media view of older people is consistent with the demographic picture presented here.
5. List stereotypical views you held or that you have heard your friends say and draft possible ways to respond next time you hear such myths.
6. Do the statistics outlined in this chapter accurately define the elders you know? How do your friends or relatives differ? Discuss some of these facts and figures about elders with your friends and family. Which ones were surprising? Which of these statistics reinforced or disspelled your stereotypes of elders?
7. The median income in 1985 for an older woman living alone was $6,313/year. Use this figure to develop a monthly budget. Be sure to include cost of $1,059/year for out-of-pocket health care costs. What expenses could not be covered in your budget? List the ways her income might interfere with the quality of her life.
8. Interview an elder and write a brief case history. How do demographic characteristics (e.g., marital status, income, family support) contribute to his/her health status? How does s/he report personal health in comparison with others his/her age?
9. Given the expected increase in the proportion of elders in 2050, project how society will have to change to better meet the health care needs of our future selves.
10. Complete the self-test for age discrimination questionnaire on page 12. Discuss your responses with your classmates.

Bibliography

Applewhite, S. R. 1983. Disadvantaged elderly. In Ernst, N. S. and H. R. Glazer-Waldman, eds. *The aged patient: a sourcebook for the health professional.* Chicago: Yearbook Medical Publishers 65–83.

Bell, D., P. Kasschaur, and G. Zellman. 1976. *Delivery services to elderly members of minority groups: A critical review of the literature.* Santa Monica, CA.: Rand Corp.

Comfort, A. 1976. *A good age.* New York: Simon and Schuster.

Comfort, A. 1979. *The biology of senescence.* New York: Elsevier.

Dancy, J. 1979. *The black elderly: A guide for practitioners.* Ann Arbor: University of Michigan.

Elderhostel. 1985. *Annual report.* Boston: Elderhostel.

Epstein, C. 1977. *Learning to care for the aged.* Reston, MD.: Reston Publishing Company.

Evaneshko, V. 1984. Ethnic and cultural considerations. In Steffl, B. M., ed. *Handbook of gerontological nursing.* New York: Van Nostrand-Reinhold.

Hendricks, J. 1983. Higher education's pursuit of the lifelong learner. *Gerontology and Geriatrics Education* 3(4):253–8.

Johnson, E., and B. Bursk. 1977. Relationships between the elderly and their adult children. *Gerontologist* 17(1):90–96.

Keefe, S. E. 1979. Urbanization, acculturation, and extended family ties: Mexican Americans in cities. *American Ethnologist* 6(2):349–65.

Kovar, M. G. 1986. Aging in the eighties, age 65 and older and living alone: Contacts with families, friends and neighbors. Preliminary data from the supplement on aging to the National Interview Survey: U.S. Jan.–June, 1984. *Advance data from Vital and Health Statistics.* National Center for Health Statistics. No. 116, May 9, 1986.

Kovar, M. G. 1986. Aging in the eighties: Preliminary data from the supplement on aging to the National Health Interview Survey: U.S. Jan.–June, 1984. *Advance data from Vital and Health Statistics,* no. 115, May 1, 1986.

Lacayo, C. G. 1980. *A national study to assess the service needs of Hispanic elderly.* Final Report. Los Angeles: National Association for Hispanic Elderly.

Leukoff, S., C. Pratt, R. Esperanza, et al. 1979. *Minority aged: A historical and cultural perspective.* Corvallis: Oregon State University.

Lum, D. 1983. Asian Americans and their aged. In McNeely and J. H. Cohen, eds. *Aging in minority groups.* Beverly Hills, CA: Sage Publ. 85–94.

Maldonado, D. 1975. The Chicano aged. *Social Work* 20:213–216.

National Center for Health Statistics. 1984. Health indicators for Hispanic, black, and white Americans. Vital and Health Statistics, Series 10, no. 148. Wash., D.C.: U.S. Govt. Printing Office.

National Council on Aging. 1981. Survey of Lou Harris, *Aging in the eighties: America in transition,* November.

Reyenson, T. A., and J. L. Johnson. 1984. *Social and demographic correlates of loneliness in later life,* Am. J. Comm. Psch. 12(1):71–85.

Siegal, J. S., and S. L. Hoover. 1982. *Demographic aspects of the health of the elderly to the year 2000 and beyond.* World Health Organization. WHO/AGE 82.3. July.

Sterns, H. L., and R. E. Sanders. 1980. Training and education of the elderly. In R. R. Turner and H. W. Reese, eds. *Life span developmental psychology: Intervention.* New York: Academic Press. 307–30.

U.S. Bureau of the Census. 1981. Supplementary Reports: 1980 census of population. PC–80–s1–1. Wash., D.C.: U.S. Govt. Printing Office.

U.S. Bureau of the Census. 1985a. Estimates of the population of the United States by age, sex and race: 1980–1984. *Current population reports,* series P-25, no. 965. Wash., D.C.: U.S. Govt. Printing Office.

U.S. Bureau of the Census. 1985b. Persons of Spanish origin in the United States: March, 1982. *Current population reports,* series P-20, no. 396. Wash., D.C.: U.S. Govt. Printing Office.

U.S. Department of Health, Education and Welfare 1977. *Characteristics, social contacts and activities of nursing home residents: U.S. 1973–1974.* National Nursing Home Survey, Vital and Health Statistics, Ser. 13, DHEW Publ. No. HRA 77–1778. Washington, D.C.: U.S. Govt. Printing Office.

U.S. House of Representatives, Subcommittee on Health and the Environment. 1984. *Indian health care: An overview of the federal government's role.* Wash., D.C.: U.S. Govt. Printing Office.

U.S. Senate Special Committee on Aging 1978. *America in transition: An aging society, 1984–85 edition.* Washington, D.C.: U.S. Govt. Printing Office.

Villers Foundation. 1987. *On the other side of easy street: myths and facts about the economics of old age.* A report from the Villers Foundation, 1334 G. Street NW, Washington, D.C.

Williams, G. C. 1980. Warriers no more: A study of American Indian elderly. In C. L. Fry, ed. *Aging in culture and society.* N.Y.: Bergen Publ. 101–11.

Chapter 1

Biologic Aging Theories and Longevity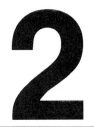

Introduction

Research on the cellular and genetic basis of aging is relatively new, although interest in why we age and ways to increase longevity has been documented throughout human history. For ages, humans have been intrigued with the aging process and have attempted to extend their length of life in a number of unique ways. As in the past, current research on the process of aging is often directed at uncovering processes that can be altered to extend life. Although the methods differ and the experiments are more sophisticated and scientific, the how and why of aging is yet to be answered. In fact, each new discovery is likely to raise more questions than it answers.

The following sections will outline the major theories of how humans grow old. Further, various therapies that attempt to extend the length of life will be examined. The chapter will conclude with a discussion of the many factors that have been correlated with long life.

Biologic Theories of Aging

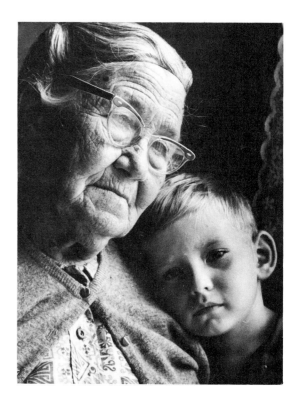

> There is probably no area of scientific inquiry that abounds with as many untested or untestable theories as does the biology of aging.
>
> Leonard Hayflick

One of the basic concerns of gerontologists is to answer the question, "What is the underlying mechanism that alters our physiology and determines our deterioration and eventual death?" Most theories are highly technical and focus on only one aspect of the aging process that reflects that researcher's expertise or point of view.

Following is a summary of several of the most plausible theories of biologic aging. These theories are often called by different names by different authors. The theories are grouped under two main subheadings: damage theories and programmed aging theories. As you study these theories, note that many overlap and some complement one another. It is not yet known if any of these theories correctly explain the aging process.

Almost every theory gives genes an important role as they have been shown to be important in limiting the life span of individual cells. Although early experiments seemed to show that cells could live forever, later experiments demonstrated conclusively that cells have a finite lifetime. In the early part of this century, Dr. Alexis Carrel, a French surgeon and scientist, showed that cells grown in a flask in a laboratory setting did not age; if given the proper nutrients and environment they would divide indefinitely. Consequently, the accepted theory of aging at that time was that aging was not initiated within the cell but by interactions between cells or a central mechanism within the organism (1912).

However, Hayflick (1961) found that Carrel's experiments were flawed. He conclusively demonstrated that cells grown in the laboratory did not divide *ad infinitum,* but have a predictable life span. For instance, human embryo cells may divide no more than forty to sixty times before death. Further, cells have the capacity to remember their maximum life span: the older the cell donor, the fewer times it divides before it dies (Hayflick 1975). Even if a cell has divided twenty times, is frozen and thawed, it continues to reproduce about thirty more times before death. Interestingly, most people die well before they reach the replicative limit of their cells. Hayflick hypothesizes that as the cells approach the end of their lifetimes, a number of biochemical decrements occur that decrease cell function and reproductive capacity. Hayflick's classic experiments changed the basic assumptions of the cause of aging and prompted researchers to explore the mechanisms originating within the cell that might explain why cells age and die.

Overview of Cell Reproduction and Repair

Because many theories of aging focus on the genetics of cells, a basic understanding of cell reproduction and repair is necessary. The body is composed of millions of cells, each specialized for a particular function (figure 2.1). Some cells (neurons) conduct electrical messages from one part of the body to another, some cells (blood cells) serve to carry oxygen to body tissues and some cells (somatic) combine with other cells to form tissues and body organs.

Most cells in the body can reproduce by dividing in two, a process called *mitosis.* After growth and development are completed, mitosis is the usual process for the body to replace damaged cells. Mitosis results in two cells that look identical to the parent cell. If one cell dies, another can divide and make a new one just like it. Cells that can divide are called *mitotic cells.* However, some cells in the body cannot divide after the individual reaches maturity (called *postmitotic cells*). This is true of all neurons and muscle cells. Once these cells die, they are never replaced. However, postmitotic cells have complicated mechanisms to repair cellular damage.

Almost every cell in the body has an identical and complete set of genetic information. Thus a nerve cell in the brain and a cell in the kidney are identical genetically, even though they have very different function. Although every cell contains all the information for development and maintenance of the body, only that section of the information that is applicable to a particular cell is used and the rest of the genetic information is ignored.

Pieces of information to direct cell function, called *genes,* are located on *chromosomes* inside each cell nucleus. Humans have 23 chromosome pairs, one of each pair contributed by each parent. Chromosomes are often called DNA because they are composed of deoxyribonucleic acid. Chromosomes carry genetic messages, which direct the cell's assembly of amino acid building blocks into proteins that are ultimately used in the cell for growth, maintenance, and repair. The directions are in a chemical code composed of four types of nucleotides A, C, T, G, each of which stands for a different chemical. These letter *nucleotides* are arranged on the chromsome in precise three-letter word combinations called *codons* that are interpreted by a compound called ribonucleic acid or RNA. The RNA molecule reads a group, or sentence, of these codons within the cell nucleus. It then moves to the cytoplasm where it directs the synthesis of a specific protein, following the directions specified in the genetic code.

A *mutation* is any alteration in the genetic code. It can be caused by a number of factors including radiation and chemical exposure. Mutations may be insignificant if they affect a part of the genetic code that is not used by that particular cell or if the cell can easily repair the damage. However, mutations can be lethal to a cell if they affect a gene that is crucial to cell function.

Figure 2.1 Diagram of a cell. (From Hole, John W., Jr., *Human Anatomy and Physiology,* 3rd ed. Copyright © 1978, 1981, 1984 Wm. C. Brown Publishers, Dubuque, Iowa. All Rights Reserved. Reprinted by permission.)

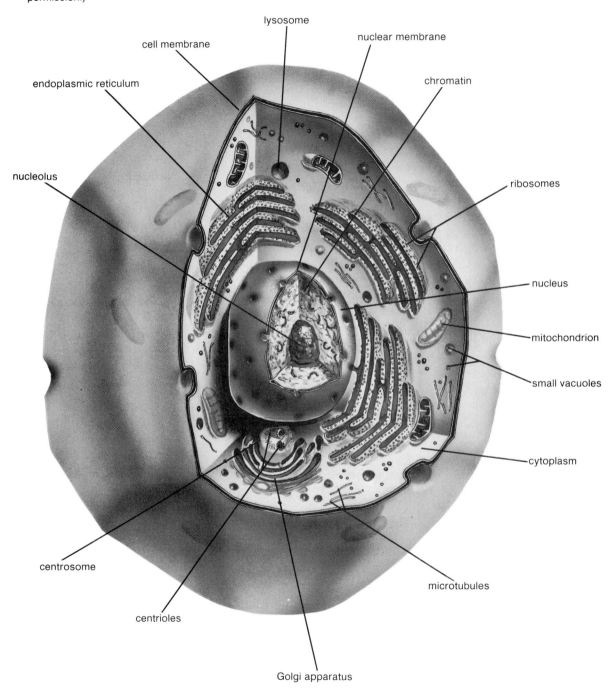

lysosome

nuclear membrane

cell membrane

chromatin

endoplasmic reticulum

nucleolus

ribosomes

nucleus

mitochondrion

small vacuoles

cytoplasm

centrosome

microtubules

centrioles

Golgi apparatus

Damage Theories

This group of theories asserts that cells function less efficiently with age because they become damaged. Damage to cell parts, accumulation of waste products, and build-up of deleterious chemicals within the cell eventually cause cells to function less effectively, leading to cellular aging. These theorists cite as major evidence the fact that with age the number of functional cells decreases and the material between cells accumulates. Damage theories to be discussed in this section include free radical, waste product accumulation, cross-linkage accumulation, and error accumulation theories.

Free Radical Theory

Harman (1968; 1984) proposes that gradual cellular aging is caused by damage from free radicals, which are produced within the cell. Free radicals are parts of molecules that have either an extra or missing electron that makes them highly reactive and likely to combine with and destroy essential cell components. Free radicals are the normal by-products of the reactions in the cell as it produces energy. They also occur when the cell is exposed to environmental chemicals such as tobacco smoke or radiation.

Although free radicals are unstable and short-lived, they can significantly damage cell components, especially the mechanism for cell maintenance and reproduction (DNA and RNA). Free radicals can also damage cell membranes, impeding their ability to transfer wastes and nutrients and eventually killing the cell. Fortunately, organisms have developed ways to counteract free radical damage by producing chemicals that seek out and deactivate them. Antioxidants, such as vitamins E and C and some minerals can capture free radicals. Also, some cells have mechanisms to repair the damage.

According to this theory, with age there is an accumulation of damage from free radicals that has escaped the cell's protective mechanisms. This accumulated damage contributes to cell malfunction and eventual cell death. It is hypothesized that free radical damage is the greatest in nerve and muscle cells that do not divide after maturity as the cell repair mechanisms may become less effective with age (Fleming et al. 1982).

Waste Product Accumulation Theory

Proponents of this theory assert that aging is caused by a time-related accumulation of inert or deleterious substances within cells that eventually impair cell function (Hochschild 1973). Even if the substances are not deleterious in themselves, the effect of waste product accumulation can take up essential space needed for cell function. Increased accumulation can be likened to a person doing jumping jacks in an increasingly crowded elevator: the more crowded it becomes, the harder it is to do the exercises correctly.

Although a number of waste products are known to accumulate in cells with age, lipofuscin has been extensively studied and is often called the age pigment. Lipofuscin is a dark colored residue that accumulates mainly in postmitotic cells (nerve and muscle cells). It is a waste product of normal cell activities. In some cells it displaces a significant volume of cell material and is believed to reduce the ability of the cell to make proteins (Mann and Yates 1974). However, as of yet, lipofuscin has not been found to impair cell function.

Cross-Linkage Accumulation Theory

Proponents of this theory hypothesize that the accumulation of cross-linked molecules in the cell is the primary cause of aging (Bjorksten 1963; 1968). With time, an increasing number of molecules within the cell connect to themselves or others to form cross-linkages. These cross-linkages may or may not impair the function of the molecule. Cross-linkages can have critical effects if they occur within the DNA or connective tissue of the cell. Free radicals and other reactions in normal cell metabolism are the primary contributors to cross-linkages.

When cross-linkages occur in the DNA molecule, the cross-linked portion cannot replicate during cell division (Brash and Hart 1978). The information on a cross-linked DNA molecule cannot be read by the RNA molecule and important chemicals may not be produced for cell maintenance. Although cells have mechanisms to repair this damage, cross-linkages in postmitotic cells are known to increase with age (Curtis and Miller 1971). This finding implies that the cellular repair mechanisms cannot keep up with the damage.

The effects of cross-linkages upon connective tissues (collagen and elastin) are well-documented. Collagen and elastin are long strands of protein that are maintained throughout life and are not renewed. They comprise 30 to 40 percent of body proteins and are present in all body cells. Cross-linkages in connective tissue cause rigidity and decreased elasticity of cells. Cross-linkages in elastin may contribute to increased rigidity of blood vessels and lung tissues and wrinkling of the skin. Cross-linkages in collagen may restrict lung movements and may interfere with cell membrane permeability, making it more difficult for cells to uptake nutrients and expel wastes.

Error Accumulation Theories

A number of theories attribute the cause of aging to an accumulation of mistakes in one or more steps of the DNA-RNA mechanism responsible for making needed proteins. The amount of active RNA and DNA within the cell has been reported to decrease with advancing age (Curtis and Miller 1971). This could be the result of deletion of key genes that eventually leads to reduced cell efficiency and cell death if the cell cannot make important proteins. The breakdown of the cellular informational system may occur at one or more critical points. The DNA itself could be faulty, errors could occur in copying the information from DNA to RNA, or mistakes may be made during the steps of protein synthesis. In any case, accumulation of mistakes reduces cell function. Three error accumulation theories will be discussed: mitotic arrest, DNA misrepair, and redundant message.

Mitotic Arrest

Strehler (1980) believes cellular aging occurs primarily in cells that do not replace themselves after maturity (postmitotic cells). He hypothesizes that *mitotic arrest,* or the inability of the muscle and nerve cells to divide after maturity, is an evolutionary adaptation to enable an organism to reach optimum body size and to establish semipermanent connections within the brain so it can carry out complex functions. Thus, the inability of nerve and muscle cells to divide is advantageous during growth and reproduction, but disadvantageous in later life because worn-out cells cannot be replaced, only repaired. Because the DNA of postmitotic cells is not replenished by cell division, the cell progressively loses its ability to synthesize needed proteins. As more cells become dysfunctional, they ultimately affect proper integration of the neuromuscular and neuroendocrine systems (Strehler 1979). Strehler estimates that 95 percent of age-associated physiological decrements can be attributed to an accumulation of errors and waste products in those cells that do not divide. He hypothesizes that those cells that do not divide lose 1 percent of their function each year after age thirty (Strehler 1977).

DNA Misrepair

Errors may accumulate because the cell's mechanism to repair DNA is damaged, allowing errors in the genetic code to accumulate. Generally, mistakes occurring in the DNA are easily repaired by specific enzymes. However, if the repair mechanism is damaged, the cell will be unable to repair its DNA, and some genes crucial to the function of the cell may be lost or misinterpreted.

Redundant Message Theory

It is known that some genes that direct production of particular proteins needed for cell function are duplicated many times along the DNA strand. These redundant, or extra genes are repressed until called into action when the active gene becomes faulty from free radical attack or cross-linkages. Soviet scientist Medvedev (1972)

Chapter 2

hypothesizes that aging occurs when the cell runs out of duplicate copies of important genes. As errors accumulate in the functional gene, the reserve sequences take over until all the genes that code for a particular protein are used up. At that time, the cell loses its capacity to function. Therefore, those genes with few or no back-up copies would be the most vulnerable. Support for this theory comes from documentation that animal species who live longer have more back-up copies of genes than animals with shorter life-spans. Further, Strehler and Johnson (1972) found that the presence of back-up copies were more important in cells that do not divide after maturity than those that continued to divide. They documented that postmitotic cells in old dogs had 30 percent fewer back up copies of a particular gene sequence than cells in young dogs, but the differences were not noted in cells that continued to divide after maturity.

Programmed Aging Theories

The programming theories assert that the processes of growth, development, and decline are written in the genetic code. Thus, the cell carries out the aging processes as directed by the DNA. Three theories of this type will be discussed. The codon restriction theory asserts that individual body cells are programmed to die while immunological and neuroendocrine theorists assert that the genetic programming has primary impact on the neuroendocrine or immune systems.

Codon Restriction Theory

Strehler's codon restriction theory (1977, 1979) is a highly sophisticated and complex model of aging. His theory is based on the premise that only a small part of the total information coded in the DNA molecule is used by the cell at any given time. Unlike the redundant message, each of these gene sequences have different gene messages. Throughout the life of the cell, different genes are activated or suppressed, directing the manufacture of different proteins at different times. Thus,

at any time in the lifetime of a cell, some of its genes are activated, but most are repressed; the cell is able to synthesize some proteins, but unable to produce others. However, the cell cannot reverse its development; once a gene message is used, it is no longer available.

Strehler hypothesizes that this progressive restriction of messages allows the cell to undergo the process of development and change over time in an orderly manner. Further, at a certain point in the lifetime of the cell, the genes direct the production of substances that then turn off those genes essential for cellular functioning. Strehler asserts that the progression of genetic messages throughout the life of a cell is not random, but the purposeful carry out of a program written in the genetic code (1977, 1979).

Immunological Theory

Originally proposed by Walford (1969), this theory suggests that aging is initiated in the genes that control the workings of the immune system. The immune system defends the body against foreign microorganisms and destroys its own abnormal cells by producing antibodies and white blood cells. These theorists hypothesize that, with age, the immune system is programmed to function less effectively.

At least part of the control of immune system responses is regulated by a group of genes called the major histocompatibility complex (MHC). Smith and Walford (1977) were able to demonstrate that the MHC is an important regulator of the rate of aging. In their experiments using mice with identical genes except for the MHC, they reported that differences in life span could be attributed to that particular gene cluster. This experiment provided the first direct evidence that one particular gene cluster (on one chromosome) is an important regulator of the rate of aging. Walford predicts that, aside from controlling immunity, genes near the MHC influence the cells' ability to scavenge free radicals and possibly repair DNA (1983). However, whether the MHC and associated genes fail to function in later life because of error or programmed decline is not known.

Neuroendocrine Theories

A number of gerontologists believe that the neuroendocrine system is the central mechanism that controls the aging process. The neuroendocrine system is the communication system of the body and includes the brain, spinal cord, and nerve cells as well as the glands and hormones they release. The brain controls most cell and organ functions in the body, either directly through nerve-to-nerve transmission or indirectly through hormones of the endocrine system.

There is a complex interrelationship between the neural and hormonal systems. In some cases, neurons directly stimulate glands to release hormones. In other cases, neurons in the brain trigger the production of releasing factors that in turn stimulate hormone release. The neural and hormonal systems are similar in that both exert their effect through similar chemical messengers— neurons use neurotransmitters and glands release hormones.

As an organism ages, a breakdown in communication within the neuroendocrine system occurs. This imbalance may occur if a highly destructive hormone is programmed to appear suddenly, or it may be a gradual process, caused by programmed hormone imbalances. One of the best examples of a rapid hormonal release in animals is the Pacific Northwest Salmon. It rapidly deteriorates from youthful vigor to death shortly after spawning. This change is triggered by the release of a massive amount of hormone from the adrenal glands into the bloodstream. However, aging in humans is more likely due to a slowly developing hormonal imbalance. The hypothalamus, the center of hormone coordination, is most likely to regulate aging.

Death Hormone Theory

Denkla (1974) believes that after puberty, the pituitary releases DECO (decreased oxygen consumption hormone), which acts as a death hormone to cause the gradual destruction of the organism. He hypothesizes that the hormone exerts its effects by prohibiting the body from using thyroxin, a thyroid hormone. Even though the body continues to produce the needed thyroid hormones, DECO prohibits target cells from responding to the hormone. He cites as evidence the fact that deficiency of thyroid hormone causes symptoms that mimic the aging process. However, Denckla has not been able to isolate the specific DECO hormone.

Neuroendocrine System Failure

Finch (1975, 1977) believes that a slowly developing hormonal imbalance, caused by a decrease of brain neurotransmitters, plays a primary role in the aging process. Finch documented that older animals have a significant decrease of the neurotransmitter, catecholamine, in the area of the brain that controls hormone release. Finch believes that the decreased production of neurotransmitters is programmed in the genes. He asserts that this reduction of neurotransmitters initiates an endocrine cascade, as changes in the secretion of one hormone alter subsequent endocrine responses. This could cause widespread hormone imbalances and decreased functioning.

Conclusion

As of yet, there is no generally accepted theory to describe the mechanisms that initiate aging. Although a number of changes within the cell are known to be associated with aging, one of the greatest difficulties researchers encounter is determining which changes are the underlying causes of aging and which are only reflections of an earlier occurrence that originated elsewhere. It is likely that a combination of processes contributes to eventual biological decline and death.

Increased knowledge regarding the biological process of aging will not only satisfy our curiosity regarding how we age, but can also serve to prolong youth and forestall deterioration. The knowledge is likely to be most useful in combating common degenerative diseases that accompany aging.

Chapter 2

Earlier in the century, colon irrigation (enema) was
thought to promote health and longer life.

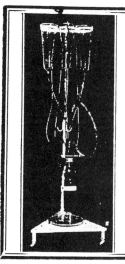
Attempts to Delay Aging

Although immortality is beyond our immediate
grasp, scientists all over the world continue to seek
ways to forestall aging. Much research on the
biologic theories of aging is motivated by a desire
to extend the human life. Researchers have not
yet discovered the magic bullet, but their attempts continue to provide a better understanding of why and how we age.

Throughout history, individuals of nearly
every culture have sought to prolong youth and
postpone the inevitable aging process. A persistent theme is a belief in a fountain of youth
that will provide immortality to its discoverer.
Perhaps the best-known seeker of immortality was
Ponce de Leon, who set sail to find the fountain
of youth, thought to exist on the isle of Bimini,
but who arrived in Florida instead.

Others have attempted to prolong youth in
other ways. Semen was once believed to be a life-
giving force by Taoists and other cultural groups.
Taoists of China believed life could be extended
if men preserved their life essence by abstaining
from ejaculation. Australian aborigines administered a semen potion to the feeble or aged to
restore their vigor (Segerberg 1974). In the late
nineteenth century, a renowned professor injected himself with an extract of crushed dog testicles and reported that it restored the strength
and vitality of his youth (Trimmer 1970). Around
the same period, vain attempts were made to graft
ape and goat testicles onto aging men to increase
virility and vitality (Walford 1983).

Other immortalists believed aging to be
caused by deleterious toxins in the intestines that
must be diluted by buttermilk and yogurt or
purged with daily enemas or strong laxatives
(Walford 1983).

These attempts to postpone aging seem foolhardy, but most modern attempts are likely as ineffective. Our magazines advertise that royal
queen bee jelly, youth tonics, negative ion gen-
erators, or oriental herb remedies will produce
miraculous results for only $29.95 plus tax. The
wistful search for eternal youth continues as it has
since the dawn of civilization; only the methods
have changed with time and culture.

This section will discuss current attempts to
extend life. It is important to understand the difference between life expectancy and life span. *Life

Would you buy this product?

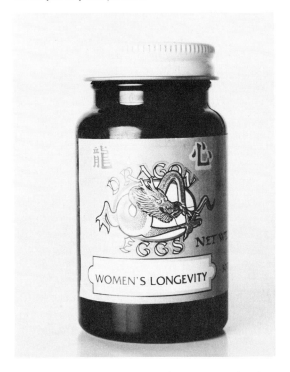

expectancy is the number of years an individual can expect to live and varies among time periods and cultures. As infectious diseases are controlled and health and sanitary conditions improve, life expectancy has increased in the United States. In contrast, *life span* is the maximum length of time an individual could live under ideal conditions. Thus, even though life expectancy has increased, life span has remained relatively constant at 110–120 years over cultures and for the past 2,000 years of human evolution. The Biblical writings of the purported age of Methusela, and, more recently, reports of extreme longevity among inhabitants of remote mountain villages have not been substantiated. A Japanese man, Shigechiyo Izumi, holds the world record for longevity—120 years, 237 days. He died in February 1986. In the U.S., the record is held by Mamie Kieth of Illinois, who lived to be 113 years old (Russell 1986).

The following attempts to increase length of life works are more likely to increase life expectancy, not life span. Further, because most experiments have been conducted on animal subjects, the effect of these treatments on human longevity remains largely hypothetical.

Dietary Manipulation: Eat Less and Live Longer?

For almost fifty years, researchers have manipulated the quality and quantity of food ingested in laboratory animals to better understand the relationship between diet and longevity. The pioneering studies of McCay and Maynard (1939) reported that underfeeding rats right after weaning significantly extended their life. One group was fed a normal, well-balanced diet while the other ingested the same vitamins and minerals, but only one-third of the calories. The rats on the restricted diet had slower growth and development and were smaller in size than the control group, but they lived 60 percent longer than those on a normal diet. Researchers subsequently reported a significant increase in life expectancy when gradual caloric restriction was initiated in adult mice. (Weindrich et al. 1982). However, researchers cautioned that diet, though restricted calorically, cannot be impoverished nutritionally.

Aside from a lengthened life, researchers report that calorie-restricted laboratory animals exhibit a significantly lower incidence of cancer, increased immune system efficiency, and a more youthful metabolism (Weindrich et al. 1982; Cheney et al. 1980). It is generally agreed that dietary restriction works because it reduces hormone secretion from the anterior pituitary secretions that consequently decreases the rate of immune system decline (Weindrich et al. 1982).

Other studies with laboratory rats show a correlation between the type of food eaten and longevity. Ross (1976) allowed rats to select their own diet throughout life. He reported that the ratio of protein to carbohydrate intake was influential in life expectancy. The shortest-lived rats chose foods low in protein and high in carbohydrates for the first few weeks after weaning. Their food preferences after that time had little relationship to their longevity.

Similarly, many individuals believe that periodic fasting is cleansing and healthful. Goodrick (*Science News* 1979) produced evidence that periodic fasting promotes vigorous and extended life in laboratory rats. In a controlled study, he observed that those rats who fasted every other day lived significantly longer than those provided continuous access to food. However, there is no documentation that fasting produces similar benefits in humans.

It is still uncertain whether studies on dietary manipulation merely allow the animals to live to the outside limits of their normal life expectancy or increase their life span. Further, the application of these results to humans is only conjecture because similar studies have not been extended to humans. The dietary regimes imposed on laboratory animals are far too severe for human subjects who might be less willing to trade stunted growth, delayed maturity, or hunger pains for the possibility of a longer life.

Body Temperature: Colder is Better?

A number of studies document a significant increase in length of life of cold-blooded animals (such as fruit flies, fish, and lizards) when body temperatures are lowered experimentally, especially in the latter half of life. Although the body temperature in cold-blooded animals may be easily manipulated by altering environmental temperature, it is very difficult to manipulate the body temperature of warm-blooded animals since a cold environmental temperature only reduces skin temperature, not internal body temperature. In fact, mammals compensate for a cold environment by increasing their metabolic rate, which may decrease their lifespan (Walford 1983).

Attempts to decrease the body temperature of warm-blooded animals by using drugs have had mixed results. Liu and Walford (1972) were able to induce mild temperature depression in mice with THC, the active ingredient in marijuana.

However, they note that after two–three doses of THC in one month, the system became resistant to the body temperature-lowering effect.

Scientists hypothesize that lowering body temperature prolongs life by slowing destructive autoimmune processes (where the immune system attacks body tissues). Although the immune system works most efficiently at elevated body temperatures (e.g., during a fever), an abnormally high body temperature may also increase the rate at which immune cells attack and destroy the body's own cells, contributing to a quickened degeneration of the organism. Thus, even though a lowered body temperature may reduce immune system efficiency, it may retard aging by reducing harmful autoimmune processes (Sohnle and Gambert 1982). Rosenberg and his colleagues (1973) hypothesize that a two–three degree lowering of human body temperature may increase length of life by twenty-five to thirty years. However, this theory will remain untested until scientists develop a safe method to reduce body temperature. At this time, the relationship between increased length of life and artificially lowered body temperature is not documented in mammals.

Antioxidant Therapy: Capturing Free Radicals

As described earlier in the chapter, free radicals accelerate aging by destroying a number of important body cell components. A widely-studied attempt to prolong longevity is to supplement the diet with antioxidants to reduce the damage of free radicals within body cells. Common antioxidants used include vitamin E, selenium, vitamin C, and BHT (a common food preservative).

Preliminary research on animals and humans indicates that antioxidant supplements may reduce the effect of free radicals and prolong life. Harman and Eddy (1978) hypothesize that vitamins E and C, selenium, and BHT decrease damaging breaks in DNA induced by cancer-causing chemicals. Harman (1968) administered antioxidant supplements to mice in a greater quantity than the normal diet, and he reported a significant increase in life expectancy. Dietary vitamin E supplements were also reported to decrease the incidence of malignant growths in laboratory mice (Packer and Walton 1977). One study on humans showed that 200 mg of vitamin E supplementation in the diets of a group of elders resulted in a significant decrease of damaging peroxides (a type of free radical) in their blood serum; after a year of supplementation, peroxide levels had fallen 26 percent (reported by Globus 1984).

Vitamin C supplementation has been noted to protect against DNA cross-linkages as well as show other health benefits such as decreasing blood cholesterol, reducing artery wall thickening, and stimulating the immune system (Anderson et al. 1980; Sokoloff et al. 1966).

Although the evidence of the usefulness of dietary antioxidants is far from conclusive, many gerontologists and laypeople supplement their diets with antioxidant vitamins just in case. However, overdoses of some vitamins and minerals (especially vitamin E and selenium) may be harmful (see Chapter 9).

Nucleic Acid Therapy: Dead End or Right Track?

It is generally agreed that with age, body cells become less able to produce and repair cell components necessary for cell maintenance and repair (especially DNA and RNA). Dr. Frank, a physician from New York, asserts that daily dietary supplementation of these metabolic building blocks (RNA, DNA, amino acids, minerals, sugars, B vitamins, and phosphates) will facilitate protein synthesis and consequent energy production within the cell (1976, 1977). He stresses that the supplements need to be ingested simultaneously to enable body cells to have all the necessary ingredients for manufacture of proteins at once. Unfortunately, the data Frank collected in experiments on both animals and humans are scanty, generally not controlled, and largely testimonial. To date, the results have not been corroborated by other gerontologists under controlled conditions.

However, experiments conducted several decades ago by other investigators indicate that RNA therapy increases lifespan in laboratory animals. Older mice receiving daily doses of RNA lived significantly longer and were hardier than the control group (Gardner 1946). Similar results were reported when rats ingested such supplements throughout their lives (Robertson 1928). A later study reported a doubling of the lives of rats when weekly injections of DNA and RNA were administered to older rats (Odens 1973). Other beneficial effects of nucleic acid therapy upon laboratory animals are immune system enhancement (Rigby 1971) and improved learning and memory (Solyom et al. 1967). However, the value of nucleic acid therapy must await further testing since there have been no controlled studies on humans.

Procaine: The Youth Drug of Celebrities

For more than thirty years, procaine-based drugs (a relative of novocaine) have been used extensively in Europe to treat age-associated symptoms (e.g., memory loss, physical weakness, skin wrinkling, and hair loss) and some degenerative diseases. Ana Aslan, a Rumanian physician, has treated thousands of patients, many of them famous, with a therapy she calls Gerovital (GH-3) (Aslan 1960). Her successes have not been scientifically documented in humans, but testimonials by her patients describe dramatic improvements in physical and mental functioning, but not length of life. Although she reported a 21 percent increase in life expectancy in laboratory animals receiving GH-3 supplements, these experiments had methodological flaws.

Controlled studies conducted in the United States to confirm her findings reported procaine to be ineffective in increasing life span, but it was significantly more successful in treating depression than a placebo or common antidepressant (Zung et al. 1974). Walford (1983) asserts that, despite its potential, the drug has never been adequately tested for life span extension in animals. As in nucleic acid therapy, until further studies document its effectiveness, any benefits are hypothetical.

Thymus Hormones and Immune Cell Transplants: The Best Bet?

As immune failure is considered by many to be a major contributor to the aging process, rejuvenation of the immune system may be a logical way to postpone aging. The thymus gland (located in the neck) is an important part of the immune system, but it atrophies after adolescence. In experimental animals, removal of the thymus accelerates decrements of the immune system. Conversely, thymus gland grafts from young animals to old animals reverse many age-associated decrements and increase their life expectancy (Hirokawa and Makinodan 1975). Although thymosin (thymus hormone) injections reverse age-associated deficiencies of this hormone in lab animals, this is generally not sufficient to restore immune system function completely. Weksler (1983) maintains that immune senescence is more complex than thymosin deficiency alone. During aging there is an excessive production of cells from the bone marrow that suppress the immune system function from the bone marrow. He believes the hormone injections need to be supplemented with bone marrow transplants from young individuals to have the greatest effect.
complex than thymosin deficiency alone.

Some scientists project that in the future, children may have some of their bone marrow and thymus tissue removed and frozen for implantation in their later years to rejuvenate the immune system to fight disease, environmental toxins, and the aging process itself. Immune system cells have already been successfully preserved in a frozen state for later use (Knight et al. 1977).

Even if thymosin injections or immune cell transplants do not increase life expectancy, their major impact may be their ability to increase immune function to resist disease. For instance, these injections may help boost the immune systems of cancer patients. In one study of cancer patients who underwent heavy doses of chemotherapy, those receiving high doses of thymosin survived almost twice as long as those who did not receive the injection (Lipson et al. 1979).

Other Drugs: Popping Pills to Stay Young

Researchers continue to seek drugs that will allow people to live longer, healthier lives. A number of drugs have already been discussed that may impact upon the deleterious effects of aging. Experimental drugs are purported to reduce lipofuscin concentration, scavenge free radicals, cool body temperature, undo cross-linkages, replace needed hormones or building blocks, and more.

One of the most promising drugs is L-dopa, a drug commonly administered to patients with Parkinson's disease. L-dopa, a synthetic precurser of the neurotransmitter dopamine, stimulates increased production of dopamine in the brain. Timiras and colleagues (1980) note that levels of dopamine decline with age in some portions of the brain. Cotzias et al. (1974) were able to demonstrate significant life extension in mice with administration of L-dopa. Although L-dopa is known to increase the life expectancy of those with Parkinson's disease, these individuals still do not live as long as the rest of the population. The drug is hypothesized to counteract the body's decreased dopamine concentration in the aging brain to enable more efficient message transmission.

Conclusion

A perusal of the most reputable methods of extending productive life reveals that, although some hold promise, none is well-substantiated

> Man's subconscious quest for a measure of immortality continues unabated; yet paradoxically, he jeopardizes his small share in the immortality of his species by his actions.
>
> Leonard Schuman

PERSPECTIVE: Consequences of Life Extension

Scientists' projections of a future in which all live to be very old are largely speculative and dependent upon many variables. Will science find a means to extend life expectancy to the current maximum of 110–120 years? Will the life span be extended to two hundred years or more? Will humans be able to retain youthful physique until death or will they age more slowly?

Not everyone believes life extension is desirable. More people living longer would strain our environmental and economic resources. More old people would mean a limited space for new arrivals, putting more pressure on food supply and energy demand. The number of people over sixty-five is rapidly increasing and by the end of the century, people over sixty-five will comprise one-fourth of the population. Under today's definition of retirement, that means one-fourth of the population will be out of the work force, supported by the labors of the working population. Even if life expectancy increased by only ten years, drastic policy adjustments would be needed for retirement, Social Security, and Medicare.

The possible consequences of life extension on our political, economic, social, and value systems are approached more often by science fiction writers than gerontologists. If we had more old people and fewer young, would this decrease the influx of creative new ideas, or would we accumulate even more knowledge on the basis of elders' wisdom? Would the government have to interfere with the freedom to bear children to curb overpopulation? If the old no longer experience the physical symptoms of aging, what effect might this have on our culture? Would people devote more energy to avoid overpopulation, pollution, and nuclear war if they personally experienced the consequences?

The goal of research on life extension is to expand the number of productive years with the highest level of physical health and mental abilities. A longer life without accompanying vitality is a foolish, even cruel endeavor. Some may consider the time and money spent on such research as futile. On the other hand, when a method to prolong our good years is discovered, which of us would turn down the opportunity?

with evidence from human subjects. At least part of the success of several treatments with human subjects may be due to faith in the treatment. We will continue to read about treatments that either promote longer life or postpone the diseases and symptoms of old age. As consumers, it is important to distinguish those commercial ventures that do nothing more than instill false hope and relieve us of our money.

Fries and Crapo (1981) assert that the quest to extend life in the laboratory is misplaced. The goals should not be to maximize the length of life, but extend the period of vitality by modifying the factors that affect the rate of aging and onset of disease (e.g., cigarette smoking). In this way, the prevalence of diseases and disorders that cause disability and early death can be reduced. As we will see in the following section, good health

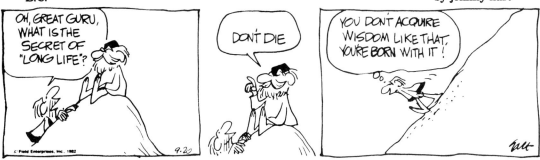

habits, social situation, and positive mental attitude are more likely to extend life than the treatments discussed above.

Factors Influencing Longevity

Gerontologists generally consider 110–120 years to be the maximum limit of human life, yet most people live less than two-thirds of that. Why do so few reach this upper limit? In an attempt to answer this question, scientists have identified a number of genetic and environmental factors correlated with long life. Some believe heredity to be the primary determinant of longevity while others hold that psychosocial and lifestyle factors are more signficant. Regardless of which determinants are most important, most agree that a variety of factors are influential. Some are beyond our control (e.g., genetics, gender), others are modifiable lifestyle choices (e.g., smoking, weight control, and physical activity). Robert Louis Stevenson's quote, "Life is not a matter of getting good cards, but of playing a poor hand well" is relevant to longevity. One individual makes the most of a poor deal while another squanders a good hand with poor playing.

Heredity and Parental Influences

Longevity has a genetic component as evidenced by a classic study by Kallman and Sander (1948). These researchers studied over one thousand pairs of twins, both identical twins (who have identical genes) and nonidentical twins (who share approximately one-half their genes). They reported that the deaths of the identical twins were separated by an average of three years while those who were same-sex fraternal twins differed in time of death by six and one-half years.

Other studies on families support the hypothesis that some components of longevity are inherited. Pearl and Pearl (1934) published a massive study that supported the adage, "the best way to live long is to choose long-lived parents." They showed that the length of life of biological parents, and to a lesser extent, grandparents, influences the child's length of life. Recently, Abbott and associates (1974) reanalyzed these data and concluded that although there was a clear genetic component to the length of life, it was slight. They also reported maternal longevity to be more important than paternal longevity in predicting life expectancy of offspring of both sexes. Whether this correlation is genetic or whether mothers have more influence over their child's lifestyle, diet, and outlook on life is still unknown. In contrast, the Duke Longitudinal Study (Palmore, 1971), reported the father's age at death, not the mother's, was significant in predicting longevity for the progeny.

It is generally agreed that in advanced age, environmental influences are more important than hereditary disposition. It is hypothesized that modern medicine has allowed those with hereditary deficits to survive whereas in earlier days they may have died sooner (Moment 1982).

Gender

There is a strong correlation between gender and longevity. In industrial countries, females have lower death rates than males in all age groups including still births and infant mortality. In those underdeveloped countries in which men live longer than women, this differential has been attributed to a high rate of maternal death during childbirth. In the United States in 1985, the average life expectancy for females was 78.2 years; for males, 71.2 years. In all races, women live longer than men. Both genetic and behavioral explanations have been proposed for this sex differential in longevity.

It is hypothesized that females have a genetic advantage that enables them to live longer than males as they have a longer life expectancy in almost all animal species. It is believed that the X chromsome (all females have two, men have one) carries the genes for immune system functioning and possibly those that repair free radical damage. This might make females more resistant to infectious diseases and cell damage (Waldron 1976). The X chromosomes may also carry genes for other survival-related mechanisms. For instance, women's natural production of estrogens may protect them against certain diseases such as atherosclerosis and heart disease. Women become more susceptible to these conditions after menopause when estrogen production is decreased (Retherford 1975).

Greater male vulnerability is thought to be influenced by the deleterious effects of testosterone on longevity. One study of mentally retarded castrated and uncastrated males reported that the castrated males (removal of the testes which produce the majority of testosterone) lived an average of 13.5 years longer than their virile counterparts and 6.7 years longer than women. Eunuchs lived even longer than women because women produce some testosterone while eunuchs produce virtually none (Hamilton 1948). Men are more prone to heart attacks in the third and fourth decade of their life when testosterone output is at its peak. This could be because testosterone promotes blood clotting, which may increase susceptibility to heart attacks. Sacher (1965) reported those with larger brain-to-body-weight ratios live longer than those with lower ratios. Even though men have a larger average brain size than women, women have a larger relative brain size because they weigh less. The larger ratio is hypothesized to enable better neural control, which increases survival value.

Gender-linked behavior has also been cited as a reason for the difference in life expectancy. Males are more apt to smoke and drink more heavily than females and these behaviors reduce life expectancy. Waldron (1976) believes that much of the sex differential in mortality is due to males' aggressive and competitive personality, which causes a higher rate of suicides, homicides, and automobile accidents. Also, women are more likely to report illness and use health services more than men. Although a number of individuals believe that the consequences of occupational equality between the sexes will increase female mortality, no evidence substantiates that prediction. For instance, the incidence of heart disease in the U.S. is not rising among women. Further, women employed outside the home are no more likely to develop coronary heart disease than full-time housewives (Haynes and Feinleib 1980).

Ethnicity

Life expectancy varies significantly among ethnic groups in the United States. For instance, blacks, Hispanics, and native Americans have a shorter life expectancy than whites, while Japanese-Americans live longer (Metropolitian Life Insurance 1977). Higher mortality rates for most nonwhite groups is not due to genetic factors. Stresses of poverty and discrimination are thought to be significant contributors to the shortened life expectancy of black, Hispanic, and native American populations in our country. Blacks, native Americans, and Hispanics have significantly lower incomes than their white counterparts, resulting in poorer diet and less access to adequate medical care.

Table 2.1 Gain in years in expectation of life if cause was eliminated (at birth).

Cause of Death	Gain in Years
Major cardiovascular-renal diseases	10.9
Heart diseases	5.9
Vascular diseases affecting the central nervous system	1.3
Malignant neoplasms	2.3
Accidents, excluding those caused by motor vehicles	0.6
Motor vehicle accidents	0.6
Influenza and pneumonia	0.5
Infectious diseases (excluding tuberculosis)	0.2
Diabetes mellitus	0.2
Tuberculosis	0.1

SOURCE: Life tables published by the National Center of Health Statistics, U.S. Public Health Service and U.S. Bureau of the Census, "Some Demographic Aspects of Aging in the United States," February 1973.

Genetic and Acquired Disease

Genetic and acquired diseases are significant determinants of life expectancy. Inherited genetic diseases such as sickle cell anemia, Down's syndrome, and insulin-dependent diabetes reduce life expectancy. It is obvious that a number of acquired health problems predispose a shorter life expectancy: heart disease, cancers, organic brain syndrome. In 1973, the National Center of Health Statistics published a table that reflects how long we would live if some of the major killers were eliminated (table 2.1). Almost twenty-three years could be added to our current life expectancy if the major diseases were eliminated.

Obesity

A number of epidemiological studies report a correlation between obesity and decreased life expectancy in humans. Obesity has long been associated with a high prevalence of a number of life-shortening diseases. Price and Pritts (1980) document the deleterious effects of obesity on virtually all body systems. They report that those who are 20 percent or more overweight have an increased risk of sudden death and are more prone to a number of diseases: diabetes, gallstones, coronary heart disease, and hypertension. Actuarials of major insurance companies have also found positive correlations between obesity and disease, disability, and death. Overweight persons tend to die sooner than average weight persons, especially those who are overweight when young. Studies based on life insurance data indicate that slightly below average weight is associated with the greatest longevity, if such weight is not due to illness, smoking, or a history of signficant medical impairment.

Obese people may have a shortened life expectancy not because of obesity itself, but because of those behaviors that often accompany it, such as overconsumption of refined sugars and fats, and lack of exercise. It is apparent from the data presented that future work defining the relationship between body weight and longevity needs to take into account such diverse variables as quality of nutritional intake, physical activity level, health status, psychological variables, and income.

Physical Activity

The most conclusive evidence thus far that exercise increases longevity is a landmark longitudinal study comparing over sixteen thousand Harvard University alumni over a period of twelve to sixteen years. Vigorous exercise such as walking, stair climbing, and sporting activities were correlated with lower mortality, especially from cardiovascular or respiratory ailments. As the physical activity increased, death rates decreased. Even when those who exercised, smoked cigarettes, were hypertensive, had gained weight, or had parents who suffered early deaths, they still lived significantly longer than the physically inactive. The researchers estimated that by age eighty, the amount of additional years attributable to regular, strenuous exercise is one to two years (Paffenbarger et al. 1986).

The value of exercise in reducing the extent of life-shortening heart disease is well-established. A number of classic studies comparing men in sedentary jobs with those in jobs that require more physical activity reported that regular patterns of physical activity reduce heart attack risk (Morris et al. 1954; Brunner et al. 1974; Paffenbarger et al. 1977). The lack of physical activity among the workers was reported to be as great a risk factor as cigarette smoking or high blood pressure.

The physiological benefits of physical activity that influence longevity are well-documented: exercise strengthens the heart, decreases the likelihood of obesity, and reduces blood clot formation. Researchers have documented that a high level of physical activity is related to increased concentrations of high density lipoproteins (HDL) in the bloodstream, which is associated with reduced heart attack risk (Hartung et al. 1980).

Anecdotal evidence supporting the value of physical activity is reported by Segerberg (1982) who studied twelve hundred centenarians in the United States. The majority of respondents reported they had done hard physical work for most of their lives.

Alcohol Use

Moderate use of alcohol (one–two ounces daily) may promote longer life. A number of health benefits from moderate alcohol consumption have been suggested. A study of heart disease in eighteen developed countries reported that increased levels of wine drinking correlated with decreased rates of heart disease (Leger et al., 1979). Klatsky et al. (1974) found that moderate drinkers were 30 percent less likely to have heart attacks than nondrinkers. In moderate dosages, alcohol increases the production of high density lipoproteins (HDL), which protect against heart disease (Johansson and Medhus 1974). On the negative side, alcohol overindulgence is associated with a number of physical and mental disorders: nutritional deficiencies, liver damage, depression, dementia, and suicide to name a few.

Although moderate alcohol consumption is associated with long life, a cause and effect relationship has not been established. It may later be discovered that moderate drinkers as a group have another lifestyle characteristic in common, other than moderate alcohol use, that predisposes them to longer life. As a group, teetotalers have a lower socio-economic status than moderate drinkers. They may also have more rigid personality structures that make them more susceptible to stress. Total abstainers in studies also include former alcoholics and those with serious health problems that may reduce their life expectancy. On the other hand, moderate alcohol consumption may produce relaxing effects that serve to reduce stress and lengthen life.

Cigarette Smoking

Experts agree that the most important action an individual can take to increase life expectancy is to quit smoking cigarettes. The link between tobacco use, serious health problems, and decreased life expectancy is well-documented. Cigarette smokers have overall mortality rates substantially greater than nonsmokers. On the average, cigarette smokers die ten years sooner than nonsmokers (Granich 1972), mainly because of increased incidence of cancers and heart disease. It is estimated that 30 percent of both cancer and cardiovascular disease deaths are caused by cigarette smoking (Report of the Surgeon General 1982, 1983).

The risk of developing and dying from coronary heart disease and cancer is directly related to cigarette smoke exposure, which includes the number of cigarettes smoked per day, total years of smoking, and degree of inhalation. The good news remains: reducing cigarette consumption or quitting altogether has been demonstrated to decrease excess mortality and premature death (Smith, et al. 1978).

The relationship between smoking and longevity is so strong that for men in their sixties, smoking is the single most accurate predictor of remaining life expectancy, making up to five years

Companionship may be one of the reasons why married people live longer than those who are not.

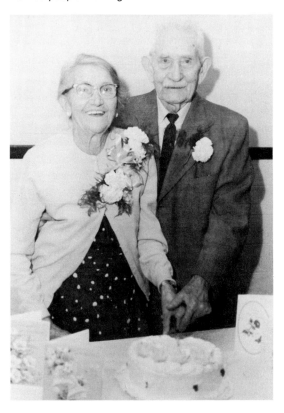

difference in longevity (Palmore 1971). Insurance companies are well aware of the higher mortality of smokers and offer reductions in premiums for nonsmokers.

Marital Status

Regardless of sex or race, those who are married live longer than those who are single, widowed, or divorced for every age past twenty (U.S. Department of Health, Education, and Welfare 1976). Pfeiffer's comparison of long and short-lived subjects in the Duke Longitudinal Study reveals that 75 percent of the women who had lived long were married, while only 29 percent of the women who had lived shorter lives were married (1970). Also, ninety-five percent of long-lived men were married, compared to 75 percent of the short-lived men.

Exactly how might marriage promote longevity? It may be that those who are married have more built-in social interaction, a better chance for care when ill, or better diets. Further, unmarried individuals (especially women) may have reduced incomes and less opportunity for social or sexual interaction. The Duke Longitudinal Study found that frequency of intercourse per week, and past and present enjoyment of sex was a significant correlate with longer life, partially explaining why married couples have increased longevity (Pfeiffer 1970). On the other hand, low sexual frequency may be a reflection of poor health status, which significantly affects longevity. Since societal mores regard married life as the ideal, the single state itself may induce stress. The stress of losing a spouse of many decades during old age may also contribute to the shortened life expectancy of the unmarried sample as that sample included those who are divorced, widowed, or were never married.

Personality

Individuals able to deal constructively with stress may live longer. Inability to deal appropriately with stress results in a number of illnesses, some of which reduce life expectancy (e.g., heart disease, hypertension). Evidence of the effect of stress on longevity is the excess mortality experienced by widowed individuals, especially men, in the two-year period after the death of their spouse (Helsing et al. 1981).

Anecdotal evidence provided by Segerberg (1982) provides support that positive coping strategies may prolong life. The majority of centenarians in his study emphasized the importance of positive attitudes and emotions and the suppression of negative ones "even to the point of appearing callous or relinquishing grief for a lifetime mate who died." A great many of them avoided strong emotions altogether. Since all centenarians he studied were hard workers, Segerberg hypothesized that such physical activity served to reduce stress by focusing their minds to block out negative mental preoccupations. He compared the mental focusing during hard labor

Can You Live to Be 100?

The following test gives you a rough guide for predicting your longevity. The basic life expectancy for males is age seventy-one, and for females it is age seventy-eight. Write down your basic life expectancy. If you are in your fifties or sixties, you should add ten years to the basic figure because you have already proved yourself to be a durable individual. If you are over age sixty and active, you can even add another two years.

Basic Life Expectancy

Decide how each item below applies to you and add or subtract the appropriate number of years from your basic life expectancy.

1. Family history

   Add 5 years if two or more of your grandparents lived to eighty or beyond   _____

   Subtract 4 years if any parent, grandparent, sister, or brother died of heart attack or stroke before fifty. Subtract 2 years if anyone died from these diseases before sixty.   _____

   Subtract 3 years for each case of diabetes, thyroid disorder, breast cancer, cancer of the digestive system, asthma, or chronic bronchitis among parents or grandparents.   _____

2. Marital status

   If you are married, add 4 years.   _____

   If you are over twenty-five and not married, subtract 1 year for every unwedded decade.   _____

3. Economic status

   Subtract 2 years if your family income is over $40,000 per year.   _____

   Subtract 3 years if you have been poor for the greater part of your life.   _____

4. Physique

   Subtract 1 year for every ten pounds you are overweight.   _____

   For each inch your girth measurement exceeds your chest measurement deduct 2 years.   _____

   Add 3 years if you are over forty and not overweight.   _____

5. Exercise

   Regular and moderate (jogging three times a week), add 3 years. _____

   Regular and vigorous (long distance running three times a week), add 5 years. _____

   Subtract 3 years if your job is sedentary. _____

   Add 3 years if it is active. _____

6. Alcohol

   Add 2 years if you are a light drinker (one to three drinks a day). _____

   Subtract 5 to 10 years if you are a heavy drinker (more than four drinks per day). _____

   Subtract 1 year if you are a teetotaler. _____

7. Smoking

   Two or more packs of cigarettes per day, subtract 8 years. _____

   One to two packs per day, subtract 2 years. _____

   Less than one pack, subtract 2 years. _____

   Subtract 2 years if you regularly smoke a pipe or cigars. _____

8. Disposition

   Add 2 years if you are a reasoned, practical person. _____

   Subtract 2 years if you are aggressive, intense, and competitive. _____

   Add 1–5 years if you are basically happy and content with life. _____

   Subtract 1-5 years if you are often unhappy, worried, and often feel guilty. _____

9. Education

   Less than high school, subtract 2 years. _____

   Four years of school beyond high school, add 1 year. _____

   Five or more years beyond high school, add 3 years. _____

10. Environment

   If you have lived most of your life in a rural environment, add 4 years. _____

   Subtract 2 years if you have lived most of your life in an urban environment. _____

11. Sleep

   More than nine hours a day, subtract 5 years.   _____

12. Temperature

   Add 2 years if your home's thermostat is set at no more than
   68° F.   _____

13. Health care

   Regular medical checkups and regular dental care, add 3
   years.   _____

   Frequently ill, subtract 2 years.   _____

                              Your Life Expectancy Total   _____

From Schultz: *Psychology of Death, Dying and Bereavement* (1978). Reprinted with permission from Addison-Wesley.

with meditation, such as the relaxation response, a well-known technique to calm individuals in time of stress.

Social Class: Education, Income, and Occupation

Because there is a high correlation among income, education, occupation, and social class, it is difficult to isolate these factors as determinants of longevity. However, it is clear that higher educational attainments and social class, more prestigious occupations, and above-average income levels contribute to greater longevity.

There is a positive relationship between longevity and education or intelligence level. Studies by the Metropolitan Life Insurance Company (1975) revealed that the life expectancy of male college graduates was significantly greater than that of the general white male population; those college graduates who were honor students lived even longer. Terman and Oden (1959) followed a group of gifted children for thirty-five years and reported that the group had less mental illness, fewer divorces, greater occupational success, and greater longevity than the population as a whole. Long-lived women in the Duke Longitudinal

Study scored about 50 percent higher on IQ testing than those who died earlier in the study (Pfeiffer 1970). It is not certain whether high intelligence or educational attainment is a direct correlate with longevity. It may be that higher educational levels are correlated with higher income and social status, which more directly affect longevity.

Pfeiffer (1970) compared long-lived and short-lived subjects from the Duke Longitudinal Study and attributed the variance in longevity to elite status. Those who lived the longest had high intelligence and sound financial status. Seventy percent of the long-lived men said they were financially comfortable, while only 20 percent of the short lived men rated themselves comfortable. Since a good income facilitates good diet, leisure time, job satisfaction, and access to high quality health care, it is easy to understand how higher financial status would influence longevity.

A related factor, social-occupational status, also affects longevity. Professionals—scientists, lawyers, architects, and physicians—live longer than people in other occupational groups. Farmers are the only nonprofessionals who also enjoy longer life expectancy (Metropolitan Life Insurance Company 1975). One sixteen-year study of more than one thousand male corporate executives from successful industrial corporations reported that these men had extremely low mortality rates, less than two-thirds that of white men in the general population (Metropolitan Life Insurance Company 1974). The higher mortality for those in low status occupations may be due to lower job satisfaction, increased stress, poor working conditions, higher occupational illness, and little control over working environment. Since low income usually accompanies low status occupations, the income variable may be the most significant.

High education level, intelligence, and occupational level are correlated with a higher income and standard of living. Those who are in the middle and upper classes live considerably longer than those in the lower classes. Whether educational level is a significant factor or whether income increases life expectancy is uncertain. Terman and Odan (1959) report not only a relationship between intelligence and educational level, but also a positive correlation between intelligence and income.

The Physical Environment

A number of factors in the external environment may affect longevity. Radiation, air pollution, water quality, and the geochemical environment have been associated with variations in life expectancy.

Humans are exposed to low levels of radiation daily. This low-level radiation can impair cell function by causing mutations in the genetic code. Higher levels of radiation can shorten life by accelerating the aging process. Radiation is thought to damage the immune system, making the body less resistant to infection. Leukemia and tumor development are more prevalent after irradiation. It has been estimated that a single radiation dose of one roentgen ages humans the equivalent of five–ten days (Hershey 1974).

Death rates in areas with dense air pollution are much higher than those in pollution-free communities (Ayres and Buehler 1970). One expert hypothesizes that if air pollution levels were reduced by half, we could reduce bronchitis cases by 25–50 percent, heart disease by 20 percent, and cancer by 15 percent (reported in Kurtzman and Gordon 1977). As the threats of groundwater pollution, acid rain, and increased pollution of air and water increase with technological advancements, it is likely that many more effects of pollution on human health and longevity will be documented.

Environmental factors such as soil, climactic factors, and drinking water quality may impact on health and longevity. The most well-studied of these variables is drinking water composition. Feder (1981) compared the composition of drinking water in selected areas of the United States and found that areas with high life expectancy had water with higher levels of important minerals such as calcium and magnesium (hard water) than low-longevity areas.

Conclusion

This section discussed the many and varied influences upon length of life. A number of genetic determinants, such as gender, familial history, and predisposition to genetic diseases have a role in determining length of life. The physical environment may have more influence than was once believed, and is becoming more important as the threats of radiation, air pollution, acid rain, and groundwater contamination become a reality. The good news is that a number of factors that influence length and quality of life are under personal control: such as controlling weight, abstaining from cigarette smoking, participating in regular, strenuous exercise, and learning to cope with stress. Alteration of these maladaptive behaviors increases the chance for a longer life—or, at the least, a healthier old age.

Summary

For centuries, people have been interested in why we age and how aging can be prevented. Old theories of biological aging have been replaced with more scientific ones, but they remain speculative. Two major types of theories were addressed: damage and programmed aging theories. Damage theories assert that cells function less efficiently with advanced age because they become damaged. Damage theories include the accumulation of free radicals, cross-linkages, waste products, and errors. In contrast, the program theorists assert that cellular decline and death is programmed in the genetic code. These theories include the codon restriction, immunological, and neuro-endocrine theories. It is unclear whether one or more of these theories will yield the true reason why we age, but research is continuing.

Interest in life extension has continued throughout history. Many current methods to prolong life have evolved from the major biologic aging theories but remain speculative since few have been documented for human subjects. Although some may affect life expectancy (the amount of time an individual can expect to live), few affect life span, the maximum time a human can live (110–120 years).

The glamorous methods to prolong life are less documented than the modification of personal health behaviors. Such factors as level of physical activity, cigarette smoking, obesity, and ability to deal with stress are much more likely to promote a longer and healthier life than any of the miracle drugs or techniques.

Activities

1. What theory of aging or combination of theories do you believe to be the most probable and why?
2. Collect and analyze five advertisements from magazines or newspapers that boast that their product promotes longevity or reduces the rate of aging. How could you determine if they are fraudulent?
3. Devise an experiment or set of experiments where you attempt to isolate one of the factors that influence longevity. Would your experiment show a causal relationship or merely a correlation between the factor and longevity? Can you see the difficulty in isolating one factor?
4. If everyone lived to be 120 years old, what would be the effect on our society—politically, socially, economically, medically, and psychologically? What might some of the consequences be and how might we surmount them?
5. How long do you want to live? Why? Would you want to live longer if you could be guaranteed good health? Do you think it would be a good idea to extend the lifespan? Why or why not?
6. Debate: Life extension studies should be supported by the United States Government.
7. Complete the exercise: Can You Live to be 100?

   List those variables that subtracted years from your life expectancy. Which can you change? Which are you willing to change? Which are you not able to change? Which factor added the most years to your life expectancy? Which factor subtracted the most years?
8. Imagine that you are given an opportunity to take an anti-aging drug guaranteed to double your life span. Will you take it? Why or why not?
9. Interview a long-lived individual who you know. What personal characteristics do they believe enabled them to live longer than their cohorts? Can you see additional positive characteristics they exhibit? Write the material up in the form of a biography.

Bibliography

Abbott, M. H., E. A. Murphy, D. R. Bolling, and H. Abbey. 1974. The familial component in longevity, a study of offspring in nonagenarians. II. Preliminary analysis of the completed studies. *Johns Hopkins Med J* 134(1):1–16.

Anderson, R., R. Sosthuizen, R. Marity, et al. 1980. The effects of increasing weekly doses of ascorbate in certain cellular and immune functions in normal volunteers. *Amer J Clin Nutr* 33:71–6.

Aslan, A. 1960. Procaine therapy in old age and other disorders (Novacaine factor H 3). *Gerontol Clin* 3:148–76.

Ayres, S. M., and M. E. Buehler. 1970. The effects of urban air pollution on health. *Clin Pharmacol Ther* 11:337–71.

Bjorksten, J. 1963. Aging primary mechanism. *Gerontologia* 8:179–92.

Bjorksten, J. 1968. The crosslinkage theory of aging. *J Am Geriatr Soc* 16(4): 408–27.

Brash, D. E., and R. W. Hart. 1978. Molecular biology of aging. In *The Biology of Aging*. J. A. Behnke, C. E. Finch, and G. B. Moment, eds. New York: Plenum Press. 57–81.

Brunner, D., G. Manelis, M. Modan, and S. Levin. 1974. Physical activity at work and the incidence of myocardial infarction, angina pectoris and death due to ischemic heart disease: An epidemiological study in Israeli Collective Settlements (Kibbutzin). *J Chronic Dis* 27: 217–33.

Carrel, A. 1912. On the permanent life of tissues outside of the organism. *Jour Exp Med* Volume 15: 516–29.

Cheney, K. E., R. U. Liu, G. S. Smith, et al. 1980. Survival and disease patterns in C57BL/6J mice subjected to undernutrition. *Exp Geront* 15:237–58.

Cotzias, G. C., S. T. Niller, A. R. Nicholson Jr., et al. 1974. Prolongation of the lifespan in mice adapted to large amounts of L-Dopa. *Proc Nat Acad Sci* 71:2466–9.

Curtis, H., and K. Miller. 1971. Chromosomal aberrations in liver cells of guinea pigs. *J Gerontol* 26:292–3.

Denckla, W. D. 1974. A time to die. *Life Sci* 16:31–44.

Feder, G. L. 1981. Contrasts in drinking water quality between the increased-longevity, low-death-rate area and the decreased-longevity high-death-rate-area in the United States. In Panel on Aging and the Geothermal Environment, ed., *Aging and the geochemical environment*. Washington, D.C.: National Academy Press. 92–103.

Finch, C. E. 1975. Neuroendocrinology of aging: a view of an emerging area. *Biosci* 25(10):645–50.

Finch, C. E. 1977. Neuroendocrine and autonomic aspects of aging. In C. E. Finch, and L. Hayflick, eds. *Handbook of the biology of aging*. New York: Van Nostrand Reinhold. 262–80.

Fleming, J. E., J. Miguel, S. F. Cottrell, et al. 1982. Is cell aging caused by respiration dependent injury to the mitochondrial genome? *Gerontology* 28:44–53.

Frank, B. S. 1976. *Dr. Frank's no aging diet*. New York: Dial Press.

Frank, B. S. 1977. *Nucleic acid, nutrition, and therapy*. New York: Rainstone.

Fries, J. F., and L. M. Crapo. 1981. *Vitality and aging*. San Francisco: W. H. Freeman.

Gardner, J. 1946. The effect of yeast nucleic acid on the survival time of 600 day old albino mice. *J Gerontol* 1:445–52.

Globus, S. 1984. Antioxidants can increase longevity by scavenging oxygen free radicals. *Health and Longevity* 2(12):8.

Granich, M. 1972. Factors affecting aging: pharmacologic agents. In P. S. Timiras, ed. *Developmental psychology and aging*. New York: Macmillan. 607–14.

Hamilton, J. B. 1948. The role of testicular secretions as indicated by the effects of castration in men and by studies of pathological condition and the short life span associated with maleness. *Recent Prog Horm Res* 3:257–322.

Harman, D. 1968. Free radical theory of aging: Effect of free radical inhibitors on the mortality rate of male LAF mice. *J Gerontol* 23:476–482.

Harman, D., and D. E. Eddy. 1978. Free radical theory of aging: Effect of adding antioxidants to maternal mice diets on the lifespan of the offspring. *Age* 1:162.

Harman, D. 1984. Free radicals and the evolution and present status of the free radical theory of aging. In D. Armstrong et al. eds. *Free radicals in molecular biology: Aging and disease.* New York: Raven Press. 1–12.

Hartung, G. H., J. P. Foreyt, R. E. Mitchell et al. 1980. Relation of diet to high density lipoprotein cholesterol in middle aged marathon runners, joggers and inactive men. *N Engl J Med* 302(7):357–61.

Hayflick, L. 1961. The limited *in vitro* lifetime of human diploid cell strains. *Exp Cell Res* 37:614–36.

Hayflick, L. 1975. Current theories of biological aging. *Fed Proc* 34(1):9–13.

Haynes, S., and M. Feinleib. 1980. Women, work, and coronary heart disease. *Am J Public Health* 70:133–141.

Helsing, K. J., M. Szklo, G. W. Comstock. 1981. Factors associated with mortality after widowhood. *Am J Public Health* 71:802–9.

Hershey, D. 1974. *Lifespan and factors affecting it.* Springfield, IL: Charles Thomas.

Hirokawa, K., and T. Makinodan. 1975. Thymic involution: effect on T-cell differentiation. *J Immunol* 114:1659–64.

Hochschild, R. 1973. Effect of dimethylaminoethyl p-chlorophenoxyacetate on the lifespan of male Swill Webster albino mice. *Exp Gerontol* 8:177–83.

Johansson, B. G., and A. Medhus. 1974. Increase in plasma alpha-lipoproteins in chronic alcoholics after acute abuse. *Acta Med Scand* 195:273–77.

Kallman, F. J., and G. Sander, 1948. Twin studies in aging and longevity. *J Hered* 39:349–57.

Klatsky, A. L., G. D. Friedman, and A. B. Siegelaub. 1974. Alcohol consumption before myocardial infarction. *Ann Intern Med* 81(3):294–301.

Knight, S. C., J. Farrant, and L. E. McGann. 1977. Storage of human lymphocytes by freezing in serum alone. *Cryobiology* 14:112–15.

Kurtzman, J., and P. Gordon. 1977. *No more dying.* New York: Dell Publishing.

Leger, A. S., A. L. Cochrane, and F. Moore. 1979. Factors associated with cardiac mortality in developing countries with particular reference to the consumption of wine. *Lancet* May 12:1017–20.

Lipson, S. K., P. B. Chretien, R. Makuch, et al. 1979. Thymosin immunotherapy in patients with small cell carcinoma of the lung: Correlation of in vitro studies with clinical courses. *Cancer* 43:863–70.

Liu, R. K., and R. L. Walford. 1972. The effect of lowered body temperatures on lifespan and immune and non-immune processes. *Gerontologia* 18:363–88.

Mann, D. M., and P. O. Yates. 1974. Lipoprotein pigments—their relationship to ageing in the human nervous system. *Brain* 97:489–98.

McCay, C. M., and L. A. Maynard. 1939. Retarded growth, life span, ultimate body size and age changes in the albino rat after feeding diets restricted in calories. *J Nutr* 18:1–13.

Medvedev, Z. A. 1972. Repetition of molecular genetic information as a possible factor in evolutionary changes of life span. *Exp Gerontol* 7:227–38.

Metropolitan Life Insurance Co. 1974. Longevity of corporate executives. *Statistical Bulletin* 55:2–4.

Metropolitan Life Insurance Co. 1975. Socioeconomic mortality differentials. *Statistical Bulletin* 56:3–5.

Metropolitan Life Insurance Co. 1977. Expectation of life among non-whites. *Statistical Bulletin* 58:5–7.

Moment, G. 1982. Theories of aging: An overview. In *Testing the theories of aging,* R. C. Adelman, and G. S. Roth, eds. Boca Raton, Fla.: CRC Press. 1–23.

Morris, J. N., and P. A. B. Raffle. 1954. Coronary heart disease in transport workers. *Br J Ind Med* 11:260–4.

National Center of Health Statistics. 1973. Some demographic aspects of aging in the U.S. Bureau of the Census, U.S. Public Health Service, February.

Odens, M. 1973. Prolongation of the lifespan in rats. *J Am Geriatr Soc* 21:450–1.

Packer, L., and J. Walton. 1977. Antioxidants vs. aging. *Chemtech* 7 (5):276–81.

Paffenbarger, R. S., W. E. Hale, R. J. Brand, and R. T. Hyde. 1977. Work-energy level, personal characteristics and fatal heart attack: A birth cohort effect. *Am J Epidemiol* 105(3):200–213.

Paffenbarger, R. S., R. T. Hyde, A. L. Wing, and C. Hsieh. 1986. Physical activity, all-cause mortality and longevity of college alumni. *N Engl J Med* 314(10):605–12.

Palmore, E. 1971. The relative importance of social factors in predicting longevity. In *Prediction of life span,* E. Palmore and F. Jeffers, eds. Lexington, Mass.: Heath Lexington Books. 237–47.

Pearl, R., and R. de W. Pearl. 1934. *The ancestry of the long-lived.* Baltimore: Johns Hopkins University Press.

Pfeiffer, E. 1970. Survival in old age: Physical, psychological and social correlates of longevity. *J Am Geriatr Soc* 18(4):273–85.

Price, J. H., and C. Pritts. 1980. Overweight and obesity in the elderly. *J Gerontol Nurs* 6:341–47.

Report of the Surgeon General. 1982. *The health consequences of smoking: Cancer.* Washington, D.C.: U.S. Dept. of Health and Human Services. Public Health Service.

Report of the Surgeon General. 1983. *The health consequences of smoking: Cardiovascular disease.* Washington, D.C.: U.S. Dept. of Health and Human Services, Public Health Service.

Retherford, R. D. 1975. *The changing sex differential in mortality.* Westport, Conn.: Greenwood Press.

Rigby, P. F. 1971. The effect of "exogeneous" RNA on the improvement of syngeneic tumor immunity. *Cancer Res* 31:4–6.

Robertson, T. B. 1928. On the influence of nucleic acids of various origins upon the growth and longevity of the white mouse. *Aust J Exp Biol Med Sci* 5:47.

Rosenberg, B., G. Kemeny, L. G. Smith, et al. 1973. The kinetics and thermodynamics of death in multicellular organisms. *Mech Ageing Dev* 2:275.

Ross, M. 1976. Nutrition and longevity in experimental animals in Winick, M., ed. *Nutrition and aging.* New York: John Wiley and Sons.

Russell, A., ed. 1986. *Guinness Book of World Records.* New York: Sterling.

Sacher, G. A. 1965. The role of physiological fluctuation in the aging process and the relation of longevity to the size of the central nervous system. In A. M. Brues and G. A. Sacher, eds., *Aging and levels of biological organization.* Chicago: University of Chicago Press.

Schultz, R. 1978. *The psychology of death, dying, and bereavement.* Reading, Ma.: Addison-Wesley.

Science News. 1979. Fasting fosters longevity in rats. 116: 375.

Segerberg, O. 1974. *The immortality factor.* New York: E. P. Dutton.

Segerberg, O. 1982. *Living to be 100.* New York: Chas. Scribner's Sons.

Smith, D. W., E. L. Bierman, and N. M. Robinson. 1978. *The biologic ages of man.* Philadelphia: W. B. Saunders.

Smith, G. S., and R. L. Walford. 1977. Influence of the main histocompatibility complex on aging in mice. *Nature* 270:727–729.

Sohnle, P. G., and S. R. Gambert. 1982. Thermoneutrality: An evolutionary advantage against ageing? *Lancet* May 15: 1099–1100.

Sokoloff, B., C. C. Sqelhof Hori, T. Wrzolek, and T. Imai. 1966. Aging, atherosclerosis and ascorbic acid metabolism. *J Am Geriatr Soc* 14:1239–60.

Solyom, L., H. E. Enesco, and C. Beaulieu. 1967. The effect of RNA on learning and activity in old and young rats. *J Gerontol* 22(1): 3–7.

Strehler, B. L., and R. Johnson. 1972. A 30 percent decrease in DNA dosage during aging of dog brain. *Fed Proc* 31:A910.

Strehler, B. L. 1977. *Time, cells, and aging.* New York: Academic Press.

Strehler, B. L. 1979. The mechanisms of aging. *Body Forum* March: 34–45.

Strehler, B. 1980. A critique of theories of biological aging. In *Aging—its chemistry* A. A. Dietz, ed. Washington, D.C.: American Association for Clinical Chemistry. 25–45.

Terman, L. M., and M. H. Oden. 1959. The gifted group at mid-life: 35 years followup of the superior child. In L. M. Terman, ed. *Genetic studies of genius* Vol 5. Stanford, Calif.: Stanford University Press.

Timiras, P., P. E. Segall, and R. F. Walker, 1980. Physiological aging in the central nervous system: Perspectives on interventive gerontology. In *Aging—its chemistry,* A. A. Dietz, Washington, D. C.: American Assoc. for Clinical Chemistry.

Trimmer, E. J. 1970. *Rejuvenation.* New York: A. S. Barner.

U.S. Department of Health, Education, and Welfare. 1976. Differentials of health characteristics by marital status: United States, 1971–1972. *Vital and Health Statistics.* Washington, D.C.: U.S.Government Printing Office.

Waldron, I. 1976. Why do women live longer than men? *Journal of Human Stress* 2 (1):2–13.

Walford, R. L. 1983. *Maximum life span.* New York: Norton and Co.

Walford, R. L. 1969. *The immunologic theory of aging.* Copenhagen: Munksgaard.

Weindrich, R., S. R. S. Gottsman, and R. L. Walford. 1982. Modification of age-related immune decline in mice dietarily restricted from or after mid-adulthood. *Proceedings of the National Academy of Science USA* 79:898–902.

Weksler, M. E. 1983. The thymus gland and aging. *Ann Intern Med* 98(1):105–7.

Zung, W. W. K., D. Gianturco, E. Pfeiffer, et al. 1974. Pharmacology of depression in the aged: Evolution of Gerovital H 3 as an antidepressant drug. *Psychosomatics* 15:127–31.

The Body and Its Age Changes: Part I 3

Cellular aging is a reality, but there is much truth in the phrase "nobody ever died of old age." In fact, we kill ourselves long before our bodies have an opportunity to wear out.

Introduction

Wrinkled skin and graying hair are obvious physical changes associated with aging. However, these changes do not affect the function of the body. There are, however, a number of changes with age that occur at the cellular and tissue level that reduce the efficiency of some body systems. After maturity, the body gradually loses functional capacity. Body processes become less efficient and functional cells are lost and replaced with fibrous or fatty tissue. In general, age-associated physiological decline is reflected in a decreased capacity to adapt to physical and emotional stress placed upon the body. As a result, the body becomes more vulnerable to disease and heals more slowly. Morbidity (illness) and mortality (death) rates increase progressively after maturity.

Although growing old is inevitable, all individuals do not age in the same manner or at the same rate. In the later years, chronological age is not a good indicator of biologic age. Some elders perform better on physiological measures than younger adults. Without a doubt, genetic, environmental, and life style differences play an important role in the rate of aging. Further, the degree of functional loss of each organ varies within an individual. For instance, a seventy-year-old woman may have excellent vision and hearing, but have poor lung capacity. The ability to adapt to those changes also varies among individuals. Some adapt easily to heavy losses and are minimally affected in their daily routine while others have minimal losses but adapt so poorly that they require major lifestyle changes. Whether an elder is debilitated or challenged by a loss of body function is dependent on the interrelationship of physiology, emotional state, and presence of social support.

These photos of George Burns illustrate that aging is a very gradual, but obvious process.

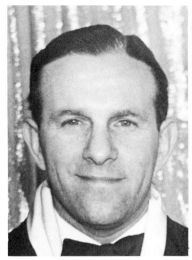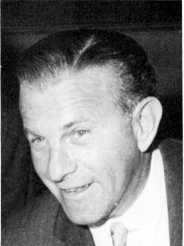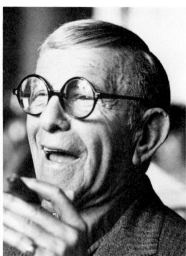

It is difficult to distinguish those physiological changes that often accompany old age from those that are due to aging itself. For a decrement to be considered the result of aging, five requirements must be fulfilled (Rowlatt and Franks 1978). The decline must be *universal,* that is, it occurs in all members of a species to a certain degree. The decline must be caused by *intrinsic* factors (such as age or genetics) and not due to environmental influences. The onset of the decline is *progressive*—a gradual process rather than a specific event. Changes due to age are *irreversible,* although it may be possible to slow the process. The change must be *deleterious,* leading to a loss of function.

Although these requirements seem clear-cut, they remain theoretical. Cross-cultural studies of physiological changes accompanying age are sparse so the requirement of universality remains unfulfilled in most cases. Additionally, it is virtually impossible for researchers to determine whether a decrement is intrinsic or caused by disease, poor diet, physical inactivity, environmental contaminants, mental state, or even decrements in another body system. For instance, a lack of physical activity is associated with a number of decrements in the body that resemble age

changes. The proportion of age-related decrements in function attributable to the aging process and those due to physical inactivity is still not clear.

It is important to be aware of the extent of physiological changes with age so that disease states can be differentiated from normal aging processes. Because elders often have chronic illnesses in addition to normal age changes, it is often difficult for health professionals and elders to determine if a somatic complaint is a symptom of disease or old age. Elders may suffer unnecessary deterioration because they do not seek treatment for many conditions. For instance, an elderly man with severe joint pain that limits his mobility may not bring his problem to the attention of his physician because he believes bone pain is a necessary accompaniment to old age. However, his pain may be due to any of several treatable conditions.

Knowledge of the physiological aging process gives us a realistic view of aging. Contrary to popular belief, the body does not completely fall apart at age sixty-five. Although some decrements are known to be caused by aging, these do not significantly affect the functioning of body systems and have little effect on lifestyle. Alex

I Hate the Way I Look

I MIND being wrinkled
And stooped and
Shaky and
Gray.
When I look in the mirror,
I feel betrayed. As if
A dear friend had turned into an ugly beast.
But that's unfair.
My body is still my friend.
It struggles valiantly to do my bidding.
I should be kinder to it.
The years have been pelting it and I haven't helped much.
I eat too much, drink too much, get angry too much,
    overwork.
Actually, my body
Has forgiven me a lot.
I should be more charitable to it now.
When young people look away in distaste, I
Should say: Never mind old friend-body,
They don't know all you've been through.
When they're old one day, too,
I just hope they take it as well as you.

do not significantly affect the functioning of body systems and have little effect on lifestyle. Alex Comfort (1976) believes that most age changes are due to sociological pressures; our youth-oriented society and ageist attitudes affect our feelings of self worth and do more to age us than the natural physiological process. As Cicero stated, "It is not old age that is at fault, but rather our attitude towards it." Although the following two chapters focus on age-related decline, it is important to realize that none of these decrements cause significant problems. The deterioration due to disease has a much more significant effect on health.

Knowledge of physiological changes with age should not be used to restrict elder's job access, intellectual pursuits, leisure activities, or to unnecessarily label them as feeble. The intent is not to categorize older people as different, but to emphasize that everyone experiences gradual changes with advancing age. Many are occurring even as you read this page. Cells are gradually lost and others do not function as effectively. Eventually those changes are interpreted as signs of aging as they become more visible to us and to those around us.

Chapters 3 and 4 provide an overview of each body system and the major changes associated with advanced age. The term *age-associated* is generally used to describe these changes because they are associated with advancing age, but not necessarily due to age itself. Chapter 3 will discuss the integument, musculoskeletal, cardiovascular, immune, respiratory, digestive, and urinary systems. Chapter 4 will discuss the nervous, sensory, endocrine, and reproductive systems.

The Body and Its Age Changes: Part I

The Integumentary System

The skin and its accessory organs comprise the integument, the largest and most visible body system. The skin protects underlying tissues from harmful environmental influences and minimizes water loss. The large surface of the skin and its capacity to sweat and shiver is important in the regulation of body temperature. Through sweating, the skin also serves to eliminate salts and other waste products. A variety of sensory receptors in the skin permit us to respond to environmental changes such as heat, cold, pain, or light touch. Upon exposure to ultraviolet light, the skin synthesizes vitamin D, important in calcium absorption. The subcutaneous fat cushions the body from injury and forms a large part of our energy reserves. The skin is also able to absorb certain drugs and dermal patches are becoming a common method to administer medication.

The skin consists of an epidermis (outer layer), dermis (inner layer), and subcutaneous layer below the skin. Dead skin cells on the skin surface are constantly worn away as newer cells are formed in the deeper layer of the epidermis. Skin cells become thickened and hardened as they are pushed toward the surface. The pigment, melanin, is produced in the epidermis and protects the body from sunlight by absorbing light energy. Skin color is dependent upon the amount of melanin in the epidermal cells. Those with dark complexions have more melanin than those with light complexions. The dermis consists of nerves, blood vessels, hair follicles, sweat and sebaceous oil glands, and connective tissue. The blood vessels supply nutrients to all skin cells as well as regulate body temperature. Specialized nerve fibers, receptive to heat, cold, touch, pressure, and pain, are found in the dermal layer. The subcutaneous layer beneath the dermis is composed of blood vessels, nerves, collagen (a supportive tissue), and fat and connects the skin to the organs beneath it. The complexity of skin structure is evidenced by figure 3.1.

Age-Associated Changes in the Integumentary System

The speed and extent of skin changes vary among individuals and are strongly influenced by heredity, hormone balance, and exposure to sun, harsh weather, and chemicals. In general, older skin tends to be more wrinkled, folded, mottled, and dry than younger skin, especially among Caucasians. Skin wrinkling can be attributed to a number of underlying physiological changes. First, it is generally agreed that the outer epidermal layer of skin becomes thinner with age because cells are not replaced at the same rate they are shed. The collagen layer in the subcutaneous tissue becomes less elastic with age and is replaced with inelastic fibrous tissue, reducing the resiliance of the skin (Thorne 1981). In addition, the action of sebaceous (oil) glands is reduced in old age, causing the skin to become drier and rougher and more likely to suffer mechanical damage when exposed to environmental agents. Because the face is most exposed to sun and wind, it is the most likely to show damage. The skin is stretched when facial muscles move in characteristic expressions. With age, the skin is less likely to return to its original shape so that, by age forty, most have creases that reflect habitual facial expressions.

Subcutaneous fat smooths out the contours of the body. With advancing age, subcutaneous fat is reduced and collects in areas of fatty deposits. Less padding, combined with diminished skin elasticity and gravity causes sagging and folding of the skin (Whitbourne 1985). This decrease in subcutaneous fat causes changes in appearance, such as making underlying bones, tendons, and blood vessels more prominent. A reduction in muscle mass further contributes to the loosening of the skin.

Age-changes in the skin can decrease elders' ability to cope with temperature extremes because the decrease in subcutaneous fat reduces insulation capacity. The age-associated loss of sweat glands and reduced capacity of heat and cold sensory receptors also contribute to difficulty in temperature regulation. Elders, especially those over eighty, are particularly susceptible to hyperthermia and hypothermia (see Chapter 6).

With age, small hemorrhages commonly occur under the skin due to thinness of skin and increased fragility of blood vessels and capillaries. Thus, wounds and bruises may heal more slowly. Fair-skinned older adults may lose some pinktones in their skin because of a reduction of blood flow to the skin surface caused by capillary loss.

Decreases in melanin production with age cause the age or liver spots commonly associated with old age. Elders have fewer melanin pigment cells and those that remain tend to be larger, appearing in areas most often exposed to the sun such as the back of hands, lower arms, face, and neck. Reduced melanin production over most of the body increases susceptibility of sunburn in older people. Black skin, which has a greater degree of melanin, resists sun damage, ages more slowly, and deteriorates much later in life than Caucasian skin. Among Caucasians, those with freckled or fair complexions, red or blond hair, and blue eyes are most susceptible to sunlight damage. Caucasians with dark or olive complexions are better protected.

Although most people consider wrinkled, loose, leathery skin a necessary accompaniment to old age, researchers report that so-called aged skin is not directly related to the aging process itself but is mainly due to exposure to sunlight. Sunlight damages elastic fibers in the skin, causing wrinkling and sagging. Sunlight also stimulates the development of age spots and pre-malignant and malignant (cancerous) skin lesions. A certain degree of irreversible skin damage occurs with each prolonged exposure and accumulates to cause what we call aged skin. The degree of skin degeneration is directly related to the amount of sun exposure.

Although wrinkling and age spots have little effect on longevity, they may profoundly affect feelings of self-worth, especially for those who

Minimizing Sun Damage

Despite the knowledge that sunlight ages the skin, individuals of all ages, especially the young, rarely protect themselves from the sun. Sunlight feels pleasurable and relaxing and many leisure activities are conducted outdoors in sunny weather. Additionally, in American culture, the suntanned look is considered to be healthful, attractive, and sexually appealing. In reality, tanning is not a sign of health, but is a mechanism to limit the amount of sun damage.

To maintain healthy skin, it is critical to protect it from the harmful effects of the sun. Experts recommend avoiding prolonged exposure to sunlight. Sun damage can also occur on cloudy or foggy days as the ultraviolet rays penetrate cloud cover. If one must be in the sun for long periods, long sleeves and hats with brims should be worn. Sunscreen lotions containing PABA (para-aminobenzoic acid) offer protection against sunburn. Sunscreens are classified by number according to SPF (Sunlight Protection Factor): the higher the SPF number, the greater the protection. Extra precautions should be taken when some drugs (such as tetracycline) are used because they increase photosensitivity of the skin.

strive to look youthful. Society places more pressure on women than men to maintain a youthful appearance. Thus, women are a receptive market for a lucrative cosmetic industry that offers formulas to delay wrinkling, age spots, and loosening of skin. Some middle-aged individuals resort to plastic surgery or collagen injections to temporarily rid themselves of wrinkled and baggy skin.

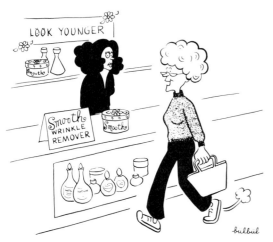

"Wrinkle remover! Are you kidding, I earned all my wrinkles fair and square."

Change of hair color and distribution commonly occur with advanced age. A reduction in the amount of hair pigment causes graying, which usually begins in the late thirties or early forties.

About half the male population can expect some degree of baldness, which may begin as early as the late teens or not until the late forties. Although both males and females may carry the gene for baldness, the gene must be activated by the male hormone testosterone so only males are affected. Typically, hair loss begins when hair follicles shrink and produce finer and shorter hair, eventually resulting in a ring of hair above the ears and around the back of the head. Females with the genetic trait do not exhibit baldness, although their hair may become thinner.

The pattern and texture of hair growth on other parts of the body changes in the later years. As hair of the scalp, underarm, and pubic area is lessened, hairs in the ears, nostrils, and eyebrows become coarser, especially in males. In women, facial hair may also coarsen under the nose and on the chin because of changes in the balance of sex hormones.

With age, nails become more furrowed and nail growth slows, probably due to diminished blood supply. Some elders, especially those with deteriorating vision, poor coordination, or arthritis, may be unable to cut their own toenails and referral to a podiatrist may be necessary to prevent foot discomfort, infections, and mobility problems.

The Musculoskeletal System

Muscles and bones work together to protect and support the organs of the body, preserve body shape, posture, and stability, and enable body movement. The skeleton consists of over two hundred bones as well as cartilage and ligaments that bind bones together at the joints. Bones are very active tissues as they are the storage site for calcium and other necessary minerals. When the body needs calcium for muscle contraction, nerve conduction, blood clotting, and other functions, it is extracted from the bones. Some bones also produce red blood cells and white blood cells.

Muscles are important for support of the skeleton and account for almost one-half the body weight. Active muscles release a large amount of heat that is conducted to other body tissues by the blood to maintain body temperature.

Muscles can be divided into three categories based on their structure: skeletal (or striated), smooth, and cardiac. Skeletal muscles are primarily attached to the skeleton and act upon the bones to produce voluntary actions such as those needed for posture, facial expressions, and locomotion. In contrast, smooth muscles are mainly involuntary and line the walls of the digestive tract, windpipe, bladder, and blood vessels. The movement of smooth muscles is slow and sustained, often wavelike. Cardiac muscle is comprised of a network of fibers that contract as a unit. These muscles initiate their own contraction and are responsible for the continual pumping action of the heart.

Muscles act by contraction and relaxation. When one muscle group contracts, an opposite muscle group relaxes. When skeletal muscles contract they pull on the ligaments that are attached to the bones, stimulating the bones to thicken and strengthen. Physical exercise increases bone mass by causing stress on the bones. Without physical activity the bone tissue becomes weaker and thinner. Similarly, skeletal muscles become strengthened by use. A muscle that is not used decreases significantly in size and strength.

Vigorous physical activity in later life retards many physiological decrements associated with aging.

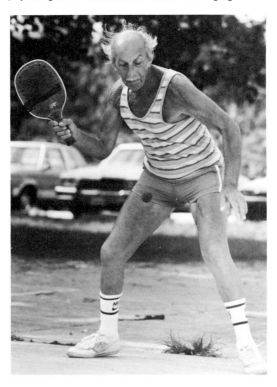

Age-Associated Changes in the Musculoskeletal System

It is generally assumed that elders lose muscular strength with advancing age. Although muscle strength remains constant through adulthood, strength begins to decrease at about age sixty (deVries 1980). Persons in their seventies and eighties suffer more rapid rates of muscle strength loss—up to 40 percent (Grimby and Saltin 1983). Loss of muscle strength is greater in the legs than in arms and hands (Shephard 1981). Progressive loss of muscular strength with age is related to a loss of muscle mass with age. In elders, individual muscle fibers may be atrophied or the number of fibers may be reduced.

Studies measuring loss of muscle strength may not have controlled for decline due to inactivity. High levels of activity can prevent muscle deterioration. Elders who maintain high levels of activity have less deterioration of muscle mass and strength than those with lower activity levels (Asmussen 1981). In contrast, those who are immobile show very high rates of muscular atrophy. Even when activity is initiated late in life, deterioration can be slowed or reversed. In one study of sixty-nine–seventy-four year old men, muscle gains of up to 22 percent were reported following initiation of an exercise regimen (Aniansson and Gustafsson 1981).

Joints become less flexible with age, creating minor stiffness and limited movement. Although joint degeneration is associated with old age, the aging of the joints begins even before skeletal maturity. Thus, joint problems may occur in all adults and increase in frequency as aging progresses. Calcification, fraying, or cracking in the cartilage and ligaments contribute to joint movement difficulties. Cartilage may become eroded in heavily-used joints causing bone pain, stiffness, and loss of flexibility. Limitations in limb and neck joints may cause moderate alterations in posture, gait, and balance. Although extremely common, joint problems are not inevitable in old age. Like muscles, joint problems decrease with regular exercise.

A decrease in bone strength and mass is associated with advancing age. The bones lose mineral content and become more porous and susceptible to fractures. This is thought to occur because the rates of bone rebuilding do not keep pace with the rates of bone breakdown. Bone loss is more severe in elder women than men. Women lose 20–30 percent of their bone mineral density over the adult age span (Avioli 1982), while men lose only about 10–15 percent of their bone mineral density (Mazess 1982). Some describe osteoporosis (a chronic disease) as an accelerated version of normal, age-related bone loss. While some bone thinning is thought to accompany old age, osteoporosis is characterized by excessive bone loss and increased susceptibility to fracture (see Chapter 5).

Since bone density increases when bones are stressed, and atrophy with disuse, it is generally agreed that physical inactivity plays a significant role in bone-thinning. Other variables such as a diet deficient in calcium, fluoride, or low levels of vitamin D and estrogen seem to play a role in the bone-thinning process.

Loss of bone mass affects elders by increasing minor aches and pains as well as increasing the incidence of fractures. When older bones are injured, they may take longer to heal. Ironically, the immobility needed for the healing process can further exacerbate bone loss. Brittle bones may markedly affect activity level as elders become overly cautious about any activity, inadvertently promoting further decline.

Alterations in posture may occur with advanced age. Elders commonly assume a stooped posture—head and neck held forward, bent or stooped shoulders, and slight bending of the hips and knees. These changes may be caused by compression of the vertebral disks in the spinal column, a decrease in elasticity of joints and ligaments, a loss of strength and shortening of tendons or muscles, or degenerative changes in the central nervous system. Gravitational compression of the vertebral disks in the spinal column also lead to a gradual shortening of stature. However, osteoporosis, spinal deformity or injury, foot problems, obesity, poor nutrition, emotional stress, or low self esteem also affect posture.

Poor posture affects a number of bodily functions. It interferes with stability and balance, increases back problems, and may also impede movement. Curvatures of the back may reduce lung capacity or compress internal organs. Lastly, poor posture detracts from general appearance, contributing to a decreased sense of self-worth. It is important to note that good posture can be maintained with exercise and is not inevitable in old age.

The Cardiovascular System

The cardiovascular system transports nutrients and wastes through the body. The system includes the heart, blood vessels, (arteries, veins, and capillaries) and the blood. The heart is a

Figure 3.1 Diagram of heart. (From Hole, John W., Jr., *Human Anatomy and Physiology*, 3rd ed. Copyright © 1978, 1981, 1984 Wm. C. Brown Publishers, Dubuque, Iowa. All Rights Reserved. Reprinted by permission).

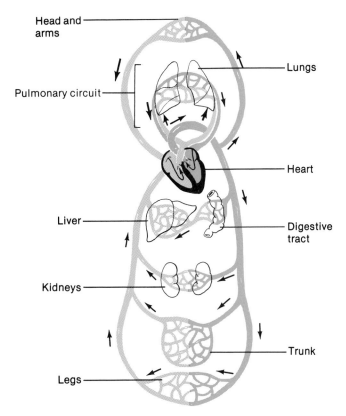

muscular pump that rhythmically moves blood through the body through a closed network of transport vessels—the arteries, capillaries, and veins. Through this network, blood and dissolved substances are carried to every cell in the body. Oxygen from the lungs, nutrients from the digestive system, hormones from the endocrine glands, and antibodies from the immune system are transported to body cells. Waste products are moved to the lungs and kidneys for removal through the blood. Blood also maintains body temperature by transferring the heat generated by the skeletal muscles to the rest of the body.

The heart muscle consists of four chambers, two upper (atria) and two lower (ventricles) (figure 3.1). The atria and the ventricles are separated by valves that control the timing and amount of blood flow in each of the chambers and between the large arteries and the ventricles. The right side of the heart receives deoxygenated blood from the veins and pumps it to the lungs to be oxygenated. Oxygen-laden blood returns to the left side of the heart to be pumped to the rest of the body via the arterial system. The heart beats about seventy-two beats a minute and pumps about 170 gallons of blood in an hour.

Unlike other types of muscle, the muscle fibers in the heart wall initiate contractions that spread through specialized fibers to all parts of the heart. Some heart fibers (pacemaker cells) are specialized to initiate a rhythm of contraction that signals the other heart muscle fibers to contract. Although heart rate can be altered by neural impulses that can speed or slow its rate, these neural signals are not necessary for the heart to contract.

When the heart contracts, it pushes blood into muscular, elastic arteries that carry blood away from the heart. Since heart tissue also needs a steady blood supply to function, several coronary arteries deliver oxygenated blood to the heart muscle. In order for the blood to get to all tissues of the body, blood passes through arteries, into smaller branches (arterioles) and into the capillaries where nutrient and waste exchange with body cells takes place. Deoxygenated blood then flows into the venules and into the veins. Blood must flow uphill to return to the heart, a slower process than the blood flow rate in the arteries as venous walls are thinner and less muscular. Some veins contain one-way valves to assist blood in returning to the heart and prevent back flow. Skeletal muscle movements and the muscle contractions in respiration are important in helping blood to return to the heart.

Capillaries connect the smallest arterioles and venules and consist of a single layer of cells. These highly permeable walls allow substances in the blood to be exchanged with other substances in the fluid surrounding the body cells. Oxygen, nutrients, and hormones pass out of the capillaries. The surrounding cells uptake these essential nutrients and release carbon dioxide and metabolic waste products into the extracellular fluid. The carbon dioxide and metabolic waste products are eventually excreted by the lungs and kidneys.

The lymphatic system returns the extracellular fluid lost from the circulatory system back into the bloodstream. Excess tissue fluid moves into small lymph capillaries located in the spaces of most body tissues. This fluid, called lymph, is then carried to lymphatic vessels, lymph nodes, larger lymphatic collectors and finally to a large collecting duct that empties into blood-carrying veins in the neck. The lymphatic system has no pump and lymph movement depends on contraction of surrounding skeletal muscles. The lymphatic system also serves a protective function since the lymph nodes inactivate bacteria and filter foreign matter from body fluids.

Age-Associated Changes in the Cardiovascular System

Both longitudinal and cross-sectional studies have documented a decrease in maximum heart rate and maximum oxygen consumption with age (Robinson et al. 1975). These reductions are noticeable during heavy exercise. The decline in heart rate occurs at a constant rate from birth. Maximum heart rate is estimated to be 220 minus one's age. The loss in maximum oxygen consumption is also linear through adulthood (McArdle et al. 1981) and is estimated to amount to a loss of 30 to 40 percent from young adulthood to age 60 (Shepard 1978). A decrease in maximum oxygen consumption and heart rate with age results in less oxygen available to body tissues during heavy exertion. The decline in maximum oxygen consumption may be due to age-related decrements in the heart muscle and respiratory and musculoskeletal systems. On the other hand, the decreased maximum oxygen consumption may be due to decreased oxygen needs as elders commonly have less muscle mass than younger groups. However, the degree of loss attributed to age vs. lack of activity has not yet been fully explored.

Reduction in the efficiency of the heart is highly variable. Data on healthy elders who have maintained exercise programs throughout their lives show that cardiovascular performance is much higher in elder subjects who have high physical fitness levels. Most age-related alterations in cardiovascular efficiency do not affect the ability to carry out daily activities. However, maximum exercise performance decreases almost

Chapter 3

universally with age. Decreases in maximum aerobic capacity, heart rate, stroke volume (the volume of blood expelled with each heart beat), and cardiac output (volume of blood pumped per minute) affect ability to sustain heavy exertion (Brandfonbrener et al. 1955).

Changes in the arteries also contribute to the reduced cardiovascular efficiency in elders. Arterial walls progressively become less elastic with age due to calcification and the build-up of collagen connective tissue. This decrement is called arteriosclerosis, or hardening of the arteries. Arteriosclerosis occurs whether or not vascular disease is present and is considered to be age-related and independent of lifestyle. In contrast, atherosclerosis, the buildup of cholesterol within the walls of the arteries, is a disease process associated with lifestyle. Atherosclerosis will be explored more fully in Chapter 5.

Effects of age upon the venous system have not been studied as extensively as the arterial system. It is known that the veins become thicker and more twisted and some of the larger veins increase in capacity due to decreased elasticity of the walls. Deterioration of the venous valves creates an increase in venous pressure and pooling of blood in some areas causing varicose veins in some elders.

Amount of blood flow to the internal organs diminishes with age. Capillary number and density decreases in many body organs. However, many body organs decrease in mass with age so that decreased blood flow to the organs may be in response to a decreased need for oxygen and nutrients.

The Immune System

The immune system protects the body from invasion of bacteria, viruses, fungi, and its own defective body cells. The major components of the immune system are the thymus gland, spleen, lymph nodes, bone marrow, and leucocytes. The skin prevents foreign agents from entering the body, and stomach acid destroys bacteria that enter the digestive tract. In contrast, five types of leucocytes (immune cells) circulate in the bloodstream and are specialized to search out and destroy specific types of invaders.

The most-studied leucocyte is the lymphocyte (white blood cells). Like other leucocytes, they are manufactured in the bone marrow. Colonies of these cells establish in the spleen, thymus gland, and lymph nodes and continually reproduce. The lymphocytes that mature in the thymus gland are called T cells and comprise the majority of all lymphocytes. Lymphocytes that mature elsewhere are called B cells. Both B and T cells are very specific in the type of foreign invaders they will attack. The B cells combat bacterial and some viral infections by secreting highly-specific antibodies into blood and body fluid that deactivate invaders. Antibodies will continue to be produced until all the invaders have been destroyed. When another similar invader enters the bloodstream, even years later, some of these cells (memory cells) can produce more of these unique antibodies. In contrast, T cells directly attack body cells that have become infected by viruses or bacteria, cancerous cells, or invader cells. T cells do not secrete antibodies directly, but kill cells by attaching directly to them. However, for B cells to work, they need T cells to trigger them.

The major sites of lymphocyte defense activity are the lymph nodes and the spleen. The lymph nodes are enlargements in the lymph circulatory system vessels. The lymphatic system extracts fluid from the bloodstream and cleanses it as the fluid passes through lymph nodes. The B and T cells, as well as other types of leucocytes housed in the lymph nodes, inactivate foreign substances in the fluid. The cleansed blood is then returned to the bloodstream. The spleen also serves a similar function. Some endocrine glands may also affect the function of the immune system. Thymosin, a hormone secreted by the thymus gland, is thought to stimulate activity of the lymphocytes. Further, the thyroid and pituitary glands affect immune processes.

Age-Associated Changes in the Immune System

It is thought that with age, immune system function declines and the ability to destroy foreign bodies and aberrant cells of the body is reduced. There is evidence of a reduction in T cell production with advancing age. However, data are sparse on the exact mechanism. It is impossible to attribute elders' increased susceptibility to disease to any one deficiency in their immune systems. With age, the production of antibodies in response to a foreign agent decreases. This may explain elders' greater susceptibility to some diseases such as cancer, tuberculosis, and pneumonia. Further, with advancing age and peaking around age seventy, the body has an increased number of antibodies against its own cells in the blood (Hill and Stamm 1982). However, there is no evidence that these antibodies are actually attacking the body tissues since there is no increase in autoimmune disease with age. After adolescence, the thymus gland, responsible for T cell formation, shrinks and the hormone thyroxin decreases. How or whether this affects immune system function is not yet known.

The Respiratory System

All body cells require oxygen to survive. Since cells and tissues are unable to store oxygen, a new supply must be delivered continuously by the bloodstream or they will die. The waste product of oxygen metabolism, carbon dioxide, is excreted from the body cells into the circulatory system. The major function of the respiratory system is to transfer oxygen from the air into the bloodstream and to remove carbon dioxide from the bloodstream into the environment. Figure 3.2 illustrates the structure of the respiratory system.

Air enters the nostrils and is filtered, warmed, and moistened in the nasal cavity. First, air passes through the pharynx, a flexible tube that also carries food to the esophagus. Air then moves through the larynx (voicebox) to the trachea (windpipe). The trachea divides into two bronchi in the upper part of the chest cavity and these continue to divide and subdivide into smaller and smaller cartilage-ringed branches that reach deep into the right and left lungs. The smallest tubes have muscular walls and are called bronchioles. Each bronchiole ends in a tiny air sac called an alveolus. Nearly a billion microscopic balloon-like alveoli are housed in the lungs, giving the lungs a spongy appearance. The walls of the alveoli are one cell thick and covered with capillaries; they are the site for oxygen and carbon dioxide exchange. Oxygen from the airway is exchanged in the alveoli, then is transported through the blood via hemoglobin molecules inside red blood cells. Carbon dioxide, the waste product of oxygenization dissolved in the blood, moves through the alveoli walls to be exhaled.

The mechanism of breathing is very complex. The rate and depth of breathing is regulated by a respiratory control center in the brain. Exercise, high levels of carbon dioxide, or low levels of oxygen in the blood can trigger an increase in breathing rate or depth by altering muscle contractions. The diaphragm (a sheet of muscles acting as a partition below the rib cage) and intercostal muscles (muscles between the ribs) are the primary moving forces in breathing. Upon inhalation, the muscles in the diaphragm contract, causing the diaphragm partition to lower. This creates a decreased pressure inside the lungs that causes air to enter the respiratory passages. Upon exhalation, the diaphragm muscle relaxes, bowing upwards again. This constricts the lungs and forces the air out. Movement of the intercostal muscles increases the depth of inhalation or expiration by lifting the chest.

The bronchial tubes are lined with cells that produce and secrete a mucus that lines the airway. Protruding cells with hair-like projections (cilia) trap foreign particles that are inhaled and move them upward to the pharynx. Once in the pharynx, mucus and foreign material pass through the esophagus and into the stomach to be neutralized by stomach acid.

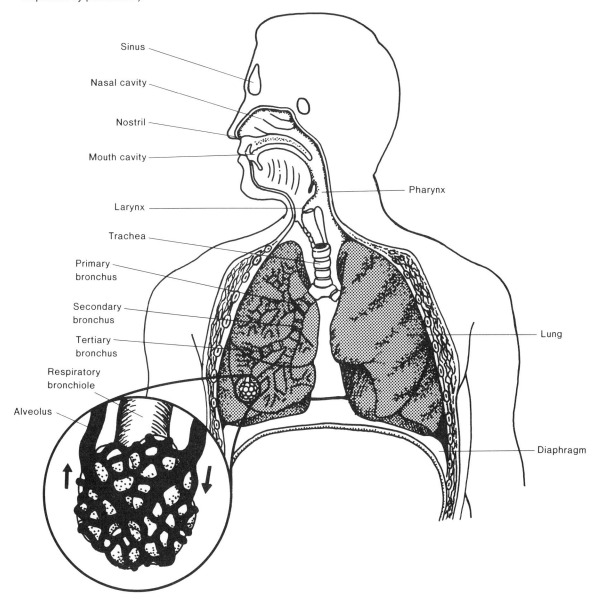

Figure 3.2 Respiratory system—problem. (Source: Hole, John W., Jr., *Human Anatomy and Physiology*, 3rd ed. Copyright © 1978, 1981, 1984 Wm. C. Brown Publishers, Dubuque, Iowa. All Rights Reserved. Reprinted by permission).

Sinus

Nasal cavity

Nostril

Mouth cavity

Pharynx

Larynx

Trachea

Primary bronchus

Secondary bronchus

Tertiary bronchus

Respiratory bronchiole

Alveolus

Lung

Diaphragm

Age-Associated Changes
in the Respiratory System

Respiratory structures are constantly exposed to environmental pollutants. Because of this, it is extremely difficult to differentiate the extent of respiratory deterioration due to age from that caused by an accumulation of damage by pollutants. Although there are noticeable decrements associated with age, the degree and rate of loss is also highly dependent upon the state of the cardiovascular, nervous, and musculoskeletal systems, overall health status, and degree of physical activity.

The main effect of age on the respiratory system is the reduction of the amount of oxygen taken up from the environment by the blood (Whitbourne 1985). With age, air tends to distribute unevenly within the lung, lowering the efficiency of gas exchange in older people. This occurs because lung tissue becomes less elastic with age, which decreases the amount of time the airways in the lungs are kept open. This decrease in elasticity affects the amount of oxygen-containing air that can fill the alveoli, especially those in the lower portion of the lung. As the lower lungs are most important in supplying oxygenated blood to body tissues, this significantly decreases the oxygen available to the tissues, especially during times of heavy exertion (Bode et al. 1976; Whitbourne 1985).

Gas exchange is also limited by other age-related factors. Alveoli are enlarged and flattened, reducing the area for gas exchange (Thurlbeck and Angus 1975). In addition, the chest wall muscles and skeleton become more rigid, which increases the amount of effort to breathe and reduces the ability of the lungs to expand during inspiration and compress during exhalation (Brooks and Fahey 1984). Because of this, maximum breathing rate decreases with age.

The most consistent change in breathing capacity with age is a decrease in vital capacity. Vital capacity is the amount of air that is moved in and out of the lungs when the person is inhaling and exhaling as hard as possible. It is estimated that vital capacity decreases about 40 percent between age twenty and seventy (Lynn-Davies 1977). An increase in residual lung volume is commonly noted with age (Asmussen et al. 1975). Residual volume is the amount of air left in the lungs after a maximal exhalation. The air that stays in the lungs is not replaced with each breath and therefore is not available for oxygen-carbon dioxide exchange.

Decreased pulmonary efficiency with age has little effect on daily functioning. However, maximum exertion levels or the length of time older people can sustain heavy physical activity may be affected. Elders may need more rest periods during heavy physical exertion because they tire more easily and take longer to recover. Decreased pulmonary efficiency can lower metabolic rate and decrease oxygen supply to body tissues, especially during heavy physical exertion. Elders also have decreased capacity to cope with environmental pollutants and are more susceptible to pulmonary distress or death during periods of high pollution. However, there is great variation among elders in pulmonary efficiency. Cigarette smoking and duration and physical fitness have a significant impact.

The Digestive System

The digestive system is a modified, muscular tube (called the alimentary canal) that extends from the mouth to the anus (figure 3.3). Portions of this tube are specialized for different functions. Each plays a role in the breakdown of food into usable nutrients, absorbing them into the blood and temporarily storing the waste products until elimination. Accessory structures release chemicals into the canal to facilitate digestion and absorption. Other body systems affect the workings of the digestive system. The nervous system regulates the contractions of the muscles in the wall of the alimentary canal and the blood flow to these organs. Digestion also involves the secretion of enzymes and hormones by the endocrine system. The cardiovascular system transports food molecules from the digestive system to body cells.

Figure 3.3 Digestive system. (Source: Hole, John W., Jr., *Human Anatomy and Physiology,* 3rd ed. Copyright © 1978, 1981, 1984 Wm. C. Brown Publishers, Dubuque, Iowa. All Rights Reserved. Reprinted by permission.

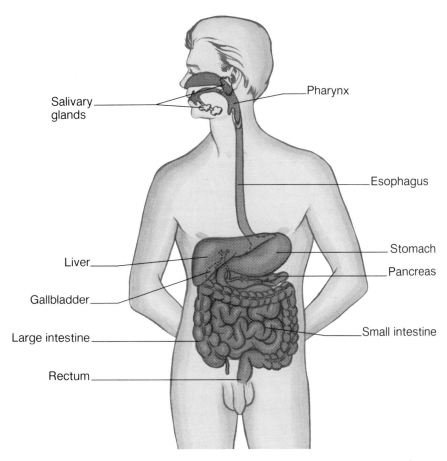

Digestion begins in the mouth where teeth mechanically break down the food particles. Saliva, secreted by three major pairs of salivary glands, moistens the food and secretes an enzyme that breaks down complex sugar molecules. Salivary secretions also facilitate taste bud functioning and keep the oral cavity clean. The tongue mixes food with saliva and also moves food from the mouth into the passageway of the esophagus.

When food is swallowed, rhythmic muscular contractions of the esophagus push food towards the stomach. When the esophagus contracts, a valve (cardiac sphincter) opens at the entrance to the stomach. As the sphincter closes, the muscular stomach wall churns, mechanically working on the food. Some digestion happens in the stomach, but its major function is storage. In the stomach, an enzyme (pepsin) and hydrochloric acid initiate the digestion of proteins. Gastric juice also contains other enzymes, one of which aids in the absorption of vitamin B-12. This mixture of partially digested food and secretions then passes from the stomach through the pyloric sphincter into the first part of the small intestine, the duodenum.

The Body and Its Age Changes: Part I

The small intestine is the main site for absorption of nutrients, water, and salts. Two pancreatic secretions pass through the pancreatic duct into the small intestine. One assists the break-down of carbohydrates, fats, and proteins; the other neutralizes the acidic food mixture from the stomach. Bile, produced by the liver and stored in the gallbladder, also empties into the duodenum. Bile emulsifies fats and enhances absorption of fatty acids and certain fat-soluble vitamins. The lining of the duodenum also secretes a number of different enzymes that further break down proteins, complex starches, sugars, and fats.

As the food moves through the small intestine, fingerlike outgrowths (villae) of the internal wall with hairlike projections (microvillae) absorb the water, salts, sugars, proteins, and fats into the blood and lymph capillaries. Most food energy is absorbed as it travels through the small intestine.

After four to six hours in the small intestine, the remaining material empties into the large intestine through another valve. The large intestine consists of the colon, the rectum, and the anal canal. The appendix is a nonfunctional tubular appendage that extends from the entrance of the large intestine. Although it has little significance in absorbing nutrients, the large intestine absorbs water and salts and forms and stores solid feces. When the muscular terminal portion of the colon (the rectum) is filled, feces are eliminated through the anal sphincter. Feces usually contain 50–75 percent water, undigestable plant matter, dead cells, and bacteria.

Age-Associated Changes in the Digestive System

The digestive system has a high turnover of cells and a substantial reserve capacity, enabling it to withstand considerable decrements before any effect is noted on digestive functioning. However, some age-associated alterations in structure and function of the alimentary canal and associated organs has been documented.

Perhaps the most obvious changes in the digestive system associated with advancing age is tooth loss. However, tooth loss is not considered a true age-change. Factors influencing tooth loss are poor oral hygiene, malnutrition, and gum disease. Teeth do wear down with age, but the rate of wear is insignificant. There is also some evidence that gums recede from the teeth with advancing age, but whether this is a true age change or the result of poor dental hygiene is not known.

With age, there is a reduction of secretion of gastric juices. One report found that the normal volume of stomach secretions decreased by 25 percent by age sixty (Bernier et al. 1973). The reduction in pepsin may impair protein digestion (Fikry 1965). The decrease in hydrochloric acid and the enzyme needed to absorb Vitamin B-12 may reduce digestion of calcium, iron, vitamin B-12, and folic acid as well as increase bacterial growth in the intestinal tract (Bowman and Rosenberg 1983).

There are some structural age changes in the intestine. The weight of the small intestine decreases with age as does the surface area (Minaker and Rowe 1982). These age effects have little effect because the surface cells throughout the digestive system are numerous and constantly being replaced. There are no significant functional changes in the structure or function of the liver, gall bladder, or pancreas.

The Urinary System

As each body cell breaks down food into molecules necessary for cell growth and energy, waste products are formed and are transported away from the tissues by the lymph and blood. The respiratory system eliminates one waste product, carbon dioxide, from the body. The urinary system rids the body of other waste products and toxic substances. Aside from its excretory function, the urinary system also regulates acid-base balance, volume of body fluids, and salt concentration in the body.

The urinary system is composed of a pair of kidneys each attached to a muscular tube, the ureter, which transports urine from the kidneys to the bladder. The bladder stores the urine until

Figure 3.4 Urinary system. (Source: Hole, John W., Jr., *Human Anatomy and Physiology,* 3rd ed. Copyright © 1978, 1981, 1984 Wm. C. Brown Publishers, Dubuque, Iowa. All Rights Reserved. Reprinted by permission).

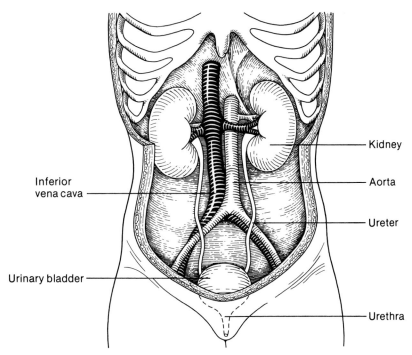

the urethra, a narrow tube connected to the bladder, transports the urine outside the body (figure 3.4).

The kidneys are located on the posterior wall of the upper abdominal cavity and measure about 4 inches in length. Each kidney houses about one million tiny structures called nephrons, which filter reusable water and minerals from the blood. Blood flows from the renal artery into the capillaries within each nephron. Almost 99 percent of the water and nutrients are selectively removed from the nephron back into the bloodstream while waste materials and a small amount of water and salts (urine) pass through the entire nephron into collecting ducts, through the ureters and into the bladder. The urinary filtration system is very efficient: the entire volume of blood in the body is filtered almost fifty times a day.

The bladder, an expandable muscular sac, stores the urine. When the bladder is about half full, sensory receptors in the bladder wall signal the brain, resulting in the urge to urinate. Urination is dependent on voluntary relaxation of the bladder sphincter and contraction of the bladder muscles. From the bladder, the urine flows through the bladder sphincter to the urethra. In males, the urethra is about 8 inches long; in females, 2 inches. The urethra in the male also serves a reproductive function as it carries semen.

Age-Associated Changes in the Urinary System

Cross-sectional data show that the kidney becomes gradually less efficient at filtering the blood beginning in the mid-thirties until around age seventy when there is a sharp drop in efficiency

(Rowe et al. 1976). A number of age-associated structural changes in the kidney may contribute to this reduced efficiency. Between ages forty and eighty, the kidney loses about 20 percent of its weight (McLachlan 1978). Renal blood flow starts to decrease in the fifth decade, then declines 10 percent per decade (Epstein 1979). This decreased blood flow may be due to reduced cardiovascular efficiency or to a decreased need for blood by the kidney because of its reduced mass. Some nephrons change in structure and it is hypothesized that many become nonfunctional with advancing age. However, kidneys have a large reserve capacity.

This decrease in filtering efficiency has little effect on normal function of the kidney because the organ has a great reserve capacity. However, reduced kidney efficiency may be noticeable during stress or dehydration. Reduction in filtration rate with age affects excretion of some drugs. If an elder is taking drugs that are excreted by the kidney, they may remain in the body longer. To account for reduced kidney efficiency in elders, physicians should adjust the dosage of drugs normally excreted by the kidney.

Although age-related decrements in kidney efficiency have been reported many times in cross-sectional studies, one longitudinal study reported that kidney decrements are not as great as earlier reported. Reports for the Baltimore Longitudinal study of healthy older people indicate that many subjects maintained stable kidney function over long periods of time and some older adults actually improved kidney function (Shock et al. 1978). This brings into question the health of the populations studied earlier. It is known that those with other diseases, especially cardiovascular and diabetes, have reduced kidney function. In addition, these data demonstrate that, like most other body systems, some decline is expected, but the severity and rate of decline is highly variable.

With age, the bladder becomes less able to store a large amount of fluid and more urine remains in the bladder after voiding. As a result, older people may need to urinate more often. Incomplete emptying can predispose elders to bladder infections. Older men and women are more likely to wake up at night to urinate; however, this increased frequency was found to occur independently of any structural changes in the kidney or bladder (Goldman 1977). Whereas younger adults generally receive a neural message that their bladder is becoming full when it is only half full, the message in elders may be delayed or absent. The reduced time differential between awareness and involuntary urination produces anxiety in elders, especially in unfamiliar environments. However, again, there is great variability in loss of bladder efficiency.

Summary

The majority of structural changes occurring in body systems with age have little effect on normal function. The speed and extent of age-associated changes in the integumentary system are highly variable and affect appearance. Skin becomes more wrinkled and less elastic, the body loses subcutaneous fat, and hair may thin, become gray or coarsen. Age-associated changes in the musculoskeletal system are also highly variable and are much more severe in elders who are physically inactive. Elders may lose some muscular strength, joint flexibility, and bone strength and mass. In the cardiovascular system, maximum heart rate and maximum oxygen consumption decrease with age and the system becomes less efficient. However, these reductions are only noticeable during heavy exertion. Although it is thought that immune system function becomes less efficient with age, the exact mechanism is still undetermined. The main effect of age on the respiratory system is a decreased elasticity of lung tissue, reducing the rate of oxygen-carbon dioxide exchange. Again, this reduction in efficiency is only apparent when the individual is exercising at maximum exertion. Because the digestive system has high reserve capacity, age has little effect on its function. With age, the kidneys becomes less efficient at filtering wastes from the blood. Further, structural changes in the bladder may cause decreased fluid capacity and urinary retention after voiding.

Activities

1. List the health behaviors you currently practice that may hasten your aging process. Which systems do these behaviors affect? How might these behaviors affect your functioning ten years from now? Twenty?

2. Make a list of physiological changes you believe are inevitable with aging. Which of these changes are valid for all elders you know? How are the elders you know affected by these aging processes? How do they adjust?

3. Assuming you will be alive, draw or describe your appearance and lifestyle at age eighty. What physiological changes did you illustrate? Which may be lessened with changes in health behaviors?

4. The phrase, "I must be getting old," is commonly repeated by individuals of all ages. What were the circumstances in which you or others have said this? Was it a valid feature of aging or was it due to disease or environmental factors?

5. Select a characteristic you believe to be a true age change. Using the criteria given and recent literature, gather information that leads to your conclusion that the decrement is due to age itself.

6. Design a commercial, printed advertisement or radio spot advocating sunscreen use and aimed at younger people. How did you convince the public to take care of their skin before they notice damage?

7. Many companies prosper from products designed to make the public feel or look younger. Collect advertisements that promote this theme and share them with your classmates. Might their claims be valid? If not, write a letter to one of the companies protesting their practices.

Bibliography

Aniansson, A., and E. Gustafsson. 1981. Physical training in elderly men with special reference to quadriceps muscle strength and morphology. *Clin Physio* 1:87–98.

Asmussen, E. 1981. Aging and exercise. In S. M. Horvath, and M. K. Yousef, eds. *Environmental physiology: Aging, heat and altitude.* New York: Elsevier. 419–28.

Asmussen, E., K. Fruensgaard, and S. Horgaard. 1975. A follow-up longitudinal study of selected physiologic functions in former physical education students—after 40 years. *J Am Geriatric Soc* 23:442–50.

Avioli, L. V. 1982. Aging, bone and osteoporosis. In S. G. Korenman, ed. *Endocrine aspects of aging.* New York: Elsevier Biomedical. 199–230.

Bernier, J. J., N. Vidon, and M. Mignon. 1973. The value of a cooperative multicenter study for establishing a table for normal values of gastric secretions as a function of sex, age and weight. *Biologie et Gastro-Enterologie (Paris)* 6:287–96.

Bode, R. J., J. Dosman, R. R. Martin, et al. 1976. Age and sex difference in lung elasticity and in closing capacity of nonsmokers. *J Appl Physiol* 41:129–35.

Bowman, B. B., and I. H. Rosenberg. 1983. Digestive function and aging. *Hum Nutr Clin Nutr* 37C:75–89.

Brandfonbrener, M., M. Landowne, and N. W. Shock. 1955. Changes in cardiac output with age. *Circulation* 12:557–66.

Brooks, G. A., and D. Fahey. 1984. *Exercise physiology: Human bioenergetics and its applications.* New York: Wiley.

Comfort, A. 1976. *A good age.* New York: Simon and Schuster.

deVries, H. A. 1980. *Physiology and exercise for physical education and athletes.* Dubuque, Iowa: W. C. Brown.

Epstein, M. 1979. Effects of aging on the kidney. *Fed. Proc.* 38:168–72.

Fikry, M. E. 1965. Gastric secretory functions in the aged. *Gerontologica Clinica* 7:216–26.

Goldman, R. 1977. Aging of the excretory system: kidney and bladder. In C. E. Finch, and L. Hayflick, eds. *Handbook of the biology of aging.* New York: Van Nostrand Reinhold. 409–30.

Grimby, G., and B. Saltin. 1983. The aging muscle *Clin Physiol* 3:209–18.

Hill, C. D. and W. E. Stamm. 1982. Pneumonia in the elderly: The fatal complication. *Geriatrics* 37:40–50.

Lynne-Davies, P. 1977. Influence of age on respiratory system. *Geriatrics* 32:57–60.

Mazess, R. B. 1982. On aging bone loss. *Clin Orthopaedics and Related Res* 165:239–52.

McArdle, W. D., F. I. Katch, and V. L. Katch. 1981. *Exercise physiology: Energy, nutrition and physical performance.* Philadelphia: Lea and Febiger.

McLachlan, M. S. 1978. The aging kidney. *Lancet* 2:143–46.

Minaker, K. L., and J. W. Rowe. 1982. Gastrointestinal System. In J. W. Rowe, and R. W. Besdine, eds. *Health and disease in old age.* Boston: Little-Brown. 297–315.

Robinson, S., D. B. Dill, S. P. Tzankoff, et al. 1975. Longitudinal studies of aging in 37 men. *J Appl Physiol* 38:263–67.

Rowe, J. W., R. A. Andres, N. D. Tobin, et al. 1976. The effect on creatinine clearance: cross sectional and longitudinal study. *J Gerontol* 31:155–63.

Rowlatt, C., and L. M. Franks. 1978. Aging in tissues and cells. In Brocklehurst, J. C., ed. *Geriatric medicine and gerontology.* New York: Churchill and Livingstone. 3–17.

Shephard, R. J. 1978. *Physical activity and aging.* Chicago: Yearbook Medical Pub.

Shephard, R. J. 1981. Cardiovascular limitations in the aged. In E. L. Smith, and R. C. Serfass, eds. *Exercise and aging: The scientific basis.* Hillside, N.J.: Enslow. 19–30.

Shock, N. W., R. Andres, A. H. Norris, and J. D. Tobin. 1978. Patterns of longitudinal changes in renal function. *Proc. XII Intl. Congress of Geront., Tokyo, August 20–25.* Amsterdam: Exerpta Medica. 525–27.

Thorne, N. 1981. The aging of the skin. *Practitioner* 225:793–800.

Thurlbeck, W. M., and G. E. Angus. 1975. Growth and aging of the normal human lung. *Chest* 67(2):3s–6s.

Whitbourne, S. K. 1985. *The aging body: Physiological changes and psychological consequences.* New York: Springer-Verlag.

The Body and Its Age Changes: Part II

4

Introduction

The nervous, sensory, and endocrine systems are the communication networks of the body that allow the body to adapt its physiology to the environment. Any alteration in these systems with age have important consequences for older people. Some age-related alteration in sensory function, especially vision and hearing, is apparent; however, the majority of other age-associated changes in structure and function of these body systems are minimal and do not cause restriction of daily activities. This chapter will continue the discussion of alterations in function with age in the nervous, endocrine, sensory, and reproductive systems.

The Nervous System

Cells, tissues, organs, and body systems must act together to maintain orderly function. The nervous system coordinates body functions through central integrators (brain and spinal cord) and nerve networks that control muscles and endocrine (hormone) glands. The neuron (nerve cell) is the basic unit of the nervous system. Millions of neurons combine to form the brain, spinal cord, and associated nerve pathways called peripheral nerves. Neurons vary in size, shape, and function, but all carry electrochemical messages in the form of nerve impulses. Some are specialized sensory receptors that gather information about the internal and external environment and transmit it to the spinal cord and the brain. Neurons within the spinal cord and brain interpret and act upon the information received from the receptors. Others transmit messages from the brain or spinal cord to stimulate muscles or glands to respond. Another type of cell common in the brain and spinal cord is the neuroglial cell. These cells, the connective tissue between neurons, provide support, protect, and nourish the neurons. They outnumber nerve cells ten to one (Whitbourne 1985).

The mechanism of nerve transmission is complex, but a simplified description is presented here. Specialized receptor neurons detect any significant internal or external changes in temperature, pressure, chemical concentration, or electrical condition, and initiate an electrical impulse. This message transmitted from neuron to neuron along complex nerve pathways to the brain or spinal cord to be interpreted. Because individual neurons are not connected, the electrical impulse must jump from nerve to nerve across a gap called a synapse. The impulse is transmitted across the synapse by chemicals called neurotransmitters. When the message reaches its destination (brain or spinal cord) it is interpreted and an action message travels along a different nerve pathway to direct the response of other body parts.

The nervous system includes the brain, spinal cord, and peripheral nerves. The brain consists of approximately 100 billion neurons that transmit information within the brain and to nerves in other parts of the body. The brain is divided into three parts, each with specialized functions. The cerebrum is responsible for such intellectual functions as speech, thought, learning, memory, and reasoning. The cerebrum also interprets impulses from sensory receptors and controls voluntary muscle action. The cerebellum coordinates voluntary muscle movements and maintains muscle tone, posture, and equilibrium. The brain stem controls heart beat, blood pressure, respiration, temperature, and some hormones. The brain stem also relays sensory impulses to the cerebellum.

The spinal cord is a bundle of nerves situated within the vertebral bones of the spinal column. Spinal cord neurons receive messages from various body parts and transmit directions to the brain or other parts of the body. Neurons that branch out from the spinal column and brain constitute the peripheral nervous system. Some of these peripheral nerves regulate voluntary actions (such as movement of the skeletal muscles in the arms and legs). Others regulate involuntary actions such as heart beat, breathing, digestion, and release of some hormones.

Age-Associated Changes in the Nervous System

Because the nervous system controls and coordinates other body functions, decrements in the nervous system have a significant impact on body and cognitive function. However, there is little documentation that nervous system function declines with advancing age. Some structural changes in the nervous system with age are well-documented. However, the effect of these changes on the function of the nervous system is speculative.

Reduction in brain volume and size is thought to accompany aging (Ordy 1975). However, this decrease may be due to other factors as healthy individuals experience less brain weight loss (Tomlinson et al. 1968). The loss of brain volume is due to a reduction of neurons. With advancing age, neurons die and are not replaced. The greatest nerve loss is within the cerebrum, the

Contrary to popular belief, intellectual ability and creativity do not decline with age.

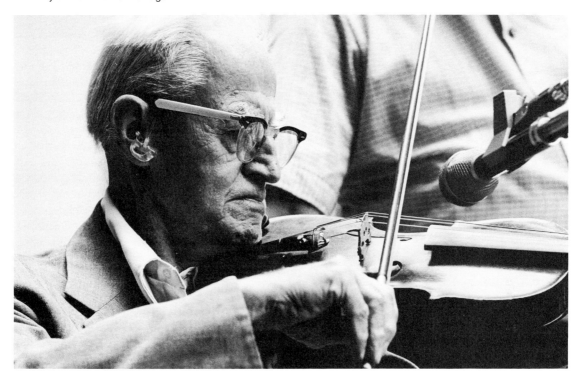

center of sensory processing, and the motor cortex, the movement center. However, there is no evidence that this nerve cell loss causes reduced intelligence, memory, or learning capacity. There is a great deal of redundancy in neurons: even though some may be lost, others remain. Further, it seems that neurons have the ability to regenerate new connections (Buell and Coleman 1979). There is a reduction in some neurotransmitters at the nerve synapse in certain parts of the brain with age; however, this decrease does not occur at all synapses and its effect on function is unclear.

Other structural changes occur in some neurons and neuroglial cells, although the functional consequences are unknown. Neuroglial cells increase in number in some parts of the brain and decrease in others with advancing age. Further, neurons accumulate lipofuscin, an age-associated pigment. After age sixty, tangles begin to appear in some neurons in the cerebrum and

small numbers of plaques (deposits of fat and connective tissue) occur among the neuroglial cells (Tomlinson et al. 1968). These plaques may affect mental function as they are common in those with organic brain syndrome such as Alzheimer's Disease.

Blood supply to the brain is decreased in older persons as compared to younger persons (Frankowiak et al. 1980). The decrease is believed to be a compensation for the decreased brain mass. There is evidence that blood flow to the brain may be increased with exercise (Spirduso 1980).

A number of studies have demonstrated that reaction time decreases with age. The decrease in visual and auditory reflexes and time to complete a physical or mental task decreases 20 percent or more from youth to old age, depending on the study (Hicks and Birren 1970). Those with disease exhibit even slower reflexes. This decrement may be due to physiological alterations in the neural pathway, alterations in vision or hearing, difficulty with testing situations, or increased cautiousness with age. Even though there is a statistically significant reduction in reaction time, in real life this translates into a reduction of only hundredths of a second, and is not functionally important.

Although popular opinion asserts that cognitive function decreases with age, studies on the nervous system show very little physiological alteration. It has tremendous reserve and compensatory ability and can continue to conduct impulses effectively even with the loss of neurons. Although some individuals may exhibit decrements in nervous system functioning, the differences are highly variable and affected by other factors besides age itself.

The Sensory System

The nervous system depends on its specialized sensory receptors to gather information about the internal and external environment. The receptors include those needed for vision, hearing, smell, taste, touch, equilibrium, temperature, and pain sensation. Although each sensory receptor responds to only one kind of environmental stimulus, all convert the stimulus received from the environment into nerve impulses that are transmitted along nerve fibers to the brain and spinal cord for processing.

Sensory decrements are the most crucial physiological changes associated with the aging process because they affect an individual's perceptions and response to the world. Since visual and hearing changes are gradual, elders may not seek medical attention because they adapt to the deficits.

Vision

The eye is a hollow sphere about one inch in diameter (figure 4.1). Eyelashes, eyelids, tear glands, and tear ducts protect the eye from dirt, injury, or dryness. The sclera is the white, outer layer of the eyeball. The cornea is a transparent membrane that covers the front of the eyeball.

The iris is the circular, colored part of the eye that lies behind the cornea and in front of the lens. The opening at the center of the iris is the pupil. When the light is dim, the pupil opening expands to allow more light to stimulate the receptors. When the light is bright, the pupil contracts to protect the receptors from damage from intense light.

The lens is located behind the pupil and is suspended by ligaments. It focuses light rays entering the pupil so they merge to a point on the retina, located on the back of the inside of the eye. The lens does this by flattening or bulging its shape with the help of supporting ligaments and muscles. This capacity allows for sharp vision at any distance. In some people, the shape of the eyeball or lens focuses light rays at a point beyond the retinal surface, which causes farsightedness (an inability to focus on near objects). In others, light rays come to a focus at a point in front of the retina instead of directly on it causing nearsightedness or myopia (an inability to focus on distant objects). Both disorders can usually be corrected with eyeglasses or contact lenses.

Vision receptors are located in the retina and consist of rods to distinguish general outlines and cones for color vision and sharp outlines. The rods and cones connect with neurons to form the optic nerve. The blind spot, where the optic nerve connects to the retina, has no visual receptors. Viscous fluids (the aqueous humor in front of the lens and the vitreous humor behind it), maintain proper eye pressure and fluid balance to allow the eye to function properly.

Age-Associated Changes in Vision

A number of structural changes occur in the eye that affect vision in the middle and later years. One of the most well-documented is the thickening of the lens with age. The lens triples in mass by age seventy, making the lens more dense (Paterson 1979). The lens also becomes less elastic, decreasing its ability to alter its shape to view close objects. Starting at age forty, the eye becomes less able to focus on objects at close distance, and by age sixty, the lens is incapable of

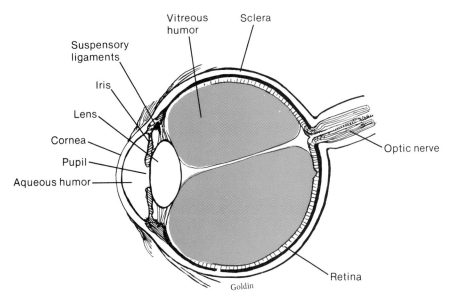

Figure 4.1 Structure of the eye. (Source: Hole, John W., Jr., *Human Anatomy and Physiology,* 2nd ed. Copyright © 1978, 1981 Wm. C. Brown Publishers, Dubuque, Iowa. All Rights Reserved. Reprinted by permission.

focusing at close distance. This change is a universal condition called presbyopia. A common symptom of presbyopia is the tendency to hold reading material farther and farther away in order to read it. Interestingly, the development of presbyopia seems correlated with environmental temperature; those people in warm climates manifest the condition earlier (Weale 1981). Presbyopia responds very well to corrective lenses or a magnifying glass for reading and close work. Some people may need bifocals: glasses that incorporate one prescription for close focus and another for distant focus. Bifocals can be ground to look like ordinary glasses.

The thickening of the lens also reduces the amount of light that can pass through the lens, causing blurred or dim vision (Spector 1982). Further, the lens becomes yellowed with advanced age (Warwick 1976). This reduces light passage to the retina and impairs the ability to differentiate blues, greens, and violet colors. Because more light is necessary to stimulate the light receptors in the retina, night vision is impaired. The amount of light entering the eye is also reduced because of age-related reductions in the size of the pupil. This is caused by atrophy of the muscle that dilates the pupil (Carter 1982). As the pupil becomes less responsive, the eye loses its ability to adapt to abrupt changes from light to darkness.

Visual clarity is further reduced by clouding of the lens. Any clouding of the lens is considered to be a cataract, whether or not it interferes with vision. Cataracts are the most common visual problem among elders. Most cataracts are associated with age, but medical disorders, chemicals, radiation, or injury can also cause cataract formation. In our country, three-fourths of all adults over sixty have some degree of cataract formation, but less than one of ten is legally blind

The photo on the right illustrates the effect of the aging process of visual acuity. Because age changes are gradual, elders may not realize their vision is declining.

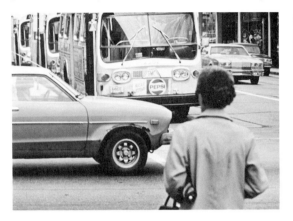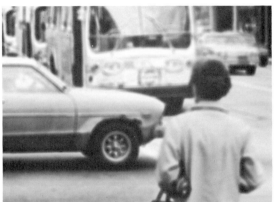

from them. Only 15 percent experience a significant vision loss and only 5 percent will need surgery (National Society to Prevent Blindness 1980). One national survey found that about 20 percent of elders reported they had cataracts. Both age and sex were related to cataract prevalence. Ten percent of the men between ages sixty-five and seventy-four reported cataracts while 32 percent of men over eighty-five did so. A higher proportion of elder women reported cataracts: 15 percent of those between ages sixty-five and seventy-four and 41 percent of those over age eighty-five. Approximately 10 percent reported they had a cataract operation (Havlik 1986). No drugs reverse cataract growth, but drugs to dilate the pupil will enable an elder to see better. Surgery involves removal of the lens and substitution of eyeglasses, contact lenses, or transplants. Contrary to popular belief, a cataract does not have to be ripe before it can be removed. The decision to operate depends on the influence of the cataract on the person's life style.

The cornea also becomes thicker and less transparent with age. The thickened lens and cornea can cause light to scatter inside the retina, decreasing visual clarity. This scattering of light rays makes it very difficult for elders to see clearly at night or when there is glare. The ability to

Experts in Vision Care

Three types of health professionals deal with eye care. An *ophthalmologist* or oculist is a physician with special training in eye diseases who can diagnose eye disease, perform eye surgery, and prescribe correction for inadequate vision. An *optometrist,* though not a physician, is trained to examine for visual defects and prescribe proper correction. If a disease is suspected or surgery is required, the client is referred to an ophthalmologist. An *optician,* following the directions of the ophthalmologist or optometrist, grinds and fits the lenses.

detect details at a distance decreases in the twenties, holds steady until the forties, then progressively declines (Pitts 1982). By age eighty-five, there is an 80 percent loss of visual acuity compared to the forties (Weale 1975). About 95 percent of older people wear eyeglasses and almost all have little or no trouble with vision when eyeglasses are used (Havlik 1986). To increase visual

Chapter 4

My Eyes are Failing

For quite a while now, I've been pretending.
That it was just that I was tired,
That the light was bad.
But my eyes really are getting worse.
I'm afraid to go to the doctor because I'm afraid of what
  he'll say.
Which is silly. Either there is something to be done. Or
  there is not.
If it's glasses, hallelujah, and let me find the money. If
  it's an operation, see me through. If I'm going blind,
  hold me. Help me put down the terror that rises in
  my gut at the word.
Blind. There. I've said it. The ghost word that has been
  haunting me.
Help me remember if I have to walk in the dark, that I
  have had a lot of years of seeing clean and clear. I
  know the slender shape of a birch tree. I know the
  color of irises and dawn. I have seen thousands and
  thousands of things in my life, I can conjure them in
  my mind's eye.
No matter what happens, I shall not be without beautiful
  sights.
It is just that I may have to settle for the ones I have already seen.

acuity in elders, the amount of light in the environment should be increased and glare should be minimized.

Some age-associated changes, which do not affect vision, occur in the structure of the eye. A gradual loss of muscle elasticity and orbital fat may cause the eyelids to droop, which affects appearance. Secretions of tear glands, which continually cleanse and lubricate the eye, may also be reduced with advancing age but it is likely that drugs, air pollution, and dehydration are responsible, not age.

Because most of the visual decrements accompanying aging occur gradually, elders adapt and their lifestyle is relatively unaffected. Elders can adapt to visual changes by altering their environment, altering their behavior, and purchasing corrective lenses. Yearly eye examinations, although expensive, will keep vision defects to a minimum and help an elder retain independence. Unfortunately, neither vision examinations nor corrective lenses are covered by Medicare, the national health insurance for those over sixty-five, although treatment of eye diseases is reimbursed. However, for those who qualify, Medicaid (or MediCal in California) may pay all or part of the expense of eye examinations and corrective lenses. In some communities, the Lion's Club assists individuals with costs related to vision problems.

Figure 4.2 Structure of the ear. (Source: Hole, John W., Jr., *Human Anatomy and Physiology,* 3rd ed. Copyright © 1978, 1981, 1984 Wm. C. Brown Publishers, Dubuque, Iowa. All Rights Reserved. Reprinted by permisison.

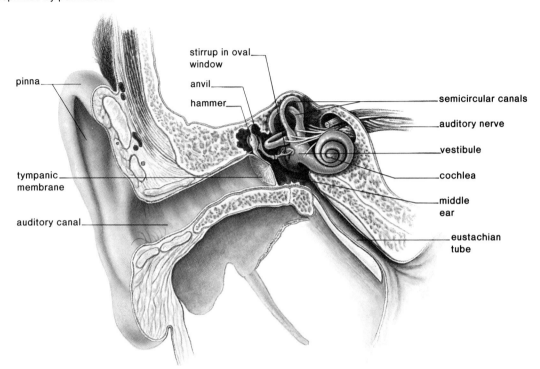

Hearing

The ear is composed of three distinct parts that act together to transmit sound waves. Sound waves enter the outer ear, are conducted into the middle ear, and are translated into nerve impulses in the inner ear. Specialized receptor cells in the inner ear transmit neural sound messages to the brain for processing. A mechanism within the inner ear is also important in maintaining body equilibrium as special fluid-filled canals signal the brain whenever they sense motion (see section on balance).

The most visible structure of hearing is the cartilaginous outer ear. Inside is an auditory canal lined with hair and wax-secreting glands. The funnel-shaped canal collects sound waves and guides them to the eardrum, which separates the outer from the middle ear (figure 4.2).

In the middle ear, three small bones, the hammer (malleus), anvil (incus), and stirrup (stapes) work together to transmit sound vibrations from the eardrum through the middle ear. In the middle ear, the eustachian tube connects the throat and ear. This connection serves to maintain equal pressure outside and inside the head, permitting the eardrum to vibrate normally. This explains why swallowing can relieve pressure in the ears during an airplane flight since this equalizes the pressure on both sides of the eardrum. Extreme pressure differences may cause the eardrum to rupture.

Sound waves are transformed into nerve impulses in the inner ear. The inner ear is completely filled with fluid and houses the cochlea, a snail-shaped tunnel also filled with fluid. The Organ of Corti is the inner lining of the cochlea

Chapter 4

I Don't Hear as Well as I Used to

I don't hear as well as I used to, God,
People have to shout and repeat things.
Frankly, a lot of what they have to say
Isn't worth repeating,
And the world's too noisy anyway.
The important thing is, I can hear,
Not with my ears, but with my heart,
What I really want to:
The children, when they were little,
Saying, "I love you, Mama."
Dan, when we lost all our savings,
Saying "Hold me, Anne,"
Stephen in front of all those people,
Saying "My mother should be receiving this honor
Instead of me."
My father-in-law, dying, laying his hand on my hair,
"You're a good gal, Annie. Carry on."
It's no fun going deaf,
But there are a lot of worse things,
And I do have a lot of good memories
To listen to.

and contains rows of receptor cells with specialized hairlike projections. The receptor cells transform sound into electrical impulses and transmit them on sensory nerve fibers to the auditory nerve and finally to the brain. These cells respond selectively to sounds of different frequencies, depending on their location on the membrane within the cochlea.

Age-Associated Changes in Hearing

In our country, hearing sensitivity decreases gradually with age beginning in adolescence and becoming increasingly evident with advanced age. Among men, 30 percent of those ages sixty-five to seventy-four and 60 percent of those age eighty-five and older report a hearing impairment. The percentage is lower in women: 18 percent of women ages sixty-five to seventy-four and 44 percent age eighty-five and older report deafness in one or both ears. Despite these high numbers, only 8 percent of both groups report they use a hearing aid (Havlik 1986).

Even though hearing loss is associated with advanced age, it is hypothesized that most hearing loss is not due to age itself, but to lifelong bombardment by environmental noise. This hypothesis is supported by the fact that elders in less technologically advanced cultures do not exhibit hearing loss to the extent of those in our society (Rosen et al. 1964). Many authorities predict even more widespread hearing difficulties because of the increasing noise in our country. Further decline in hearing can also be caused by disease, drug use, social setting, and diet.

The term used to describe the hearing loss associated with aging is presbycusis. Hearing loss is most noticeable in the high frequencies and the ability to hear high frequency sounds progressively decreases with advancing age.

The Body and Its Age Changes: Part II

There are several kinds of presbycusis, each with a different structural cause in the inner ear and different effects on hearing. *Sensory presbycusis* is caused by an atrophy of the receptor cells in the Organ of Corti. *Mechanical presbycusis* is caused by a decreased ability of the cochlea to conduct vibrations. Both affect the ability to hear high sounds, not the ability to differentiate speech sounds. *Neural presbycusis* is caused by a loss of neurons, especially in the auditory nerve. Similarly, *central presbycusis* results from a loss of neurons in the part of the brain that interprets sound. In these latter two types, elders have diminished ability to differentiate speech. *Vascular presbycusis* is caused by a lack of blood supply to the cochlea and affects hearing at all frequencies. For details on each of these types, see Anderson and Myerhoff (1982).

Those with presbycusis experience difficulty in comprehending speech. The high frequency consonant sounds such as f,g,s,z,t,sh, and ch are more difficult to differentiate. Older people also find it more difficult to screen out interfering noises. Further, elders are less able to comprehend extremely fast speech than their younger counterparts (Bergman et al. 1976).

Individuals with presbycusis may exhibit any or all of the following behaviors:

1. Prefer radio or television at a higher volume than others in the room.
2. Complain that others are not speaking clearly or loudly enough.
3. Consistently turn one side of head toward speaker or cup ear with hand.
4. Commonly ask others to repeat phrases or words or say "What?" or "Huh?"
5. Have difficulty hearing at large gatherings with background noise: lectures, church sermons, social events.
6. Have difficulty in locating the origin of sounds.
7. Confuse words or make silly mistakes.
8. Understand men's voices better than women's.

Types of Hearing Specialists

A number of health professionals can assist elders with hearing problems. Physicians, either an *otologist* (ear specialist) or an *otolaryngologist* (ear, nose, and throat specialist), can diagnose the problem and determine if surgical or medical treatment is necessary, or if a hearing aid is indicated. *Audiologists* are highly trained, nonmedical specialists who can evaluate hearing problems and counsel a patient on hearing aids and rehabilitation. A *hearing aid dispenser* measures hearing loss, helps to select the proper aid, custom-fits the apparatus and explains proper use and care techniques. Hearing aid dispensers must be licensed by the state to perform these tasks, but they are not qualified to diagnose hearing problems or to prescribe medication.

In addition to presbycusis, elders may suffer hearing loss due to other age-associated changes in the ear. The wall of the outer cartilaginous portion of the auditory canal collapses inward with advancing age, narrowing the passage and making the canal less efficient in receiving and channeling sound waves to the middle ear. Further, earwax tends to thicken with age. Accumulation of earwax may occlude the auditory canal and may contribute to hearing difficulty. It is estimated that one-third of the hearing loss in elders is due to build-up of earwax (Fisch 1978).

Reduced hearing acuity may cause psychological effects. Decreased hearing sensitivity may limit enjoyment of social activities and the stimulation that other people and television provide.

By far the most popular hearing aids are in the ear and over the ear (A and B). A few individuals wear those designed as part of the temple of eyeglasses (C) and body aids that fit in breast pockets with wire into the ear (D)

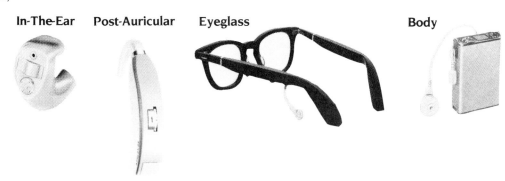

In-The-Ear   Post-Auricular   Eyeglass   Body

Tips in Communicating with the Hearing-Impaired Individual

1. Speak clearly, distinctly, and slowly; do not shout.

2. Face individuals when talking and look them in the eyes. If the person to whom you are speaking is in a wheelchair, lower yourself to eye level.

3. Be sure there is enough light for the person to see you speaking.

4. Screen out as much environmental noise as possible.

5. Give visual cues such as hand movement and facial expression in addition to your verbal message.

6. If you are asked to repeat, find other words to say the same thing.

7. In a group situation, sit in a circle so everyone can see one another's lip movement and expressions.

8. Be patient. Don't create the feeling that you are in a hurry.

9. Learn to read the individual's reaction to be certain s/he heard and understood what was said.

10. Make an attempt to discuss topics other than what is absolutely necessary even though it is harder to communicate those little things. Don't resort to curt, necessary exchanges.

Paranoid ideas and behavior, withdrawal from other people, depression, suspiciousness, and lack of contact with reality may occur in those with gradual hearing loss. Family members and friends may also withdraw from the hearing-impaired because of frustration engendered by efforts to communicate. Instead of the wide range of conversation topics, communication may be reduced to the necessities. Further, people who are hard of hearing are commonly misjudged as senile because they appear unattentive or withdrawn. Family members may overreact to reduced hearing, mistakenly believing the hearing-impaired person cannot handle personal affairs.

A number of specialists can assist those with hearing impairments. Professionals can distinguish age-related hearing loss from that caused by disease or earwax buildup.

Hearing aids are designed to reduce age-related hearing loss. The most common type of hearing aid goes behind the ear, although some can be inserted in the ear or built in the temple of eyeglasses. For severe hearing loss, a hearing aid that straps to the chest is worn. Hearing aids do not restore hearing to a normal level, rather they amplify all sounds. This can be annoying because both background noise and the human voice are amplified. Unfortunately, hearing aids are often fitted incorrectly. Because of incorrect fit or annoying background noise, elders may refuse to wear a hearing aid. In addition, some may refuse to wear a hearing aid for cosmetic reasons or because they believe it to be a sign of growing old. Further, some elders cannot afford to purchase a hearing aid as neither the examination nor the appliance is covered by Medicare. However, as in eyeglasses, Medicaid may pay for all or part of the cost if the individual qualifies.

Taste and Smell

The sensory organs of taste (taste buds) are located predominantly on the tongue, although a few may be found in other places in the mouth. Taste receptors are activated by chemicals from food that must be dissolved in saliva to be perceived. When a taste bud is stimulated, it triggers an impulse on an adjacent nerve fiber that relays the taste message to the brain.

Various taste sensations occur at different sites on the tongue. Sweet and salt receptors are located on the tip of the tongue, sour receptors are found on the sides, and bitter are located toward the back of the tongue. Although there are only four types of taste receptors, a large variety of taste sensations are possible because one food stimulates a combination of receptors. Further, the sense of smell influences taste.

Most mammals have a highly developed sense of smell because this sense is crucial in their ability to find food, select a mate, and detect danger. However, humans depend on other senses to a greater extent and their sense of smell is not as highly developed. Dogs, for instance have forty times more olfactory surface area than humans. Little research has been conducted to determine the type of smell receptors or the variety of odors humans can differentiate, perhaps because it is difficult to quantify odors.

Humans sense smells through a group of olfactory receptor cells (about ¼ inch in diameter) located high in the nasal cavity. The receptor cells have small hair-like projections that are bathed in watery fluid. The receptors transmit nerve messages to the brain. Olfactory receptors are very easily fatigued; a receptor can accommodate to a particular smell after only a minute of exposure. Significant alterations in olfaction can have profound effects on life-style. The sense of smell influences the ability to taste and enjoy food, to be aware of dangers (such as escaping gas fumes, burning electrical wires, smoke, or spoiled or burning food), and to detect body odors or pleasant smells.

Age-Associated Changes in Taste and Smell

It appears that elders retain the sense of taste and smell with advancing age. Worn out taste buds are continually replaced, thus the number of taste buds does not alter significantly with advancing years (Davidson 1979). Some studies report minor decrements in sensitivity to different tastes, but no overall reduction in taste acuity. However, studies conflict on which taste sensations decline with age. The ability of older people to detect salt and sweet tastes may decline slightly with age, but no change is noted in their ability to detect sour (Moore et al. 1982; Grzegorczyk et al. 1979). Although about 10 percent of elders experience a decrease in taste acuity (Baum 1981), this is attributed to factors other than age, including: smoking habits, dentures, poor oral hygiene, nutritional deficiencies (especially vitamin A, niacin, and zinc), and medication side effects.

Many cross-sectional studies report older people are less able to detect smells than younger adults (Doty et al. 1984). However, as in taste, these decrements may be attributed to illness or medication effects, rather than age. There seems to be wide variation in smell acuity with age and even some reports that elders have increased olfaction abilities (Rovee et al. 1975). Overall, it seems that the sense of smell in the later years is adequate for daily functioning.

Balance and Equilibrium

The major sense organ of balance is the vestibular system, located in the semi-circular canals of the inner ear (figure 4.2). Three jelly-filled canals lie on each side of the head. Inside each canal are numerous receptor cells with hairlike projections imbedded in the jelly. When the head moves, the fluid moves and presses against hairlike projections of receptor cells. These cells then send a message to the brain that the head is changing position. The brain reacts by sending motor impulses that either contract or relax particular involuntary muscles to maintain balance. Even though these canals sense only movement of the head, the information signals sent to it enable the brain to determine the position of the whole body in space.

Age-Associated Changes in Equilibrium

No conclusive results have been reported on the effect of age on the function of the vestibular system, although some structural changes have been reported. For instance, older people have fewer sensory cells lining the semi-circular canals and have some degeneration in the nerves that relay messages about body equilibrium to the brain (Bergstrom 1973). Elders commonly experience vertigo (sense that the surroundings are spinning) and dizziness (lightheadedness and unsteadiness). However, these changes are not attributed to physiological alterations with age, but to drug reactions, postural changes, diseases, or mental state.

Somatic Receptors

Somatic receptors are distributed throughout the body and alert the organism to respond to a variety of environmental changes. The structure and location of these receptors varies with the information they gather (touch, pressure, heat, cold, pain, or body equilibrium). However, most consist of free nerve endings located in the skin and internal organs. Upon stimulation, the receptors send impulses through nerve pathways to the spinal cord and brain for processing.

Touch and pressure receptors are commonly found in the skin. The hairless portions of the skin (lips, fingertips, palms, genitals, and soles of the feet) are particularly sensitive to touch because they have a higher concentration of touch receptors. Some receptors respond to heavy pressure and are located deep in the skin tissues.

Thermoreceptors respond to either cold or heat. They sense changes in temperature, but once exposed to a certain temperature for a period of time they adapt or cease to respond until there is another alteration in temperature.

Pain receptors are widely distributed throughout the skin and internal organs. Unlike the cold and heat receptors, the pain receptors do not rapidly adapt to a stimulus but continue to send messages to the brain as long as the pain continues. Receptors that respond to changes in body position are located mainly around the joints. These sense changes in joint movement and relay the message to the brain.

Age-Associated Changes in the Somatic Receptors

It is difficult to measure changes in somatic senses with age as studies must rely on subjective responses to pain or temperature change rather than objective criteria. However, it is thought that somatic receptors, like other receptors, become less sensitive with age. Therefore, elders may need a greater stimulus before the nerve endings fire and send a message to the brain. It is documented that the number and quality of specialized receptors for light touch and heavy pressure decrease in the hand with advancing age (Thornbury and Mistretta 1981). Interestingly, sensitivity to touch in the hair-covered parts of the body is maintained into later life.

It is generally assumed that elders experience a decreased sensitivity to pain with advancing age. However, there is no convincing evidence to document this phenomenon. Elders may be less likely to report pain, have a higher threshold for pain, or feel less pain because of age-changes in the receptors. The perception of pain is very individual and varies among cultural groups, situation, sex, and personality. For instance, people who are anxious or neurotic may report greater sensitivity to pain than individuals who are more social or stoic. A decreased ability to feel pain may carry both positive and negative consequences. Elders may be better able to cope with common, painful chronic diseases (e.g., arthritis). On the other hand, since pain signals danger, an elder with decreased pain sensitivity may be unaware of disease symptoms or minor injuries.

Although not documented as an age change, many elders exhibit a decreased perception of heat and cold. It is believed that reduced sensitivity to heat may contribute to the high incidence of burns among older people. Elders are more susceptible to extremes in temperature and recover more slowly after exposure to temperature stress.

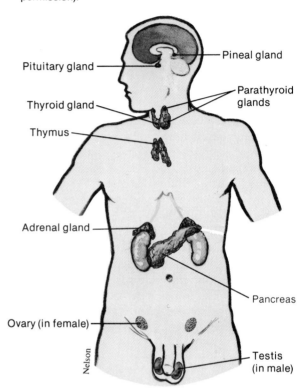

Figure 4.3 Endocrine glands. (Source: Hole, John W., Jr., *Human Anatomy and Physiology,* 3rd ed. Copyright © 1978, 1981, 1984 Wm. C. Brown Publishers, Dubuque, Iowa. All Rights Reserved. Reprinted by permission).

Pineal gland

Pituitary gland

Parathyroid glands

Thyroid gland

Thymus

Adrenal gland

Pancreas

Ovary (in female)

Nelson

Testis (in male)

The Endocrine System

Body functions are regulated and coordinated through the interdependent workings of the nervous and endocrine systems. As previously described, the nervous system rapidly transmits electrochemical impulses across nerve fibers that send messages to and from the brain and spinal cord. The endocrine system, on the other hand, transmits its chemical messages (hormones) much more slowly through the blood and its effects last longer.

Endocrine glands, located in the brain and other parts of the body, manufacture and release chemical messengers or hormones. Figure 4.3 illustrates the locations of the major endocrine glands. Each hormone has a different molecular

Table 4.1 Major hormones and functions of selected endocrine glands*

Name of Gland	Location	Major Hormones	Function
Pituitary	attached to base of brain (front)	growth (GH)	increases size and reproduction of body cells
		adrenocorticotropic (ACTH)	controls adrenal cortex hormone manufacture and secretion
		thyroid stimulating (TSH)	controls thyroid hormone secretions
		follicle stimulating (FSH)	growth and development of ova in ovaries and sperm cells in testes
		leutinizing (LH)	promotes secretion of sex hormones
	attached to base of brain (back)	antidiuretic (ADH)	regulates water reabsorption by kidneys
Thyroid	neck area, two lobes below larynx and in front of trachea	thyroxine and triiodothyronine	increases metabolic rate
		calcitonin	lowers blood calcium level by inhibiting releases of calcium from bones
Parathyroid	back surface of thyroid gland	parathyroid hormone	increases blood calcium level and decreases phosphate levels in blood
Adrenal	above each kidney		
medulla	central portion of adrenals	epinephrine and norepinephrine	activates body in response to stress
cortex	outer portion of adrenals	aldosterone	maintains potassium and sodium balance outside the cells
		cortisol	metabolism of carbohydrates, proteins, and fats; decreases capillary permeability
		sex hormone	supplements the sex hormones produced in the ovaries and testes
Pancreas	behind stomach and attached to small intestine	glucogen	stimulates liver to break down sugar stored for use by the body
		insulin	promotes uptake of glucose into cell, causing drop in blood sugar; helps liver store sugars
Thymus	behind sternum and between lungs	thymosin	affects production of certain white blood cells
Ovaries	pelvic cavity	estradiol and progesterone	development and maintenance of genital tract; promotes secondary sex characteristics in females
Testes	within scrotum behind penis	androgens, including testosterone	development and maintenance of secondary sex characteristics in males; needed in sperm development

*The pineal gland, digestive glands, and hormones directing pregnancy, childbirth, and lactation are not included.

structure and function although all generally slow or speed a particular metabolic process. Hormones travel through the bloodstream until they reach their specific target tissue. There, a specialized molecule attaches to the hormone and facilitates its entry into the cell. Those hormones that do not combine with a receptor are usually inactivated by the kidneys or liver and released as waste. Table 4.1 lists the major endocrine glands and their function in the later years. Note the variety of metabolic activities mediated by the endocrine system.

Age-Associated Changes in the Endocrine System

Comparatively little is known about the endocrine system and even less is understood about the effect of aging on the function of each gland. As in other systems, changes due to age are difficult to distinguish from those brought about by disease, malnutrition, stress, and inactivity. The complicated interrelationship between endocrine glands and the circulatory and nervous systems make distinction even more difficult.

The most-studied organ of the endocrine system is the pancreas and its associated hormone, insulin. Insulin is released into the bloodstream after a meal to enable glucose to enter body cells to produce energy. The ability to metabolize glucose decreases progressively with age. Some estimate that 50 percent of those over sixty have impaired glucose tolerance. This decreased tolerance is due to the inability of body cells to respond to the insulin in the bloodstream—not a decreased production of insulin. Because of the high prevalence of glucose intolerance among elders, researchers hypothesize that some decrease in ability to metabolize glucose is a normal accompaniment to old age and not a disease. Thus, standards of normal glucose tolerance should be adjusted for elders, rather than over-diagnosing them as diabetic based on young adult standards of normality. On the other hand, some assert that decreased sensitivity to insulin with age is more likely due to obesity and inactivity than aging itself (Kalant et al. 1980).

In general, the function of endocrine glands does not change significantly with age. Although the thymus gland shrinks significantly after maturity, thymosin levels remain constant throughout adulthood. Further, there appears to be no age-related differences in thyroxin, a hormone released by the thyroid to control metabolism (Blichert-Toft et al. 1975). Although levels of hormone released by the adrenal cortex decrease with age, the function of the gland seems well-maintained in the later years. The decrease in function seems to be a natural compensation for the body's decreased need (Wolfsen 1982). The only hormonal decrease in the later years is the female sex hormone estradiol, which decreases significantly after menopause. Changes in male and female sex hormones will be discussed in the next section.

The Reproductive System

In both sexes proper functioning of the reproductive system depends on a complex interrelationship between the hormones of the pituitary, hypothalamus, and testes or ovaries. These hormones control development of secondary sex characteristics, sexual arousal and activity, sperm and egg production, and for women, the ability to bear and nurse children. In the later years, the primary function of the system is sexual arousal and activity. After menopause, women lose the capacity to reproduce, and older men, although still capable, are rarely interested in fathering children. This section will describe the male and female reproductive systems and their age-associated physiological changes. Psychological and social aspects of aging and sexuality, changes in sexual response with age, sexual dysfunction, and therapy will be discussed in Chapter 11.

The Female

The hypothalmus, ovaries, and anterior pituitary glands secrete hormones that modulate the female's menstrual cycles, pregnancy, and the development and maintenance of secondary sexual characteristics. A pair of ovaries are located in

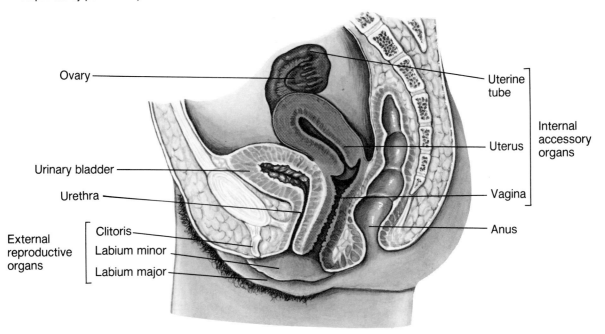

Figure 4.4 Female reproductive system. (Source: Hole, John W., Jr., *Human Anatomy and Physiology,* 3rd ed. Copyright © 1978, 1981, 1984 Wm. C. Brown Publishers, Dubuque, Iowa. All Rights Reserved. Reprinted by permission).

the lower abdomen and produce estrogens (female hormones) and ova (figure 4.4). Each monthly cycle, the mature ova are channeled out through uterine tubes enroute to the uterus. If the ova encounters sperm in these oviducts, fertilization may occur. The uterus is a muscular, pear-shaped organ held in place by four ligaments and located in front of the rectum. Its function is to receive the fertilized egg and nourish the development of a fetus. If the egg is not fertilized, a complex hormonal sequence triggers the breakdown of the lining of the uterus and the woman menstruates. The cervix is the neck of the uterus and extends into the upper part of the vaginal canal. Through the cervical opening, the monthly menstrual flow passes into the vagina. The vagina is a muscular tube that also serves as the birth passageway and receives the erect penis during sexual intercourse.

The external genital organs include the vulva, composed of the outer and inner lips (labia majora and labia minora), the organ of sexual arousal (clitoris), and the vestibule at the vaginal opening. During excitation, the labia and the clitoris become engorged with blood and are sensitive to tactile stimulation. When sexually stimulated, the veins around the vagina become engorged with blood resulting in a pressure that forces a mucus-like liquid to pass from the veins through the surface cells of the vagina. The liquid provides a coating for the entire vagina. Although not nearly as significant, a pair of Bartholin's Glands, located on either side of the vaginal opening, secrete mucus, that facilitates the insertion of the penis into the vagina.

The Body and Its Age Changes: Part II

Age-Associated Changes in the Female Reproductive System

Menopause is the most well-known age change in the female reproductive system. Throughout their forties, women experience a gradual reduction in fertility and ability to bear children until, at approximately age fifty, fertility decreases altogether. The climacteric refers to the period of decreasing fertility. Menopause is the cessation of menstruation for one year. Associated with this period are alterations in hormone levels that are thought to affect female reproductive anatomy and secondary sex characteristics.

During the climacteric, the menstrual cycle decreases in length and regularity due to a decreased production of estradiol, one of the most potent of the estrogen hormones, by the ovaries. After menopause, estradiol production drops even further and there are no longer cyclical variations in hormone production (Judd and Korenman 1982). However, this does not mean that the body no longer produces estrogens. In fact, androstenedione, a hormone secreted by the ovaries and the adrenal glands, can be converted into estrone by fat and other selected tissues. Estrone is a less potent form of estrogen that can compensate somewhat for the decreased estradiol production (Suiteri and MacDonald 1973).

It is hypothesized that a decrease in production of estradiol causes changes in the female reproductive organs. The organ systems responsible for reproduction—the uterus, ovaries, and uterine tubes—atrophy from disuse following menopause. Genitalia may lose subcutaneous fat and pubic hair. These changes also include a thinning of the vaginal walls, decrease in elasticity, reduced vaginal lubrication, and a decreased acidity of the vaginal environment with age (Schiff and Wilson 1978). However, some of these changes may be related to a lack of sexual activity, rather than aging. Masters and Johnson (1966) found no difference in the vaginal elasticity or lubrication between older, sexually active women and younger women. However, they reported that the vaginal walls of older women were thinner. Thin walls may cause the vagina to be more prone to irritation or infection with age. All evidence documents that clitoral sensation remains throughout life so that older women retain the capacity for orgasm through their later years.

The Male

The male reproductive system consists of the penis, testes, scrotum, and accessory ducts and fluid-producing glands (figure 4.5). Two oval shaped testes that produce sperm and secrete testosterone (the male sex hormone) are contained within the scrotum. Under the control of the anterior pituitary, the testes produce viable sperm and male secondary sex characteristics. Each testis contains a number of tightly coiled seminiferous tubules that produce immature sperm. In the epididymis, another convoluted tube emerging from the top of each testis, sperm cells mature and are stored. Each epididymis moves upward to form the muscular tube of the vas deferens, which is connected to a seminal vesicle near the base of the bladder. The seminal vesicles contribute fluid to aid the movement of the sperm. The prostate gland, a chestnut shaped structure surrounding the first inch of the urethra, deposits fluid in the urethra, which serves to activate the sperm.

Upon ejaculation, both the sperm and the fluid from the seminal vesicles enter the ejaculatory ducts. Semen is forcibly ejaculated from the urethra through the penis, a cylindrical shaped organ equipped to carry both urine and semen. The penis is composed of erectile tissue enabling it to enlarge with sexual excitation, permitting entry into the vagina during intercourse.

Age-Associated Changes in the Male Reproductive System

Like many other changes with age, most functional changes in the male reproductive system are highly variable and dependent on psychological status, presence of disease, and drug use. Males do, however, experience a universal, age-related decline in fertility, beginning in their forties or fifties (Harman 1978). Despite lower sperm production, men generally retain the ability to fertilize an egg into advanced age.

Chapter 4

Figure 4.5 Male reproductive system. (Source: Hole, John W., Jr., *Human Anatomy and Physiology,* 3rd ed. Copyright © 1978, 1981, 1984 Wm. C. Brown Publishers, Dubuque, Iowa. All Rights Reserved. Reprinted by permission).

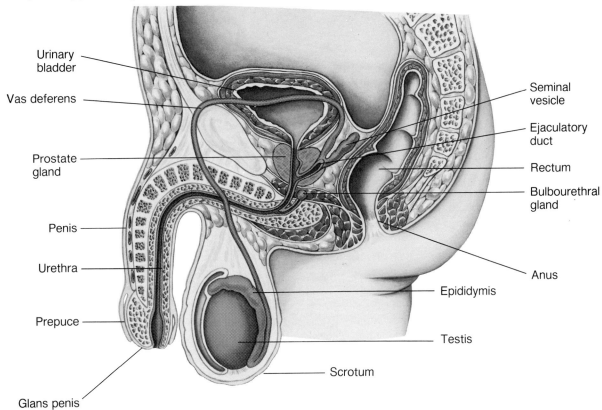

Urinary bladder

Vas deferens

Prostate gland

Penis

Urethra

Prepuce

Glans penis

Seminal vesicle

Ejaculatory duct

Rectum

Bulbourethral gland

Anus

Epididymis

Testis

Scrotum

Perhaps the most well-documented structural alteration with age is the enlargement of the prostate. The weight of the gland increases with age until, by age eighty, one-half of all men have an enlarged prostate (Whitbourne 1985). Although an enlarged prostate does not affect sexual activity, it may restrict urine flow, causing urinary problems.

Studies on healthy older men report no decrease in blood testosterone levels when compared to younger men (Harman and Tsitouras 1980; Sparrow et al. 1980). Earlier studies reported a decrease in testosterone with age. However, these studies used samples of men who were ill or institutionalized, confounding the effects of disease and inactivity with the age variable. Both disease and sexual inactivity are correlated with reduced testosterone levels (Tsitouras et al. 1982; Swendloff and Heber 1982).

Summary

Changes in the communication networks of the body—the sensory, neural, and endocrine systems—can affect an individual's ability to respond to the environment and coordinate internal function. The most significant age-associated changes occur in the visual and hearing systems. Structural changes in the eye cause presbyopia and a decreased visual acuity in low light and color discrimination. Environmental noise and structural changes in the ear result in an almost universal hearing loss with age, especially in the high frequencies (presbycusis). However, eyeglasses and hearing aids significantly reduce the impact of these changes. Some structural changes occur with age in the nervous system; however, because the system can regenerate lost connections, these changes are minimal. Similarly, alterations in taste, smell, equilibrium, and somatic receptors are highly variable, but generally minimal. Women experience menopause in the middle years, so are infertile in the later years; men remain fertile until advanced age. Healthy men and women maintain the capacity to have intercourse and orgasm throughout life.

Both Chapters 3 and 4 illustrate that although some structural alterations occur in almost every body system with age, functional effects are relatively minor and have little effect on daily life. Changes occurring in body systems are highly variable among individuals with some older individuals functioning physiologically better than some middle-aged persons. Most of the decline we associate with aging is due not to aging itself, but to disease processes, environmental factors, or modifiable behaviors such as cigarette smoking, physical inactivity, and poor nutrition.

Activities

1. A number of activities enable students to simulate age-related sensory and mobility decrements. Try some of the following and discuss the possible effects on daily routine and self-concept.

To simulate decreased touch sensitivity, put rubber cement on fingertips. To simulate decreased visual acuity, put vaseline on eyeglasses or, for those who wear glasses or contact lenses, remove them. Place cotton or plugs in ears to simulate hearing losses. A scarf tied from the neck to belt can simulate postural changes. A student may spend the whole day using a wheelchair or walker. If your college has a theatre department, ask to be made-up and dressed as an elder and then go shopping, recording your feelings and the reaction of others. Can you think of other simulation activities?

2. Interview a person you know with a degree of vision loss. How does the loss affect his or her life-style? How has s/he compensated for this loss?

3. The Lion's Club is a well-known service organization that assists people with visual decrements. Interview the president of the Lion's Club in your community to determine the services they offer. How many people are helped? In what ways? Who is eligible? Are there other organizations that assist visually impaired citizens in your area?

4. Collect fliers, booklets, and newsletters geared for elder use. Bring to class and discuss suitability of paper color, size of type, and layout. Then get input on these materials from elders and share with classmates.

5. What loud sounds have you been exposed to that may have permanently affected your hearing? List sounds that are common in your home and community that may cause hearing loss. Would you be embarrassed to wear a hearing aid? Talk with your parents and grandparents about their attitude about hearing loss and hearing aids.

Bibliography

Anderson, R. G., and W. L. Meyerhoff. 1982. Otologic manifestations of aging. *Otolaryngol Clin North Am* 15:353–70.

Baum, B. J. 1981. Current research on aging and human health. *Spec Care Dent* 1:105.

Bergman, M., V. G. Blumfield, D. Cascardo, et al. 1976. Age-related decrement in hearing for speech: Sampling and longitudinal studies. *J Gerontol* 31:533–38.

Bergstrom, B. 1973. Morphology of the vestibular nerve II. The number of myelinated vestibular nerve fibers in man at various ages. *Acta Otolaryngol* 76:173–79.

Blichert-Toft, M. L. Hummer, and H. Dige-Peterson. 1975. Human serum thyrotrophin level and response to thyrotrophin-releasing hormone in the aged. *Gerontologica Clinica* 17:191–203.

Buell, S. G., and P. D. Coleman. 1979. Dendritic growth in the aged human brain and failure of growth in senile dementia. *Science* 206:854–56.

Carter, J. H. 1982. Predicting visual response to increasing age. *J Am Opto Assoc* 53:31–36.

Davidson, M. B. 1979. The effects of aging on carbohydrate metabolism: A review of the English literature and a practical approach to the diagnosis of diabetes mellitus in the elderly. *Metabolism* 28:688–705.

Doty, R. L., P. Shaman, S. L. Applebaum, et al. 1984. Smell identification ability: Changes with age. *Science* 226:1441–43.

Fisch, L. 1978. Special senses: The aging auditory system. In J. C. Brockelhurst, ed. *Textbook of geriatric medicine and gerontology*. New York: Churchill-Livingstone. 276–90.

Frankowiak, R. S., T. Jones, G.L. Lenzi, and J. D. Heather. 1980. Regional cerebral oxygen utilization and blood flow in normal man using oxygen-15 and positron emissiontopography. *Acta Neurol Scand* 62:336–44.

Grzegorczyk, P. B., S. W. Jones, and C. M. Mistretta. 1979. Age-related differences in salt taste acuity. *J Gerontol* 34:834–40.

Harman, S. M. 1978. Clinical aspects of the male reproductive system. In E. L. Schneider, ed. *Aging, vol. 4. The aging reproductive system.* New York: Raven Press. 29–58.

Harman, S. M. and P. D. Tsitouras. 1980. Reproductive hormones in aging men. I. Measurement of sex steroids, basal luetinizing hormone and leydig cell response to human chorionic gonadotropin. *J Clin Endocrinol Metab* 51:35–40.

Havlik, R. J. 1986. Aging in the eighties, impaired senses for sound and light in persons age 65 years and over. *Advance Data from Vital and Health Statistics*. No. 125, Sept. 19, 1986. Bethesda, Md.: Public Health Service.

Hicks, L. H., and J. E. Birren. 1970. Aging, brain damage and psychomotor slowing. *Psychol Bull* 74:377–96.

Judd, H.L., and S. G. Korenman. 1982. Effects of aging on reproductive function in women. In S. G. Korenman, ed. *Endocrine aspects of aging*. New York: Elsevier Biomedical. 163–97.

Kalant, N., D. Leiborici, T. Leiborici, and N. Fukishima. 1980. Effects of age on glucose utilization and responsiveness to insulin in the forearm muscle. *J Am Geriatr Soc* 28:304–07.

Masters, W. H., and V. Johnson. 1966. *Human sexual response*. Boston: Little Brown.

Moore, L. M., C. R. Nielson, and C. M. Mistretta. 1982. Sucrose taste thresholds: Age-related differences. *J Gerontol* 37(1):64–69.

National Society to Prevent Blindness. 1980. *Vision problems in the United States: A statistical analysis*. New York.

Ordy, J. M. 1975. The nervous system, behavior and aging. An interdisciplinary approach. In J. M. Ordy, and K. R. Brizzee, eds. *Neurobiology of aging*. New York: Plenum Press. 85–118.

Paterson, C. A. 1979. Crystalline lens. In R. E. Records, ed. *Physiology of the human eye and visual system*. New York: Harper and Row.

Pitts, D. G. 1982. Visual acuity as a function of age. *J Am Optom Assoc* 53:117–24.

Rosen, S., D. Plester, A. El-Mofty, et al. 1964. High frequency audiometry in presbycusis. *Arch Otolaryngol* 79:18–31.

Rovee, C. K., R. Y. Cohen, and W. Shlapack. 1975. Lifespan stability in olfactory sensitivity. *Dev Psychobiol* 11:311–18.

Schiff, I., and E. Wilson. 1978. Clinical aspects of aging of the female reproductive system. In E. L. Schneider, ed. *Aging, vol 4. The aging reproductive system*. New York: Raven Press. 9–28.

Sparrow, D., R. Bosse, and J. W. Rowe. 1980. The influence of age, alcohol consumption and body build on gonadal function in men. *J Clin Endocrinol and Metab* 51:508–12.

Spector, A. 1982. Aging of the lens and cataract formation. In R. Sekuler, D. Kline, and K. Dismukes, eds. *Aging and human visual function*. New York: Alan Fiss. 27–43.

Spirduso, W. W. 1980. Physical fitness, aging and psychomotor speed: A review. *J Gerontol* 35:850–65.

Suiteri, P. K., and P. C. MacDonald. 1973. Role of extraglandular estrogen in human endocrinology. In R. O. Greep, and E. B. Astwood, eds. *Handbook of physiology (vol. 2, part 1)*. Baltimore: Williams and Wilkins.

Swendloff, R. S., and D. Heber. 1982. Effects of aging on male reproductive function. In S.G. Korenman, ed. *Endocrine aspects of aging*. New York: Elsevier Biomedical. 119–35.

Thornbury, J. M., and C. M. Mistretta. 1981. Tactile sensitivity as a function of age. *J Gerontol* 36:34–39.

Tomlinson, B. S., G. Blessed, and M. Roth. 1968. Observations on the brains of non-demented old people. *J Neurol Sci* 7:331–56.

Tsitouras, P. D., C. E. Martin, and S. M. Harman. 1982. Relationship of serum testosterone to sexual activity in healthy elderly men. *J Gerontol* 37: 288–93.

Warwick, R. 1976. *Eugene Wolff's anatomy of the eye and orbit*. Philadelphia: Saunders.

Weale, R. A. 1975. Senile changes in visual acuity. *Trans Opthamol Soc U K* 95:36–38.

Weale, R. A. 1981. Senile ocular changes and ambient temperature. *Br J Ophthalmol* 65:869–70.

Whitbourne, S. K. 1985. *The aging body: Physiological changes and psychological consequences*. New York: Springer-Verlag.

Wolfsen, A. R. 1982. Aging and the adrenals. In S. G. Korenman, ed. *Endocrine aspects of aging*. New York: Elsevier Biomedical.

Chronic Illness 5

When a new disability arrives, I look around to see if death has come and I call quietly, "Death, is that you? Are you there?" So far, the disability has answered, "Don't be silly, it's me."
Florida Scott Maxwell (1968)

Introduction

Although more people are surviving to old age, their later years are often accompanied by mildly to severely disabling chronic illnesses. The reduction of infectious disease has placed chronic illnesses as the main cause of premature death and disability in the United States. In contrast to acute, infectious diseases that are brief and curable, chronic diseases must be dealt with throughout life since they are irreversible and progressive in nature. Chronic disease is also more likely to be accompanied by long-term social and psychological consequences. Such complexities of chronic diseases require cooperation between the individual, the family, and health and social service providers. This chapter will discuss the nature of chronic illness and will provide an overview of a number of chronic diseases common in the later years. The ability of those who work with elders to recognize these diseases and their consequences will lead to an improved approach to the care of elders, whether they live in community or institutional settings.

The Nature of Chronic Illness

In children and young adults, being sick is more often associated with conditions from which one expects to recover: the common cold, flu, strep throat, or pneumonia. These acute diseases have an abrupt onset and are generally caused by a bacteria or a virus. With advancing age, however, the most troublesome health problems are due to chronic conditions such as arthritis, heart disease, stroke, and cancer. These are long-lasting and often cause irreversible physiological changes. The causes are multiple. Some are caused by lifestyle or environmental agents (e.g., physical inactivity, dietary patterns, cigarette smoking) while others are due to unknown factors. Physicians cannot cure chronic conditions, but can only reduce the symptoms and deterioration caused by the progression of the condition. Because chronic illnesses last a lifetime and require medical supervision, the expense for the elderly and for the government is considerable. Table 5.1 compares the differences between chronic and acute illness (Adapted from Kart et al. 1978).

More than four of five elders have at least one chronic disease and many manifest multiple chronic conditions. The percent of elders affected increases with advanced age. Although most illnesses cause only minor alterations in daily routine, these illnesses account for the majority of disability among the middle-aged and elderly. A high rate of chronic illness results in a higher bill for medications, more visits to the physician and hospital, and increased need for long-term care for elders. Chronic illness is also responsible for the majority of deaths in the older population. See table 5.2 for a comparison among adult age groups of the ten leading causes of death.

Because chronic illness may cause discomfort, disability, and death, it is important that it be properly diagnosed and treated. Diagnosing chronic illness is extremely complicated in elders. First, elders may manifest disease differently than younger groups. They may feel less pain or have mental manifestations of physical problems (such as depression or confusion). They may not exhibit symptoms, or their symptoms may be diffuse, such as generalized weakness, lack of appetite, or confusion. Secondly, because elders are likely to have more than one chronic disease, the symptoms of one disease may be mistakenly attributed to an already existing one and ignored.

Table 5.1 Difference between chronic and acute illness		
	Chronic	**Acute or Infectious**
Length of Illness	Lifetime	Brief
Cause	Often unknown, multiple, environmental	Known, often a virus or bacteria
Treatment	Treat symptoms, limit further damage	Kill microorganism, surgery
Prognosis	Generally progressive	Self-limiting, improves with treatment
Physical Consequences	Irreversible	Usually reversible
Goal of Care	Control, maintenance, rehabilitation	Cure
Duration of Care	Long, often lifetime	Brief
Cost of Care	Expensive, may involve long-term drug and physician therapy and medical supervision	Often costs less because treatment is short-term

Table 5.2 Ten leading causes of death in specified age groups: United States, 1985

25–44 Years
1. Accidents and adverse effects
2. Malignant neoplasms (cancers), including neoplasms of lymphatic and hematopoietic (blood-forming) tissues
3. Diseases of heart
4. Suicide
5. Homicide and legal intervention
6. Chronic liver disease and cirrhosis
7. Cerebrovascular diseases (stroke)
8. Diabetes mellitus
9. Pneumonia and influenza
10. Congenital anomalies

45–64 Years
1. Malignant neoplasms, including neoplasms of lymphatic and hematopoietic (blood-forming) tissues
2. Diseases of heart
3. Cerebrovascular diseases
4. Accidents and adverse effects
5. Chronic obstructive pulmonary diseases and allied conditions
6. Chronic liver disease and cirrhosis
7. Diabetes mellitus
8. Suicide
9. Pneumonia and influenza
10. Homicide and legal intervention

65 Years and Over
1. Diseases of heart
2. Malignant neoplasms, including neoplasms of lymphatic and hematopoietic tissues
3. Cerebrovascular diseases
4. Chronic obstructive pulmonary diseases and allied conditions
5. Pneumonia and influenza
6. Diabetes mellitus
7. Accidents and adverse effects
8. Atherosclerosis
9. Nephritis, nephrotic syndrome, and nephrosis (kidney disease)
10. Septicemia (blood poisoning)

[Rates per 100,000 population in specified group]
National Center for Health Statistics 1987. Advance report of final mortality statistics, 1985. *NCHS Monthly Vital Statistics Report* 36 (5) Suppl., Aug. 28, 1987. pp. 20–21.

Accurate diagnosis is required for effective treatment of any health problem.

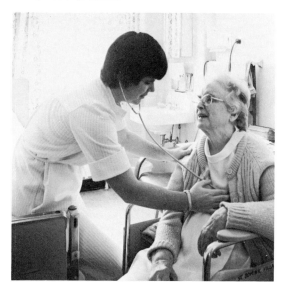

Third, if they are taking medication for one condition, the side effects of medication may be misinterpreted as another condition. Finally, symptoms of chronic illness may be incorrectly attributed to normal age changes.

Elders are likely to exhibit more complications with chronic disease than younger groups. Age changes in body systems reduce the ability to respond to the stress of illness, and drug side effects become more common. Older people may also have more complications because they are often reluctant to report conditions to the physician until they are severe. This may be due to the mistaken belief that the symptoms are caused by old age and nothing can be done, their fear of diagnosis and treatment, or their inability to pay for treatment. A number of factors affect treatment or rehabilitation success in elders. Past medical and social history, psychological status (cognitive functioning, personality, self concept, outlook on life), social supports, and the availability of funds are important considerations.

A discussion of the multiple chronic illnesses that affect older people is not intended to paint a portrait of debilitated, disabled old age. Rather, it is important to remember that despite the high

Problems of Daily Living for the Chronically Ill*

1. *Preventing medical crises and managing them when they occur.*

   Some chronic diseases are characterized by potentially fatal medical crises (e.g., diabetic coma, heart attack, epileptic seizure, stroke). To prevent a crisis, the person's life must be organized for crisis management. The signs of impending crisis must be recognized and appropriate action is necessary when they occur.

2. *Controlling symptoms.*

   Although the physician prescribes a regimen intended to control symptoms, the individual must rely largely on personal judgement to control symptoms. This task requires awareness of the present capacity of the body and coming to terms with its reduced capability. Even minor symptoms may require a change in behavior, and major symptoms may call for redesigning daily life.

3. *Carrying out prescribed regimen and managing the problems associated with it.*

   The physician usually prescribes a treatment regimen to control the symptoms and progression of the disease, but the individual must learn the regimen, and to a greater or lesser degree, must organize the day around it. Some treatments are simple, such as ingesting a pill; others may take up a significant portion of the day. Whether or not a regimen is followed depends on a number of factors: Is the regimen easy to learn? How much time and energy does the regimen take? Is it painful? Are there side effects? Is it effective? Is it expensive? Does it lead to social isolation? When an individual has more than one chronic illness, the regimen often becomes more complicated and requires considerable juggling of time and energy.

4. *Preventing or coping with social isolation.*

   Many chronic illnesses are accompanied by lessened energy and mobility, impairment of sensory processes, visible physical disfigurement, or deficits that may result in lessened social contact and increased isolation. In some cases, the sick person withdraws from social activities, in others, former social contacts withdraw. The more serious the disease, the higher the probability that the sick person will feel increased isolation. However, both the sick individual and significant others can develop tactics to reduce social isolation.

5. *Adjusting to changes in the course of the disease.*

   Both the sick individual and the family, if present, need to cope with the downward course of the illness. Every downward step requires the sick person to reassess health status and make arrangements to manage symptoms, social interactions, and activities of daily living. Those close to the sick person may also need to be involved in such arrangements since it is likely that dependence will increase as the illness progresses. The impact of the downward course of illness upon personal identity depends upon the illness. If the downward course is predictable, preparation is possible in advance of each new downward phase; if it is unexpectedly quick, then adjustment is more difficult.

6. *Attempting to normalize lifestyle and interaction with others.*

    The chief task of one who is chronically ill is to live as fully as possible despite the symptoms and the disease. How normal life can be depends on the extent of symptoms, disability, and the regimen required to keep the disease under control. The task of normalization is most difficult when the disease is fatal.

7. *Financing treatments and survival.*

    As chronic illness is usually lifelong, it almost certainly is accompanied by financial problems. One important characteristic of chronic disease is the cost of required treatment, especially drugs, machinery, physician visits, and home-based health services. In some cases, health problems can wipe out life savings and other funding sources need to be sought. The problem of seeking adequate funds for treatment and survival becomes more complex when one is also dealing with physical disability.

*Adapted from Strauss 1975

prevalence of chronic illness, these conditions do not usually restrict an older person's ability to complete daily tasks. Although chronic disease and disabilities accumulate with age, a good proportion of elders are in good health, especially those from sixty-five to seventy-five years of age. Further, despite the high prevalence of disease in old age, it is not inevitable. Many chronic illnesses can be prevented by changes in lifestyle such as improving diet, eliminating drug or tobacco use, or increasing physical activity levels. Further, if a chronic disease is detected, a treatment regime can be initiated to control many symptoms and reduce the progression of the disease.

Psychosocial Aspects of Chronic Illness

To effectively work with those who are chronically ill, knowledge of their medical problems is primary. Awareness of how the disease and symptoms impact upon a person's everyday life is also crucial for treatment and rehabilitation. Although chronic illnesses affect individuals differently, those who are chronically ill share many of the same problems. Strauss (1975) developed a framework to look at the psycho-social problems of the chronically ill and their families (above). He asserts that unless one understands how the chronically ill handle their illness on a daily basis, one cannot give effective care. Unfortunately, medical professionals are more likely to address the medical management of chronic illness than the attendant social and psychological problems of daily living arising from the illness.

One of the greatest psychological effects of chronic illness is that the professional and family may unconsciously promote dependence by allowing the chronically ill person to misuse the "sick role." Parsons (1958) described the sick role as behavior undertaken by the sick person for the purpose of getting well. The role entails certain rights and responsibilities by the sick person and the caretaker. The sick person is allowed to be dependent and is relieved of normal responsibilities as a family member and a member of society. For example, the sick person does not need to do household chores, act like a parent, or go to work. Further, the ill person is not blamed for incurring the illness. However, the ill person understands that sickness is undesirable and deviant and has the obligation to do everything possible to get well. Usually family members are supportive and the sick role is maintained until the individual is well enough to resume normal functioning.

Because chronic illnesses are not temporary and full recovery is not possible, the sick role must be modified for the chronically ill. If a chronically ill elder constantly assumed a dependent, egocentric role to cope with illness, both the chronically ill person and family would suffer. The separation from household and interpersonal duties removes the elder from those activities and roles that originally gave self-esteem. Further, primary focus of attention upon the disease may encourage further dependency. Although the sick role is sometimes appropriate when an elder needs special care, health professionals and families should be wary of supporting overly dependent behaviors of chronically ill elders. Often the family and professionals inadvertently promote dependency by excessive care, which reduces coping effectiveness and encourages further dependency (Mechanic 1960).

Common Chronic Conditions Among Elders

The remainder of this chapter will discuss selected chronic conditions that afflict middle-aged and older adults. The description of the disease, its cause, prevalence, and treatments will be discussed. Chronic mental disorders will be discussed in Chapter 8.

The following descriptions do not detail the psychosocial effects of symptoms or treatment regimen because they are highly variable and depend on extent of illness, personality, financial situation, and degree of social support. However, as you read about each of the chronic conditions, consider the impact of the illness on the affected elders and their families using box 5.1 as a framework. Some disease symptoms have little effect on life-style while others may be so debilitating that institutionalization may result.

Cardiovascular Diseases

Cardiovascular diseases (those affecting the heart and blood vessels) comprise two of the three major causes of death and disability in the United States—heart disease and stroke. Heart disease alone accounts for 43 percent of deaths among elders. The incidence increases drastically with age in both women and men. Those cardiovascular problems to be discussed that occur more often in older people are atherosclerosis, hypertension, coronary artery disease, congestive heart failure, and stroke.

Atherosclerosis

Atherosclerosis is characterized by progressive thickening of the arterial wall due to the development of fatty accumulations in the arteries. Plaques containing fats (including cholesterol), salts, connective tissue, and scar tissue reduce the opening of the artery, sometimes closing it off altogether. Atherosclerotic vessels are also more likely to burst, causing internal hemorrhage. This buildup is believed to play a major role in the development of cardiovascular diseases. Atherosclerosis is often confused with arteriosclerosis, a general term referring to hardening of the arteries. Arteriosclerosis is a progressive, age-associated condition resulting in a loss of elasticity of the arterial walls.

Advanced atherosclerosis in the legs causes a condition called intermittent claudication that is characterized by insufficient circulation in the lower extremities. Symptoms include numbness and coldness in the lower limbs and chronic leg pain when the legs are moved. The usual recommendation is to engage in a walking program to increase circulation around the occluded arteries. If the individual is not relieved of pain, surgery to bypass the obstructed artery may be necessary to get adequate blood flow to the legs.

Experts believe a number of behavioral modifications can prevent or slow the progression of atherosclerosis. Weight loss, dietary changes, systematic exercise, stress reduction, and cessation of smoking are thought to reduce the risk of atherosclerosis. However, most studies indicate that these lifestyle changes are most effective if initiated before atherosclerosis becomes severe.

Hypertension (High Blood Pressure)

Hypertension is defined as the persistent elevation of pressure of the blood against the walls of the arteries to exceed a reading of 140/90. The causes of hypertension are not clear, but stress, excessive salt intake, obesity, and heredity are associated with the disease. Hypertension is associated with atherosclerosis. When the diameter and flexibility of the arteries are reduced through atherosclerosis, the heart must work harder to maintain blood flow through the vessels. Those with hypertension are at increased risk for heart and kidney failure, strokes, and blindness. The disease is often called the silent killer because of its lack of symptoms.

Experts disagree upon what reading constitutes high blood pressure in elders. An increase in blood pressure with age is thought by some experts to be a normal compensation for decreased cardiac output. If the blood pressure were not increased, organs such as the kidney, brain, and heart would not receive sufficient blood. Thus, Anderson (1978) suggests the upper limits of normal blood pressure in elders should be altered as follows:

Age	Men	Women
70 to 79	205/104	215/106
80 to 89	215/108	230/110

Aside from the controversy of what level of blood pressure should be treated in elders is the difficulty in obtaining accurate blood pressure

Blood Pressure

Blood pressure is the force exerted by the blood against the walls of the arteries. When the heart contracts, a great volume of blood is forced into the arteries and pressure reaches a maximum point (called systolic pressure). After the heart has contracted and pushes blood out, it pauses to refill. During this time, the pressure in the arteries is at its lowest point (called diastolic pressure). Systolic and diastolic pressure can be measured by an instrument called a sphygmomanometer, commonly known as a blood pressure gauge. The highest and lowest pressures exerted on the arteries by the blood is translated into the amount of pressure able to raise a column of mercury a certain distance. Readings are commonly expressed as a fraction; the top number is the systolic pressure, while the bottom is the diastolic. The average blood pressure is 120/80.

readings. Blood pressure readings are highly variable. Anxiety, stress, physical activity, even talking during a reading, may elevate blood pressure. In addition, many borderline hypertensives exhibit a "white coat syndrome," in which their anxiety at seeing a doctor can increase blood pressure by ten to fifteen points. One report recommends blood pressure not be taken within the first ten minutes of the visit to reduce this effect (Mancia et al. 1983). A single blood pressure reading does not accurately reflect average blood pressure. To increase accuracy, readings should be repeated over a period of days. An ambulatory blood pressure moniter is sometimes used to monitor blood pressure over an extended period (Kiesling 1983). Even repeated documentation of high blood pressure readings are not sufficient to begin therapy; the effect of the high blood pressure upon the heart, brain, eye, or kidney must be demonstrated before active treatment is considered (Drayer and Weber 1985).

The first line of treatment of a hypertensive individual is to modify his/her lifestyle: restrict salt intake, reduce weight, start an exercise program, and stop smoking. Mineral supplements of potassium, calcium, and magnesium are also effective in some cases. The last line of treatment should be prescription drugs to reduce hypertension (see Chapter 7). Hypertensive drug therapy is controversial among elders as it is often accompanied by adverse effects. There is yet no convincing evidence that drug treatment of those with mild to moderate hypertension increases survival rate (except in those with pre-existing heart or kidney problems) (McAlister 1983; Kaplan 1983). In addition, reducing blood pressure too aggressively may cause decreased blood flow to vital organs, dizziness, and increased risk of falls.

Finally, the negative psychological effect of considering oneself sick and in need of daily medication outweighs any drug benefits, especially in those with mild and moderate hypertension (Kaplan 1983).

Coronary Artery Disease

Coronary artery disease (also called ischemic heart disease) is the most common type of heart disease in elders. The main contributor to coronary artery disease is atherosclerosis of the coronary arteries, the vessels that supply oxygen and nutrients to the heart muscle. A blood clot can more easily become lodged in a narrowed vessel, resulting in insufficient blood flow to the heart. The reduction in blood flow may be temporary, as in angina pectoris. However, if the deficient blood supply persists, a heart attack will result. The extent of the attack depends upon how much heart muscle dies below the coronary artery blockage (figure 5.1).

Figure 5.1 A heart attack. (Reprinted with permission. © American Heart Association).

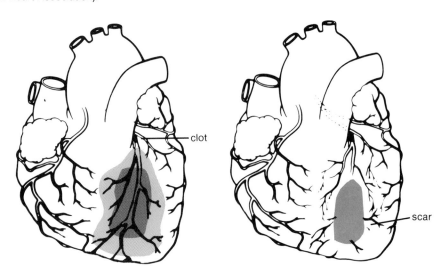

Angina pectoris is characterized by chest pain from exertion, emotional distress, or cold weather. Anginal pain typically lasts about fifteen to twenty minutes and may be relieved by rest or nitroglycerine tablets placed under the tongue to expand coronary vessels. A number of controlled studies have documented that an aspirin a day significantly reduces the risk of death and heart attack for those with angina (*FDA Drug Bulletin* 1985). If drugs do not relieve angina pain, balloon angioplasty may be used (figure 5.2). A catheter with a tiny balloon on its tip is threaded into a coronary artery from a large artery in the groin or arm. The catheter contains a fluid that shows up in an X-ray so the process can be continually visualized on an X-ray machine. When the tip gets to the narrowed portion of the carotid artery, the balloon is inflated with solution a number of times to press the fat deposits against the arterial wall, expanding the diameter of the artery. This treatment is relatively low-risk as it involves only a small incision at the site of catheter origin and requires only local anesthesia.

Coronary bypass surgery can relieve angina pain that is not responsive to less intensive therapies. In this case, a vein is taken from the leg and grafted into the heart to allow blood to flow around the blockages to nourish the heart (figure 5.3). Women and those with severe heart disease are poor risks for such surgery. Because bed rest after major surgery can pose other complications for elders, this surgery is considered a last resort. Risks of coronary bypass surgery will be discussed in Chapter 12.

Figure 5.2 Balloon angioplasty. (Source: Reprinted from the American Heart Association, *American Health,* Nov. 1984, p. 45).

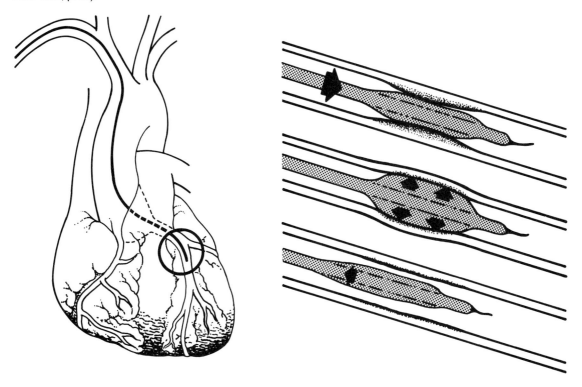

Figure 5.3 Coronary bypass. (Source: Reprinted from the American Heart Association, *American Health,* Nov. 1984, p. 44).

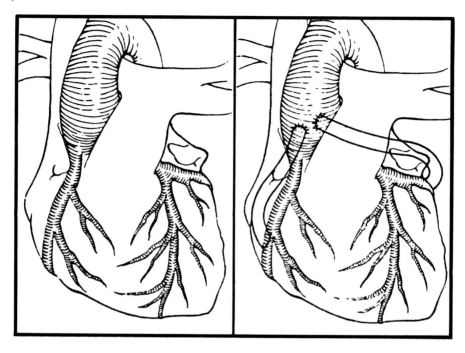

A heart attack, or myocardial infarction, includes one or more of the following symptoms: prolonged chest pain radiating to the shoulder or arm, shortness of breath, sweating, and nausea. Although the presence of chest pain is less common during heart attacks among elders, it is still the most frequent symptom of that group, occuring in about 70 percent of the cases (MacDonald et al. 1983). Treatment includes a week to ten days of rest to heal heart tissue. Chair rest, rather than bed rest is recommended because it puts less strain on the heart. After that time, the individual should be encouraged to be mobile, and eventually to develop a walking program. In addition, a number of drugs may be used after a heart attack to increase heart functioning. One aspirin daily has been shown to reduce the recurrence of heart attack and the risk of death after a heart attack (*FDA Drug Bulletin* 1985). Stress reduction, low salt and low fat diets are also recommended to reduce the threat of another myocardial infarction. Coronary bypass surgery is used for heart attack victims, although its success in reducing subsequent heart attacks is questionable.

Congestive Heart Failure

Congestive heart failure, common among elders, occurs when the heart muscle does not pump blood efficiently. Although its name implies that the heart fails, this condition arises from a decrease in pumping efficiency of the heart. This develops because one or more chronic conditions (e.g., atherosclerosis, coronary artery disease, hypertension, kidney impairment) create a strain on the heart. The heart may increase in size due to heavier demand, but eventually the overextended cardiac muscle loses its strength. Consequently, blood flow to the kidneys is reduced, decreasing urine output. The excess fluid stays in the circulatory system, creating further strain on the heart. Typical symptoms of congestive heart failure are shortness of breath upon exertion, fatigue, difficulty in sleeping when prone, and swelling of feet and ankles.

The mainstays of treatment include drugs and salt restriction. Digitalis, the most commonly prescribed drug, increases the force of heart muscle contractions. Diuretics are commonly prescribed to promote salt and water excretion. Patients are advised to reduce salt intake and to lose weight if overweight. These strategies usually improve the condition; however, recurrences are likely if the regimen is not followed. Those with congestive heart failure should be closely monitored. Sudden weight gain may indicate a dangerous level of fluid retention predisposing one to a crisis situation. Further, adverse effects are common with diuretics and digitalis therapy. Nevertheless, those with congestive heart failure are able to complete most normal activities if they allow sufficient rest periods, do not overexert themselves, and follow their prescribed regimen.

Stroke

Strokes are the third leading cause of death and the major cause of disabilities among elders (Murray et al. 1980). Strokes result when a portion of the brain is denied needed blood. A stroke may be caused by a *cerebral hemorrhage* when a blood vessel in the brain bursts, preventing blood from passing the hemorrhage to brain tissue beyond it. Cerebral hemorrhages are uncommon and occur primarily in severe hypertensives. They have no warning signs and are often lethal. The most common type of stroke in elders is *cerebral thrombosis,* in which a blood clot becomes lodged in an already narrowed artery, cutting off the blood supply to brain tissue beyond the clot. In both types of strokes, the extent of damage depends on the area of the brain affected as well as the extent of brain tissue damaged. An affected elder may be mildly disabled or have partial or total paralysis of one side of the body. Inability to express oneself verbally (aphasia) and disturbances of vision and hearing are also common following a stroke.

Strokes from cerebral thrombosis are often preceded by one or more mini-strokes or transient ischemic attacks (TIAs). TIAs are caused by a temporary blockage of the cerebral artery. They may result in transient or permanent motor weakness, blackouts, speech disturbances, or personality changes. The attacks may last from a few minutes to twenty-four hours. To prevent further attacks, an anticoagulant drug may be prescribed after a TIA. Surgical intervention may also be attempted to prevent a full-scale stroke. Because atherosclerosis of the carotid artery is responsible for most strokes (Groteboer 1978) a carotid endartectomy may be performed. This technique involves the scraping of plaques and blood clots from one or both carotid arteries. Balloon catheterization is another technique that may be employed. However, the increased survival of patients who undergo this surgery as compared with those treated with drugs alone has not been documented.

Stroke rehabilitation depends on the type and extent of the stroke as well as the client's overall health status, motivation, personality, and financial resources. An extensive physical and mental assessment should be conducted to determine sensory and motor loss, psychological state, and the victim's ability to speak and understand. It is important that rehabilitation begin immediately; almost 90 percent of all stroke victims have rehabilitation potential soon after a stroke, but it diminishes more each day rehabilitation is not implemented (Hirshberg 1976). During the acute phase following the stroke, proper positioning and bed exercises to promote circulation and minimize fluid accumulation in the tissues are necessary. As soon as possible, occupational, physical, and speech therapists should implement a rehabilitation plan. Because the emotional effects of a stroke are common (e.g., lack of motivation, depression, anxiety, or frustration) and can adversely affect recovery, psychological counseling and support are appropriate for both patient and family. Unfortunately physical rehabilitation and counseling of elders after a stroke is seldom initiated.

Cancer

Cancer is the second leading cause of death in the United States. The risk of developing cancer increases significantly with age; more than half of those with the disease are over sixty-five. Most cancer deaths among elders are caused by lung, colon and rectum, prostate, and breast cancers. Cancer is believed to be caused by aberrant body cells that multiply out of control. The cause of multiplication is still not known.

A number of factors may explain increased risk of the older age group. The aging process may reduce the ability of the immune system to reject abnormal growths. Some hypothesize that elders lack sufficient DNA for the increased repair demands of an aging body, thereby allowing defective cells to grow unchecked (Jarvick 1979). In addition, those who are old have had more time to be exposed to carcinogens such as cigarette smoke, environmental pollutants, and chemical additives.

Cancer is difficult to diagnose in elders. In younger patients, cancer is usually the only disease condition present. However, in elders, cancer symptoms are often overshadowed by symptoms of other diseases. Further, physicians may mistakenly attribute warning signals to diseases already present. For instance, the rectal bleeding characteristic of colon cancer may be attributed to long-standing hemorrhoids. Most cancers among elders are found when examining for other illnesses.

Attention to the seven warning signals of cancer is important. However, the most effective way to diagnose cancer is to get annual physical examinations—including screening for breast, colorectal, and prostate cancer—because many warning signs do not appear until the disease has progressed. Early diagnosis and treatment of cancer decreases the probability of further cancer growth. A number of health habits can reduce the risk of developing cancer. Specific preventive strategies will be discussed in each section.

Seven Warning Signals of Cancer

1. Change in bowel or bladder habits
2. A sore that does not heal
3. Unusual bleeding or discharge
4. Thickening or lump in breast or elsewhere
5. Indigestion or difficulty in swallowing
6. Obvious change in a wart or mole
7. Nagging cough or hoarseness

Surgery is a common method used to diagnose and control cancer growth in the body. However, some elders are at higher surgical risk than younger patients. Complications increase with other chronic conditions, sensory deficits, and limited mobility. Cancer may also be treated with chemicals (chemotherapy) or radiation; however, these treatments have a number of negative side effects. Age, rate of growth of cancer, type and extent of treatment, and health status are variables to consider when deciding on a treatment plan. In addition, the quality as well as the quantity of life should be considered. If surgery or chemotherapy only increases the survival slightly, if the procedure has a high complication rate, or if cancer growth is slow, it may be better to limit treatment to symptom relief (Hodkinson 1978). Cancers of the lung, prostate, colon and rectum, and oral cavity will be addressed in more detail under the heading of the body system they affect.

Breast Cancer

Breast cancer is the second leading cause of cancer death among women. It occurs infrequently in men. The incidence of breast cancer increases with advancing age in both sexes. Because it is so common, all older women are considered to be at risk and should be annually screened by a physician (Moe 1985). However, women should not depend on their physician to locate tumors. One recent sample of eighty physicians reported that on the average, less than half the lumps in a silicon breast model were detected. The percentage of lumps detected by each physician ranged from 17 to 83 percent. (Fletcher et al. 1985).

The most important method to detect breast cancer is monthly self-examination, as most breast cancer nodules are detected by women. Despite the increased risk of breast cancer in older women, one national study reported that one-third of women over sixty-five have never examined their breasts for lumps, even though three-fourths report they know the procedure. Further, almost a third of older women have either never had a breast exam by a physician or have not had one in the last five years (Thornberry et al. 1986).

In addition to breast self-exam and physician exams, mammography is the most reliable diagnostic aid. Although radiation exposure has its dangers, it is believed to be less hazardous for high risk groups than undetected breast cancer.

If a lump is found, a needle biopsy is performed to determine if it is malignant (cancerous). Malignant breast cancer is usually treated with surgery, which varies in its extent. Surgeons may remove the lump only (lumpectomy), the breast (simple mastectomy), or the entire breast, lymph nodes under the arm pits and adjacent muscle tissue (radical mastectomy). Although radical mastectomies are common, they are no more effective in preventing the spread of cancer and forestalling death than less radical means (Fisher et al. 1985). Radiation therapy is usually used as an adjunct to surgery and may also be used without surgery. The five-year survival rate for those with breast cancer is 72 percent for whites and 60 percent for blacks (National Cancer Institute 1985). There is evidence that older women are less likely than younger women to be treated with vigorous therapy for breast cancer, even when their condition is the same. A study of 374 women with breast cancer concluded that some physicians treat the disease according to chronological age, not condition. The researchers concluded that this practice may needlessly shorten the lives of older women patients (Samet et al. 1986).

Respiratory Diseases

The threat of both acute and chronic respiratory disease increases with advanced age. The increased susceptibility of older people to respiratory conditions can be attributed to many factors: decreased resistance to environmental contaminants and microorganisms, age-associated decrements that reduce pulmonary function, and length of exposure to carcinogenic substances. Cigarette smoking is by far the prime cause of chronic bronchitis, emphysema, and lung cancer. In the United States, approximately one-third of those between ages twenty-one and sixty-four smoke; this proportion is decreased by half by age sixty-five so that only one-sixth of elders smoke (Thornberry et al. 1986). This decrease is caused by the low survival rate of heavy smokers as well as the fact that many elders reduce or eliminate smoking in the later years to improve their health.

Breast Self-Examination (BSE)

Here is how to do BSE:

1. Stand before a mirror. Inspect both breasts for anything unusual, such as any discharge from the nipples, puckering, dimpling, or scaling of the skin.

    The next two steps are designed to emphasize any change in the shape or contour of your breasts. As you do them you should be able to feel your chest muscles tighten.

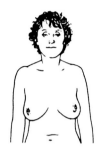

2. Watching closely in the mirror, clasp hands behind your head and press hands forward.

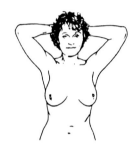

3. Next, press hands firmly on hips and bow slightly toward your mirror as you pull your shoulders and elbows forward.

    Some women do the next part of the exam in the shower. Fingers glide over soapy skin making it easy to concentrate on the texture underneath.

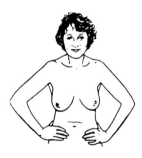

Breast self-examination should be done once a month so you become familiar with the usual appearance and feel of your breasts. Familiarity makes it easier to notice any changes in the breast from one month to another. Early discovery of a change from what is "normal" is the main idea behind BSE.

If you menstruate, the best time to do BSE is 2 or 3 days after your period ends, when your breasts are least likely to be tender or swollen. If you no longer menstruate, pick a day, such as the first day of the month, to remind yourself it is time to do BSE.

Reprinted with permission from the National Cancer Institute's brochure, "Breast Exams: What You Should Know."

Chapter 5

4. Raise your left arm. Use three or four fingers of your right hand to explore your left breast firmly, carefully, and thoroughly. Beginning at the outer edge, press the flat part of your fingers in small circles, moving the circles slowly around the breast. Gradually work toward the nipple. Be sure to cover the entire breast. Pay special attention to the area between the breast and the armpit, including the armpit itself. Feel for any unusual lump or mass under the skin.

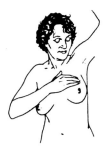

5. Gently squeeze the nipple and look for a discharge. Repeat the exam on your right breast.

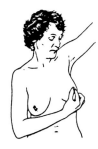

6. Steps 4 and 5 should be repeated lying down. Lie flat on your back, left arm over your head and a pillow or folded towel under your left shoulder. This position flattens the breast and makes it easier to examine. Use the same circular motion described earlier. Repeat on your right breast.

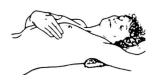

Cigarette Smoking

The vast amount of research on the relationship between smoking and disease documents overwhelming evidence of the harm of cigarette smoking. Cigarette smoking is the leading cause of preventable death in the United States. It is estimated to decrease life expectancy by five to eight years (Rogot 1978). Cigarette smoking is responsible for 90 percent of all lung cancer deaths and 30 percent of all cancer deaths. Of all the agents known to be correlated with cancer, cigarette smoking is the most important by ten-fold. Cigarette smoking is associated with lung cancer, oral cancer, cancers of the larynx, esophagus, bladder, kidney, and pancreas. Pipe and cigarette smoking also increase the risk of cancer of the lung, mouth, esophagus, and larynx (U.S. Surgeon General's Report 1982). The primary carcinogenic agent in cigarettes is the tar (Wynder 1982).

Cigarette smoking is strongly associated with a number of pulmonary dysfunctions. Those who smoke have a faster decline in pulmonary function with age than those who do not, and heavy smokers exhibit the greatest decline (Speizer and Tager 1979). They also have more frequent and more severe respiratory infections (Monto et al. 1975; Aronson et al. 1982). Chronic cough and phlegm production is strongly related to cigarette smoking (Weiss 1984). Even those who do not smoke but are around those who do (passive smokers) are known to have reduced small airways functioning (White and Froeb 1980) and increased risk of respiratory infection and lung cancer (U.S. Surgeon General's Report 1986).

In addition to the detrimental effects on the lungs, tobacco smoking markedly affects metabolism of some drugs (Dawson and Vestal 1984) and slows blood flow to the brain. Cigarette smoking also increases risk of coronary heart disease. This risk increases steadily with the number of cigarettes smoked. (U.S. Surgeon General's Report 1982). One report compared the risk of coronary heart disease of elders who currently smoked, those who had quit, and those who had never smoked. Current smokers were 1.75 times as likely to die as those who were nonsmokers, while those who quit had the same mortality rate as nonsmokers. Pipe and cigar smokers were significantly more at risk than nonsmokers (Jajick et al. 1984). Fortunately, when an individual quits smoking, the risk of heart disease, lung cancer, and acute and chronic pulmonary conditions declines.

Chronic Obstructive Pulmonary Disease

Chronic obstructive pulmonary disease (COPD) describes a syndrome of respiratory dysfunctions in which there is a chronic obstruction of air flow in the bronchi of the lungs that worsens over time. COPD is the most rapidly increasing health problem in the United States. The percentage of deaths attributed to COPD has more than doubled in the past twenty years, primarily due to cigarette smoking. The incidence of COPD increases with age (Reichel 1978).

COPD commonly includes chronic bronchitis, emphysema, and asthma. All affect the lung similarly and exhibit similar symptoms: an

Effects of Breathlessness on Life-style

A common symptom of pulmonary dysfunction—such as COPD or emphysema—is breathlessness. Coping with breathlessness and consequent lack of energy reserves is the central concern of the day for some individuals. One can better visualize the impact of breathing problems upon everyday life by reading the following:

> One woman who becomes short of breath after a few steps requires two to three hours to get dressed. She arises from bed and goes to the bathroom, rests, washes sitting in a chair with frequent rest periods, walks back to the bedroom, rests, and dresses, always needing to rest every few minutes. Another patient worked out an elaborate routing pattern to mop his kitchen every week. He gathers the cleaning paraphernalia and puts it near a chair in the middle of the room—these motions requiring frequent periods of "getting my breath back." He mops a few strokes and rests, sitting in the chair (Strauss 1975).

intermittant productive cough, difficulty in breathing, and fatigue upon exertion. Elders with COPD are easily exhausted, even with very simple tasks. Elders may have one or more of these respiratory disorders simultaneously.

The most important preventive measure is to stop, or better, to never start smoking cigarettes. Those with COPD are advised to stop smoking to reduce irritation of the bronchial tubes. In addition they are often prescribed drugs that dilate the bronchial passages, or exercises to enhance breathing. Those in advanced stages of COPD often must use an oxygen tank.

Chronic Bronchitis

Chronic bronchitis is the most common respiratory condition among elders. It is characterized by a chronic cough and abundant sputum production for at least three months a year for two consecutive years. The lining of the bronchial tubes contain mucus-producing cells that have hair-like projections called cilia that trap foreign particles and move them up the tubes towards the mouth. Chronic irritation by infections and environmental contaminants overwhelms the defenses of the respiratory tract. Consequently, the mucous cells produce excessive and thickened mucus causing a decrease in the ciliary activity in the airway. Breathing becomes even more difficult as the increase in size and number of the mucus-producing cells thicken and narrow the bronchi. A persistent cough and expectoration occur to attempt to rid the airways of excessive mucus secretions.

The best treatment is to discontinue cigarette smoking since the physiological changes are reversible when contaminants are removed. Chronic bronchitis is also treated with drugs that dilate the bronchii. Postural drainage, which places the patient on an incline board with head and chest lowered, promotes the movement of secretions to the larger airway to be expectorated. Individualized exercise programs to maximize remaining capacity may also be prescribed (see Chapter 10). In a few cases, supplementary oxygen is used. If left unchecked, chronic bronchitis may develop into emphysema.

Emphysema

Emphysema is an irreversible deterioration of the air sacs (alveoli) in the lungs that results in decreased oxygen consumption. Air becomes trapped behind mucous plugs in the narrowed airways, causing prolonged inflation of the air sacs. This prolonged inflation of stale air reduces the amount of fresh air available for oxygen/ carbon dioxide exchange. With time, the air sacs, which remain inflated by trapped air, eventually burst. Thus, the small separate air pockets merge to form larger sacs, which decreases the surface area available for oxygen/carbon dioxide exchange.

Symptoms of emphysema include shortness of breath, difficulty in inhalation and, in later stages, a barrel chest. Typically those with emphysema need to make a strong effort to exhale to rid themselves of trapped air. Reduced oxygen uptake reduces energy levels and any exertion can result in respiratory distress. The main problem to be addressed for those with emphysema is how to adapt their lifestyle to accommodate their lack of energy. Although the condition cannot be reversed, physical activity, drugs, breathing exercises, and oxygen can reduce its progression.

Lung Cancer

Lung cancer is the leading cause of cancer death in our country, responsible for 31 percent of cancer deaths in males and 12 percent in females (National Cancer Institute 1985). It is four times more common in men than women. This differential is attributed to the fact that more men smoke than women and more men are heavier smokers than women. However, because of the growing popularity of cigarette smoking among females, the lung cancer death rate among women is increasing dramatically and now surpasses breast cancer as the leading cancer killer in women (U.S. Surgeon General 1986). The average age for those newly diagnosed with lung cancer is sixty. However, it is believed that elders do not necessarily have increased susceptibility, but rather have been exposed longer to the harmful effects of cigarettes.

Ninety percent of all lung cancer incidence is attributed to cigarette smoking. The more one smokes, the greater the risk of contracting the disease. Those who smoke two or more packs a day have death rates fifteen–twenty-five times greater than nonsmokers. Those who smoke filtered, low tar cigarettes have lower lung cancer risks, but still have death rates much higher than nonsmokers. Other environmental contaminants causing lung cancer are asbestos, high doses of ionizing radiation, and possibly air pollution.

Common symptoms of lung cancer include chronic cough, coughing up blood, chest pain, wheezing, hoarseness, or breathlessness. The treatment is surgical removal of part of the lung. However, the prognosis for this cancer is poor. The five year survival rate of those with lung cancer is about ten percent, but for elders it is even lower (National Cancer Institute 1985).

Sensory Disorders

Disorders of the sensory system, primarily hearing and vision, frequently occur among elders. Vision problems increase with advancing age. Among elders living in the community, almost 10 percent of those sixty-five to seventy-four and 27 percent of those eighty-five and over report trouble with their vision (Havlik 1986). These disorders can have profound effects on the ability to perform daily activities and can cause withdrawal or depression. Chapter 4 discussed three age-associated decrements believed to be part of the aging process: presbyopia (the ability of the eye to focus at close range), cataracts (clouding of the lens), and presbycusis (loss of ability to hear high frequency sounds). The reader is directed to that chapter for details on these common neurosensory deficits. This section will address two other disorders of the eye that occur with increasing frequency in old age.

Glaucoma

Although not the most common eye disorder among elders, glaucoma is considered to be the most serious because it can cause blindness if not treated. It develops gradually between age forty and sixty-five and is caused by increased pressure within the eyeball due to a buildup of aqueous humor. Fluid is formed faster than it can be eliminated, increasing the fluid pressure in the eye. This pressure can damage the nerves responsible for vision. Glaucoma may come on suddenly (acute) or develop slowly (chronic). The symptoms of acute glaucoma include nausea, vomiting, eye pain and redness, and cloudy vision. By far, the more common form of glaucoma among

This man is being tested for glaucoma. The machine emits a short puff of air into the pupil which measures the fluid pressure within the eyeball.

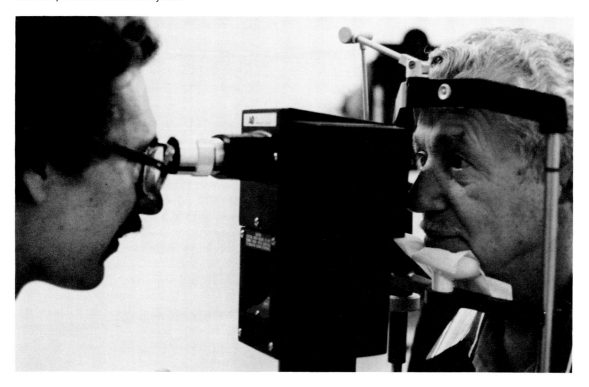

elders is the chronic type. Chronic glaucoma results in a gradual loss of peripheral vision. It is often called the "sneak thief of sight" because the vision loss is so subtle that significant damage may occur before diagnosis and treatment are sought. Warning signs are headache, nausea, blurred vision, and the appearance of halos or rainbows around lights.

There is no cure for glaucoma, but various types of drugs either eliminate excess fluid or encourage drainage of the aqueous humor to reduce pressure in the eye and subsequent nerve damage. It is imperative that medication be used regularly to be effective. Other treatments include spotheating the eye with ultrasound, which melts a portion of the tissue to initiate eye drainage (Carey 1984). Surgically opening a permanent drainage hole in the eye is used as a last resort.

Persons over forty years old should have glaucoma exams every two years as prompt diagnosis and treatment can minimize further vision damage.

Senile Macular Degeneration

Macular degeneration is a deterioration of the area of the retina responsible for central vision (macular area). The disease affects central vision by decreasing the ability to distinguish fine detail. As a result, only a grey shadow in the central visual field remains. Macular degeneration does not cause total blindness because peripheral vision is unaffected. However, it limits usual activities where detail is needed, such as sewing, reading, or driving. There is no medical or surgical treatment for this disease, but magnifying devices, hand-held or eyeglasses, can help elders read and do other detail work. Researchers are unsure what causes this disease, but diabetes and hypertension may play a role in its development.

Neurological Disorders

A number of neurological disorders occur more frequently in elders. They may be caused by other diseases, vitamin deficiency, viruses, trauma, or ineffective nerve transmission. The symptoms of neurological disorders are varied and depend on their cause. This section will address two of the more common neurological disorders, Parkinson's disease and tardive dyskinesia. Those neurological diseases affecting mental function will be discussed in Chapter 8.

Parkinson's Disease

Parkinson's disease is a slow, progressive disorder that affects the part of the brain that controls movement. It is estimated that one percent of the population over fifty has this disorder. Symptoms may include tremors of the extremities, slow movement, body rigidity, mask-like facial expression, and speech and gait disturbances. The most common symptoms are tremors in the resting state with a pill-rolling movement of the fingers and shaking of the head. Weakness or partial paralysis of the muscles in the arms, face, or tongue are preliminary symptoms of the disorder, followed by uncontrollable, unsteady movements of the face, arms, and hands. Because Parkinson's disease progresses very slowly, many individuals do not seek treatment. It is not known what causes Parkinsonism, however, it is associated with the encephalitis virus, carbon monoxide, and metal poisoning. Those who were stricken in the 1918 influenza epidemic are more likely to have the disease (Moore 1977).

Parkinson's disease is characterized by a shortage of the neurotransmitter dopamine in the brain, which interferes with efficient nerve transmission. There is no cure for the disease. However, levodopa, a precurser of dopamine, is usually prescribed. Levodopa increases the supply of dopamine levels in the brain, which reduces many of the symptoms of the disease.

Those with Parkinson's disease often suffer from depression due to their poor physical condition. Many have impaired mobility or cannot complete activities of daily living. Therapy should control symptoms and encourage maximum independence by assisting the elder to practice speaking and swallowing, promoting physical activity, and ensuring a safe environment (Wolanin and Steffl 1984).

Tardive Dyskinesia

Tardive dyskinesia is a movement disorder caused by long-standing drug treatment to control psychotic behavior. The most common drug family that causes this disabling side effect is the phenothiazides. Older patients are at an estimated 2–22 percent higher risk than younger groups of developing this disorder. One review reported that 25 percent of institutionalized elders taking antipsychotic drugs had tardive dyskinesia (Jeste and Wyatt 1981). The condition usually appears years after drug treatment is started and persists after termination of the drug. It may also appear for the first time after drug treatment is terminated.

Symptoms vary in extent and type, but all are related to involuntary use of muscles. Most commonly, the facial muscles contort into tics and grimaces, eye-blinking, lateral chewing and jaw movements, and abnormal tongue and lip motions. Leg crossing, feet tapping, and rocking back and forth while standing are also evident in many cases (Gilmore 1984).

There is no satisfactory treatment. Ironically, some of the drugs that caused the disorder in the first place may be helpful in reducing some symptoms. The best way to decrease tardive dyskinesia is to avoid long-term, high dosages of antipsychotic drugs (Gilmore 1984). The person with the disorder is usually embarrassed because of the inability to control body movement and is likely to be depressed, even suicidal, so counseling should be an important part of therapy.

Digestive disorders

Digestive complaints are commonly heard from elders. Although many symptoms are caused by dietary practices, sometimes they are associated with pathologic conditions, such as cancer. Thus, all digestive complaints should be thoroughly investigated. Gastrointestinal conditions are more common now than in the early part of this century. Some assert that most digestive disorders are associated with a highly refined diet and little dietary fiber. Although diet is not the only variable affecting gastrointestinal complaints, a diet high in fiber and complex carbohydrates and low in animal fat is likely to reduce the number and severity of problems.

Oral Cancer

Oral cancers increase drastically with age: more than 90 percent of all such cancers occur in those over forty-five (Mahboubi and Sayed 1982). Even though oral cancer is not as prevalent as many other cancers, it can be deadly. Most oral cancers begin with an ulcer or thickening in the mouth, usually on the tongue, lip, floor of the mouth, soft palate, or throat. Smokers have a six-fold increase in risk over nonsmokers, and use of alcohol in association with tobacco multiplies the risk. Although rates of oral cancer are higher among those who smoke and drink, chronic irritation by broken teeth and ill-fitting dentures is also associated with increased risk (Graham et al. 1977). Oral cancers are fast-growing, and self examinations are recommended.

Hiatal Hernia

A hiatal hernia is a displacement of part of the stomach into the chest cavity through the opening where the esophagus passes through the diaphragm. It is thought to be caused by weakness in the diaphragm. The disorder causes inflammation of the esophagus as stomach acid is regurgitated into the lower part of the esophagus. Hiatal hernia is common in elders in developed countries; some degree of hiatal hernia occurs in about half those over age sixty (Sklar 1978) and is much more common in women than men (Leeming and Dymock 1978).

Most hiatal hernias are asymptomatic. When symptoms do appear, the most common complaint is heartburn. Pain may occur when the esophagus becomes inflamed from stomach acid secretion. Overeating, lying flat, or coughing increases the discomfort. The condition is also aggravated by obesity, straining at the stool, and wearing clothes too tight at the waist. The most common drug treatment for this condition is antacids. Weight reduction is usually recommended. Elevating the head and shoulders when sleeping and modification of dietary habits, such as eating small, frequent meals, will also reduce the symptoms. If the condition is severe, surgery may be considered. The stomach is returned to its proper place, the diaphragm is repaired and a valve is constructed around the esophagus to prevent back-flow of stomach acid. However, this surgery does not have a high record of success and should only be tried when other methods have failed.

Gallstones

The incidence of gall bladder problems and gallstones increases with age; gallstones are found in 30 percent of those over age seventy and 40 percent of those in their eighties (Goldman 1979). Those at increased risk for gallstones are women, diabetics, and those who take estrogens. Most gallstones are asymptomatic, although some elders experience indigestion, nausea, vomiting, and episodes of pain when fats are ingested. The pain is usually just below the rib cage or in the right shoulder (Wolanin and Steffl 1984).

There is a debate among physicians regarding the best treatment for gallstones. Some advocate removing the gallbladder before an acute atack to prevent other complications. However, because the surgery mortality rate is significantly higher in elders (Hyams 1978), surgery is commonly employed only in acute situations. Alternative treatments include weight reduction, antacids, and avoidance of fatty foods. A drug that dissolves gallstones may also be prescribed. A nonsurgical technique that uses shock waves to dissolve the mineral deposits seems promising, but this technique is still experimental.

Diverticulosis

Diverticular disease, rare in the early part of the century, is now the most common disorder of the colon in the United States. Diverticuli are small pouches in the mucous layer of the colon. These small distended sacs increase in size and number after age fifty and are present in 40 percent of those over seventy (Knudson 1984). A low fiber diet is thought to contribute to the development of the disease (Burkitt 1971). Constipation, obesity, and emotional tension also play a role (Bartol and Heitkemper 1979).

The disorder is often asymptomatic. When symptoms are present, pain in the left abdominal region is the most common, and rectal bleeding sometimes occurs. The problem is generally not severe unless the pouches become inflamed (diverticulitis), which may lead to serious complications. A high fiber diet has been shown to both prevent and treat this condition (Almy 1985; Painter and Burkitt 1971).

Colorectal Cancer

Cancers of the colon and rectum are the second highest cause of cancer deaths among older people in the United States. The incidence of colorectal cancers increases slowly after adolescence and rises sharply after age fifty. Those over sixty-five account for three-quarters of the cases of colorectal cancer (National Cancer Institute 1985). The incidence among those aged seventy-five to seventy-nine who have colorectal cancer is more than quadruple the rate of those aged fifty-five to fifty-nine.

Because of its high incidence in elders, experts recommend yearly colorectal examinations. A number of self-administered commercial tests are available over-the-counter that detect the presence of blood in the stool, a primary symptom of the disease. The value of routine colorectal examinations in reducing deaths from the cancer has been documented (Gilbert and Nelms 1978). However, many elders find the exams embarrassing and do not request them.

A history of colorectal growths in the family is correlated with a higher probability of developing colorectal cancer. Epidemiological studies show that those with a high animal fat and low fiber intake are also more likely to have colorectal cancer.

The only common early symptom of colorectal cancer is rectal bleeding. However, constipation or diarrhea lasting two weeks or longer may be another indicator. Removal of a small segment of the large intestine followed by radiation and chemotherapy is the most effective treatment. A temporary or permanent colostomy may result if the cancer is extensive. A colostomy is a surgical procedure in which the end of the intestine is connected to a tube routed outside the body via an artificial opening in the abdomen called a stoma. The feces are then collected in a disposable plastic bag.

Colorectal cancers are relatively slow growing in elders and do not spread to other organs until later in their growth. Thus, if the tumors are discovered and removed before symptoms appear, the survival rate is enhanced. In advanced stages, the cancer penetrates the intestinal wall and spreads into nearby lymph nodes and beyond.

Musculoskeletal Disorders

Arthritis and other bone and muscular disorders are the most common disorders affecting elders. Arthritis is the number one crippler of all age groups in the United States. However, the extent of these disorders varies: some afflicted elders are crippled by them while others have little to no limitations of their daily routine. The disorders usually appear in midlife and progress slowly with age. Because most musculoskeletal disorders cause similar symptoms (aches, pains, limitations of movement, and stiffness) they are often grouped together and called rheumatism and left untreated. However, all symptoms should be investigated because many symptoms can be alleviated. These disorders have no cure so treatment consists of preventing further degeneration, controlling pain, and encouraging as much independence as possible.

Disorders of the musculoskeletal system are rarely fatal or incapacitating. However, they are among elders' most frequent complaints because they limit some daily activities. The bent stature and stiffened, sometimes misshapen, extremities associated with musculoskeletal diseases can also affect self image. Joint changes, diminished bone mass, and subsequent poor posture and immobility increase susceptibility to falls and subsequent fractures. A modification of the living environment may be necessary to allow for maximum independence.

Osteoarthritis

Osteoarthritis is a degenerative, noninflammatory joint disease that involves a gradual wearing away of joint cartilage (figure 5.4). The primary symptom is short-term stiffness in the morning and after rest. Joint pain, limitation of motion, and enlarged joints are characteristic of later stages of the disease. Almost everyone over age fifty shows some joint degeneration on X-rays, but only 20 percent have symptoms. The disease often begins in the fingers and is manifested by joint enlargement and reduced range of joint motion. The weight bearing joints of the knees and hips may be affected, causing pain upon walking. The predominant factor predisposing one to osteoarthritis is old age. Obesity and poor posture tend to aggravate the degeneration of the weight-bearing joints. Treatment includes pain-killing drugs (usually aspirin), weight loss, and devices (walkers, canes) to reduce pressure on weight-bearing joints. An individualized rest-exercise program should be prescribed to maintain joint mobility and muscle tone. In severe cases of osteoarthritis of the hip, joint replacement surgery may be needed to restore mobility.

Rheumatoid Arthritis

Although not nearly as widespread as osteoarthritis, rheumatoid arthritis is more likely to cause pain, crippling, and disfigurement. The disease

Figure 5.4 Osteoarthritis. (Source: Booklet entitled "So You Have Osteoarthritis," p. 5. Arthritis Foundation, 3400 Peachtree Road, N.E., Atlanta, GA 30326).

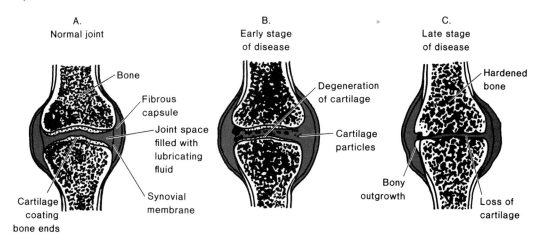

A.
Normal joint

Bone

Fibrous capsule

Joint space filled with lubricating fluid

Cartilage coating bone ends

Synovial membrane

B.
Early stage of disease

Degeneration of cartilage

Cartilage particles

C.
Late stage of disease

Hardened bone

Bony outgrowth

Loss of cartilage

may occur between age twenty and fifty, however, its prevalence increases with age. The peak of new cases of rheumatoid arthritis is from age sixty to sixty-nine in men and age fifty to fifty-nine in women (Linos et al. 1980). It is two to three times more common in women than men.

Rheumatoid arthritis is a disease of the tissue lining the joints. The joints in the small bones of the hand and foot are most often affected; however, it can also spread to the larger joints. The joint lining becomes swollen and thick and grows over the cartilage, leaving bone and scar tissue in its place. Without treatment, the joint and ligaments are destroyed, producing permanent stiffness and deformity.

The most common complaint is swelling and redness in joints. Second in importance is morning stiffness that lasts up to five hours. Weight loss, weakness, and fatigue are other symptoms. The same joint on both sides of the body is often afflicted. The disease is characterized by flare-ups and remissions. Just as the pain leaves one joint, it may reappear in another. In some cases, the disease is inactive and the individual has no symptoms. Older adults may already have deformity and permanent damage because of lack of treatment in earlier years. Today, treatment can prevent severe crippling in most cases. The cause of rheumatoid arthritis is not clear but may be related to an inappropriate response of the immune system to its own tissues. Emotional upset is known to trigger an episode of the disease.

Rheumatoid arthritis is treated by a variety of methods. Aspirin is the most common and effective drug to reduce pain and joint inflammation. Because high dosages must be used, special precautions should be taken to reduce its adverse effects (such as gastric disturbances, anemia, and ringing in the ears). Other anti-inflammatory agents are sometimes used, such as cortisone and gold salts. A balance of rest during flare-ups, and exercise several times a day during remission is recommended to achieve the fullest possible range of motion in each joint. The application of moist heat to afflicted joints temporarily reduces pain,

swelling, and stiffness and makes exercise easier. When immobility and constant pain occur, various types of surgery to repair joints and tendons and to correct deformities may be performed. Psychological support for the affected individual is important because the pain, disability, and consequent dependence cause stress that further aggravates the disease.

Gout

Gout is an arthritic disorder caused by a malfunction in either the production or elimination of uric acid. Uric acid is a waste product of the breakdown of proteins. It accumulates in the bloodstream if too much is produced or if elimination is inefficient. Excessive levels of uric acid in the bloodstream may form uric acid crystals that deposit themselves in the fluid of particular joints. The problem often appears in only one joint, commonly the big toe, periodically causing a gouty attack lasting a few days. Symptoms of an attack are excruciating joint pain and inflammation. Attacks may recur with increasing intensity and frequency or may not reappear for months or years. In severe cases, disfiguring tophi deposits composed of chalky uric acid crystals form around the ears and joints. These deposits are large and are evident through the skin.

Primary gout is caused by a hereditary metabolic disorder and is usually detected first around age fifty to sixty. The great majority of primary gout cases occur in men, although some women may get gout after menopause. When gout initially occurs in those over sixty-five, it is likely due to thiazide diuretic use that partially blocks urate excretion by the kidneys (Healy 1984) and is called secondary gout. Secondary gout may also occur with obesity, joint injury, stress, or dehydration, and it occurs equally in men and women.

Control of blood levels of uric acid is the key to effective management of gout. Two types of drugs accomplish this purpose. Anti-inflammatory agents are used during an acute attack to relieve symptoms. Other drugs lower blood levels of uric acid and must be taken throughout life. Those with primary gout should reduce intake of

Dowagers hump, common among older women, is indicative of osteoporosis.

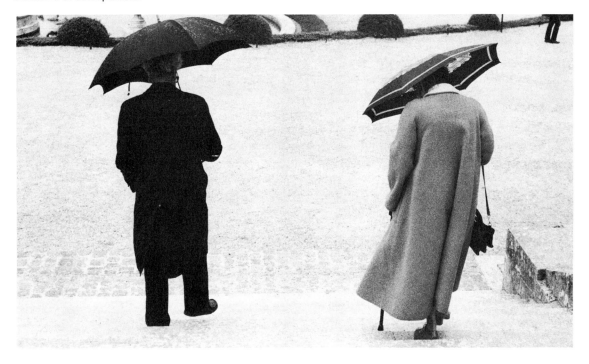

shellfish and organ meats during an acute attack because these foods are high in a specific compound that aggravates the condition.

Osteoporosis

Osteoporosis is characterized by a progressive decrease in bone mass and porosity. Generally, bone is constantly being broken down and rebuilt at the same rate. However, in osteoporosis, the rate of breakdown exceeds the build-up rate causing a net loss of bone mass. These changes significantly reduce bone strength, making bones, especially those in the back, hip, and forearm, more susceptible to fractures. Osteoporosis can also cause collapsed or wedged vertebra leading to spinal deformities such as dowager's hump, loss of height, and chronic back pain.

Loss of bone mass begins in the forties, but is seldom diagnosed until after a fracture occurs. Women are four times more likely to have osteoporosis than men. Women begin bone loss earlier and the rate of loss is faster than in men, especially after menopause. It is estimated that women lose 25–30 percent of their bone mass over their lifetime, while men lose about 12 percent. Seventy percent of older women have some degree of osteoporosis; about 25 percent of those will have fractures and deformity (Vaughn 1976). White women, especially of northern European descent, are at highest risk.

There are multiple theories of the cause of osteoporosis. It almost certainly is related to estrogens as decreases in bone mass accelerate after menopause. Some experts attribute osteoporosis to insufficient ingestion of calcium or vitamin D (which enables the body to absorb ingested calcium). Lack of physical activity, cigarette smoking, and excessive intake of proteins have also been implicated. It is likely that more than one factor is involved. The typical picture of an osteoporosis candidate is a small-framed, thin, fair-skinned woman who smokes, is inactive, and does not get sufficient calcium (Chestnut 1985).

Those with advanced osteoporosis are so fragile that even a minor fall might result in a severe fracture and subsequent disability and dependence. However, immobilizing one with a fracture is not recommended because it hastens bone degeneration (see Chapter 10). Healing of a fracture is very slow in those with osteoporosis. In advanced bone loss, joint replacement is indicated.

Vertebral fractures take long to heal but are seldom painful or require hospitalization. In contrast, hip fractures are serious. Estimates vary, but from 12 to 20 percent of elders who fracture a hip die within the year. Of those who survive, greater than 40 percent are dependent upon mechanical aids or another person. Finally, 15 to 25 percent of those with hip fractures are confined to nursing homes (*Health Letter* 1987).

There is little evidence that any therapy can reverse the bone loss associated with osteoporosis, but its progression can be retarded. Prevention and treatment measures include increased calcium intake (1200–1400 mg), Vitamin D, exercise, smoking cessation and, in some cases, estrogen therapy.

Osteoporosis screening centers are becoming more common. There are several screening techniques that detect the degree of bone loss. However, as yet, the tests cannot predict who will suffer from fractures and who will not. The procedure is costly, imprecise, and unreliable and many experts do not recommend it to screen women without symptoms. Because the common treatment for osteoporosis is estrogen supplementation, if a woman does not want to take estrogens, she should not undergo the test. Its major value is in monitoring the effectiveness of therapy in women with the disease. Osteoporosis screening is not helpful for women ten years after menopause because even if osteoporosis is noted, estrogen treatment has shown to be ineffective if started that late (*Health Letter* 1987).

Paget's Disease

Paget's disease is a progressive condition characterized by abnormal bone formation, generally occuring in only a few bones. The cause is unknown. The disease is rare before age forty-five, but by age sixty-five, one in nine has the disorder (Spencer and Lender 1979).

In Paget's disease, normal bones are replaced with Paget bone and fibrous tissue, which is larger and softer than normal bone tissue. The bones affected are usually the long bones of the arm or leg, the pelvis, or skull. The soft Paget bones are easily deformed. Thus, when weight is placed upon them, the long bones of the arms and legs bow, causing skeletal deformities. Excessive bone tissue in the skull can cause pressure on the cranial nerves, resulting in neurosensory deficits. Some people with the disease do not have symptoms, others have bone pain and localized areas hot to the touch at the Paget bone site (Caird and Dall 1978). Bed rest aggravates the disease.

Paget's disease is difficult to diagnose because it is often accompanied by osteoporosis, osteoarthritis, or other illnesses. Therapy usually involves drugs that decrease abnormal bone resorption and deposition and slow the progression of the disease. Drugs may also be prescribed to relieve neurological symptoms, if present. This disease is a precursor of bone cancer so periodic assessment is needed (Spencer and Lender 1979).

Endocrine Disorders

Endocrine disorders generally occur in early or middle adulthood and none increase in incidence after age sixty-five. Diabetes and myxedema are the most significant endocrine problems affecting elders.

Diabetes

Diabetes is a metabolic disorder characterized by a deficiency in the production or utilization of insulin, a hormone produced in the pancreas needed to metabolize glucose. There are two main types of diabetes, juvenile-onset (Type I) and adult-onset (Type II). Juvenile-onset diabetes is rapid in onset and characterized by the inability of the pancreas to produce insulin. This type of diabetes is controlled by regular insulin injections. In adult-onset diabetes, the pancreas produces insulin, but the cells become less receptive to it. This type of diabetes progresses much more slowly. The classical symptoms of Type I diabetes—thirst and increased urination—are rarely present in the Type II diabetes. Fatigue, sensory changes, and increased susceptibility to infection are more common symptoms. Overweight women are at the highest risk for adult-onset diabetes.

Almost universally, individuals exhibit an age-related decrease in glucose tolerance. However, the point at which abnormal glucose tolerance is classified and treated as diabetes is hotly debated. Because overtreatment for diabetes is hazardous, experts recommend conservative management of adult-onset diabetes in elders. The first line of treatment for elder adult-onset diabetes is weight loss and a diet high in complex carbohydrates and fiber and low in refined sugar and fat (Bierman 1981). Further, a regular exercise program will help the diabetic control symptoms and lose weight (Podolsky and El-Beheri 1980; Cusack 1981). For about 70 percent of adult-onset diabetics, dietary changes, weight loss, and physical activity can control symptoms. For the remainder, insulin or hypoglycemic agents may be prescribed.

Insulin and hypoglycemic drug therapy is extremely difficult to regulate and a number of serious consequences can arise from faulty management. With insufficient insulin, even though there is sufficient sugar circulating in the blood, the body cells cannot take it in and hyperglycemia results (sometimes called diabetic coma or ketosis). Hyperglycemia is characterized by chemical-scented breath, dry skin and tongue, low blood pressure, diminished reflexes, and thirst. The onset may take from hours to days and the patient should be hospitalized and administered insulin and fluids. In contrast, too much insulin or hypoglycemic drugs may use up too much of the blood sugar, lowering blood sugar to dangerous levels (hypoglycemia or insulin shock). Hypoglycemia is characterized by sweating, unstable gait, visual problems, unconsciousness, or tremors. Hypoglycemic shock appears suddenly. When a person is taking insulin or hypoglycemic drugs, sugar candy should be on hand to prevent hypoglycemia from progressing because the condition can cause heart attack, brain damage, coma, or death.

Diabetes is associated with a number of other complications. Atherosclerosis progresses twice as fast in diabetics. Coronary artery disease is twice as common in diabetic men and five times as likely in diabetic women than nondiabetics. Because of poor circulation and peripheral nerve damage, elders are highly susceptible to infections, especially in the foot. Diabetics have a much greater chance of becoming blind than nondiabetics because of hemorrhages of blood vessels in the retina. This condition, diabetic retinopathy, is the leading cause of blindness among elders. The nephrons in the kidneys also deteriorate, causing progressive kidney failure. It is believed that adequate control will reduce the incidence of this complication. Women with diabetes are more susceptible to vaginal and urinary infections and men may suffer erectile dysfunction due to damage to the nerves that supply the penis. (National Diabetes Advisory Board 1983). For further discussion on the effect of diabetes on male and female sexual response, see Chapter 11.

Myxedema

Myxedema is the most common thyroid condition among older people and occurs much more frequently in elder women than men. Myxedema is caused by inadequate function of the thyroid gland as a result of a deficiency of thyroid hormone in the blood. The condition progresses slowly, gradually affecting appearance and mental processes. Physical manifestations of the disease are coarsening of the skin and hair and swelling due to accumulation of fluid in the skin (edema). Mental processes become slowed and may be accompanied by depression, hallucinations, and insanity. Some exhibit decreased tolerance to cold, lethargy, and reduced metabolic rate. This problem often goes untreated because many symptoms of this disorder may be mistaken for old age. Many believe that reduced thyroid functioning contributes to many chronic problems among elders (Turnbridge 1981). Laboratory tests are effective at diagnosing the disease. Regular administration of thryoid hormone reverses the condition; however, if left untreated, the condition is lethal.

Genitourinary Disorders

Elders are at high risk for a number of chronic problems of the genital and urinary systems. Although many of these conditions are reversible, the reluctance of older people to bring these problems to the attention of the physician can result in progressive worsening of these conditions. For older women, regular visits to the gynecologist can provide an opportunity for early detection of both genital and urinary disorders. However, the percentage of women who request such care is not large. Because of the high incidence of prostate problems among men, yearly digital rectal examinations are recommended. As in other chronic illnesses, treatment of genital and urinary disorders is more successful when the problem is diagnosed before the disease is advanced.

Benign Prostatic Hyperplasia

Benign prostatic hyperplasia, or enlarged prostate, is a disease of advancing age. The prostate grows very slowly from birth to puberty, then undergoes a rapid size increase until age thirty. The gland begins to grow again at forty-five and continues to grow until death. The prevalence of prostate enlargement in men between age thirty-one to forty is 8 percent, rapidly increasing to 70

percent by age sixty-one to seventy and to 90 percent by age ninety (Berry et al. 1984). Because the prostate surrounds the urethra, its growth often compresses the urethra, leading to a gradual decrease of outflow of urine and progressing to total urinary obstruction in some cases. Common symptoms are reduced force and size of the urinary stream, dribbling of urine, and inability to empty the bladder despite increased bladder pressure. Those affected may awaken frequently during the night to pass a small amount of urine. Unfortunately many men do not seek medical care for their symptoms because they develop so gradually. Others may not seek care because of fear of cancer or that treatment will result in impotence. However, it is now known that an enlarged prostate is not related to prostate cancer.

The most common treatment for an enlarged prostate that obstructs urine flow is a simple operation, called a transurethral resection (TUR). A small loop is inserted through the urethra and the part of the prostate causing the obstruction is scraped, widening the urethra. In some cases, if the prostate is excessively large, the whole prostate gland must be removed, and the operation is more complicated (see Chapter 11 for more information on prostate surgery and effects on sexuality). It is estimated that 25 percent of those men living in the United States who survive to age eighty will have had surgery to relieve urinary obstruction from an enlarged prostate and 25 percent more will need it (Palmer and Myers 1984). If not severe, the symptoms of benign prostatic hyperplasia can also be treated by less radical means. Hot baths give temporary relief. Palmer and Myers (1984) report that a catheter inserted for four weeks eliminated the need for TUR in 75 percent of the cases.

Prostate Cancer

Prostate cancer, the third most common type of cancer for American men over fifty-five, is chiefly a disease of elder men. It rarely occurs before age forty-five, but by age eighty half the males examined in autopsy had prostate cancer to some degree (Rullis et al. 1975). Elder black men in

The odds are that three of these four men have prostate enlargement, and if all live into their 80s, two will have evidence of prostate cancer.

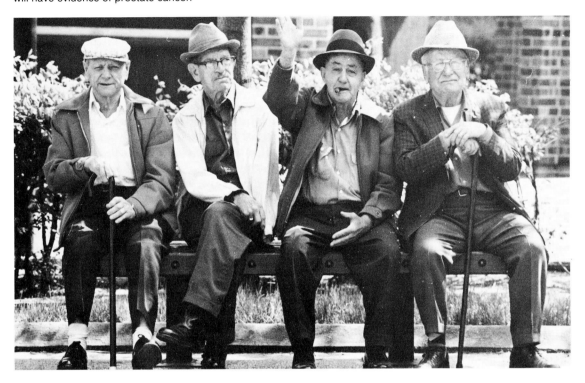

the United States have 1.5 times the rate of prostate cancer of their white counterparts. The cause of prostate cancer is not clear. The presence of testosterone plays a role because castrated men do not get the disease. It is thought that a high fat diet might increase risk of prostate cancer since fat intake affects the production of sex hormones.

Symptoms of prostate cancer are always absent when the cancer is localized and curable. A digital rectal examination is the only way to detect prostate cancer in its curable stages. Despite advantages in treatment, only 10 percent of males with the condition are detected early enough to cure (Fuchs 1985). If nodules are found, a sample of the cells taken by a hypodermic needle (called a needle biopsy) in the doctor's office can determine the presence of cancer cells. About 50 percent of detected nodules are found to be malignant (cancerous). Bone pain may occur when the cancer has progressed to bones in the vicinity. Blood in the urine and frequent urination is another late symptom (Fuchs 1985).

Before choosing a treatment strategy, the stage of the disease, survival rate of prostate cancer, the dangers of each treatment, and the health status of the patient should be taken into account (Palmer and Myers 1984). If the malignancy has not spread, removal of the prostate gland is the most effective treatment. Although in the past this treatment often resulted in impotence and sometimes urinary incontinence, new methods reduce that risk (Walsh et al. 1983). The effects of such surgery on sexual functioning is discussed in more detail in Chapter 11. Not all those with confirmed prostate cancer should undergo surgery. Because the cancer is very slow-growing, those who are very old are likely to die

Basal cell cancer is the most common type of skin cancer. It is easily removed and is not fatal. In contrast, *melanoma* is very rare, but deadly. In the later stages it may spread to other body tissues. These photos illustrate *melanoma first, intermediate and advanced stages.*

No. 1   No. 2   No. 3   No. 4

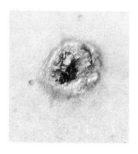 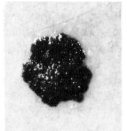 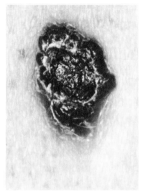 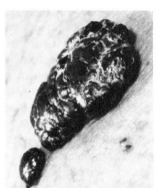

color, become ulcerated and bleed with slight injury. Its cells often spread to other parts of the body (mestasticize). They appear most often on lower legs and feet in women and the trunk in men (Jenson and Bolander 1980). In contrast, nonmelanoma skin cancers are by far the most common cancer among whites in the United States. They occur most frequently after age fifty. Despite their high prevalence, they rarely cause death. They are characterized by either a pale, wax-like, pearly nodule that may eventually ulcerate and crust, or a red, scaly, sharply outlined patch. Nonmelanoma cancers are known to be caused by exposure to ultraviolet light from the sun, but the sun's impact on melanoma is not as obvious (Urbach 1983). It is believed that UV light reduces the efficiency of the immune system. Nonmelanoma most often occurs where the skin has had the most sun exposure—the face, head, and neck. Whites, particularly those who are fair-skinned, are at the highest risk for nonmelanoma skin cancer.

Skin cancers can be easily removed by surgery, radiation, or chemicals applied to the skin. Regular examinations are necessary to ensure that new cancers are treated at an early stage. Overexposure to the sun can be carcinogenic, so it is important to learn to use sunscreens, wear protective clothing, and limit sun exposure. However, some daily sun exposure is recommended because the sun is an important source of vitamin D, needed to metabolize calcium.

Summary

Old age is often accompanied by chronic illnesses. Chronic conditions are progressive, generally irreversible, and long-term. Although chronic illnesses are widespread in elders, most cause only minor limitation of daily routine. Some, however—cancer, stroke, and heart disease are leading causes of death among elders. Rather than a cure, medical management of chronic conditions involves treating symptoms and preventing further deterioration.

The onset and severity of many chronic illnesses is often dependent on past and current health behaviors (e.g., diet, exercise, smoking). The most effective way to prevent these diseases or reduce their progression is to modify negative health behaviors. Prevention of chronic illness involves a personal, lifelong effort to improve health habits. For many, both young and old, the benefits are too distant and the costs too great. For instance, although the link between disease and cigarette smoking is widely-publicized, many continue to smoke.

Although this chapter concerns itself with causes, symptoms, and treatments of the common chronic diseases, social, financial, and emotional considerations are a critical part of coping with disease. The family and friends of those with health problems and health workers need to be attentive to such variables when dealing with those who are chronically ill.

Activities

1. Create a brief case study of an older individual with a chronic health problem or problems. Include the impact of the disease on the overall quality of life of that person. Be sure to include psychological, social, and economic aspects. Assuming the individual in the case you described above has a spouse, describe the impact upon that family member.

2. After studying the common chronic health problems of elders, which diseases will you be likely to suffer in your later years (due either to heredity or current health behaviors)? Be complete. Remember that many are extremely common. What might you do to prevent or reduce the impact of one or more of these problems? Are you working on any of these behaviors now? If, so, which ones? If not, discuss the factors keeping you from doing so.

3. Visit the campus library and peruse the recent medical journals. Choose an article that presents new information on some aspect of a common disease of elders. Write a brief summary of the findings and discuss the implications of this new information on the outcome of the disease and its effect upon the individual.

4. You have been asked to coordinate a health fair for elders in your community. You have twenty booths to fill with either agencies, screening facilities, or health education materials. Considering the information on chronic disease gathered in this chapter, list information or screening you would provide in each booth that would be most helpful to this age group.

5. Talk to the director of smoking cessation classes available in your area. What is the percentage of elders attending? In their experience, what is their success rate? How does it compare to other age groups?

6. Interview a health care worker at a local hospital. What are the common chronic health problems of older people who are hospitalized? What are the problems inherent in treating specific chronic illnesses in that age group?

7. Visit a public place (shopping mall, drug store, supermarket) and tally how many individuals have visible health problems, as well as their approximate ages. What health problem seems to be the most common? Can you detect the difference in types and numbers of problems with age?

Bibliography

Almy, T. P. 1985. Some disorders of the alimentary tract. In R. Andres, E. L. Bierman, W. R. Hazzard, eds. *Principles of geriatric medicine.* San Francisco: McGraw-Hill Book Co. 662–81.

Anderson, F. 1978. Preventive medicine in old age. In Brocklehurst, J. C., ed. *Textbook of geriatric medicine and gerontology.* New York: Churchill Livingstone. 783–90.

Anderson, K. M., W. P. Castelli, and D. Levy. 1987. Cholesterol and mortality. *JAMA* 257(18):2176–80.

Aronson, M. D., S. T. Weiss, R. L. Ben, and A. L. Komaroff. 1982. Association between cigarette smoking and acute respiratory tract illness in young adults. *JAMA* 248:181–83.

Bartol, M. A., and M. Heitkemper. 1979. Gastrointestinal problems. In Carnevali, D. L., and M. Patrick, eds. *Nursing management for the elderly.* Philadelphia: J. B. Lippencott. 311–30.

Berry, S. J., D. S. Coffey, P. C. Walsh, et al. 1984. The development of benign prostatic hyperplasia with age. *J Urol* 132:474–79.

Bierman, E. L. 1981. Diabetes mellitus—dietary management and prognosis. In M. Winick, ed. *Nutrition and the killer diseases*. New York: Wiley. 153–64.

Burkitt, D. M. 1971. Possible relationships between bowel cancer and dietary habit. *Proc R Soc Med* 64:964.

Caird, F. I., and J. L. C. Dall. 1978. The cardiovascular system. In Brocklehurst, J. C., ed. *Textbook of geriatric medicine and gerontology*. New York: Churchill Livingstone. 125–57.

Carey, J. 1984. A sound for sore eyes: ultrasound reduced blinding pressure of glaucoma. *American Health* July–August, 10.

Chestnut, C. H. 1985. Osteoporosis. In R. Andres, E. L. Bierman, W. R. Hazzard, eds. *Principles of geriatric medicine*. San Francisco: McGraw Hill Book Co. 801–12.

Clay, E. 1980. Habit training, a tested method to regain urinary control. *Geriatr Nurs* 1(4):252–54.

Cusack, B. 1981. Diabetes mellitus: The management. *Geriatric Medicine* 11(2):45–47.

Dawson, G. W., and R. E. Vestal. 1984. Smoking, age and drug metabolism. In Bosse, R. and C. L. Rose. eds. *Smoking and aging*. Lexington, Mass: DC Health. 131–56.

Drayer, J. I. M., and M. A. Weber. 1985. Hypertension in the aging: Special procedures in diagnosis and evaluation. In Codley, E. L. ed. *Geriatric heart disease*. Littleton, Mass: PSG Publ. Co. 201–07.

Fisher, B., M. Bauer, and R. Margolese. 1985. Five-year results of a random clinical trial comparing total mastectomy and segmental mastectomy with or without radiation in the treatment of breast cancer. *N Engl J Med* 312:665–73.

Fletcher, S. W., M. S. O'Malley, and L. A. Bunce. 1985. Physicians' ability to detect lumps in silicone breast models. *JAMA* 253(15): 2224–28.

Food and Drug Administration Drug Bulletin. 1985. Aspirin for myocardial infarction. Vol 15 (4). December: 35.

Fuchs, E. F. 1985. Urological disease of the aged. In Cassel, C. K., and J. R. Walsh, eds. *Geriatric medicine vol. 1: Medical, psychiatric and pharmacological approaches*. New York: Springer-Verlag. 268–79.

Gilbert, V. A., and J. M. Nelms. 1978. The prevention of invasive cancer of the rectum. *Cancer* 41:1137–39.

Gilmore, R. 1984. Movement disorders in the elderly. *Geriatrics* 29(6):65–76.

Goldman, R. 1979. Aging changes in structure and function. In Carnevali, D. L., and M. Patrick, eds. *Nursing management for the elderly*. Philadelphia: J. B. Lippencott. 53–81.

Graham, S., H. Dyal, T. Rohrer, et al. 1977. Dentition, diet, tobacco and alcohol in the epidemiology of oral cancer. *J Nat Cancer Inst* 59:1611–18.

Groteboer, J. 1978. Stroke, carotid endarectomy and the neurosurgeon. *J Neurol Nurs* 10:52–59.

Hanna, M. J. D., and A. L. MacMillan, 1978. Aging and the skin. In Brocklehurst, J. C., ed. *Textbook of geriatric medicine and gerontology*. New York: Churchill Livingstone. 626–639.

Harris, T. 1986. Aging in the eighties, prevalence and impact of urinary problems in individuals age 65 years and over. *Advance Data from Vital and Health Statistics*. No. 121, Aug. 27, 1986. Hyattsville, MD: Public Health Service.

Havlik, R. J. 1986. Aging in the eighties, impaired senses for sound and light in persons 65 years and over. *Advance Data from Vital and Health Statistics*. No. 125, September 19, 1986. Bethesda, MD: Public Health Service.

Health Letter. 1987. Osteoporosis, Part I: Screening tests. Newsletter of the Public Citizens Research Group 3(5):1–3.

Healy, L. A. 1984. Rheumatology. In C. K. Cassel, and J. R. Walsh eds. *Geriatric medicine vol. 1: Medical, psychiatric and pharmacological approaches* New York: Springer-Verlag. 289–98.

Hirshberg, G. G. 1976. Ambulation and self care are goals of rehabilitation after a stroke. *Geriatrics* 31(5): 61–65.

Hodkinson, H. M. 1978. Cancer in the aged. In Brocklehurst, J. C. ed. *Textbook of geriatric medicine and gerontology*. New York: Churchill Livingstone. 646–50.

Hyams, D. E. 1978. The liver and bilary systems. In Brocklehurst, J. C., ed. *Textbook of geriatric medicine and gerontology.* New York: Churchill Livingstone. 53–81.

Jajick, C. L., A. M. Ostfeld, and D. H. Freeman, Jr. 1984. Smoking and coronary heart disease mortality in the elderly. *JAMA* 252:2831–34.

Jarvik, L. 1979. Genetic aspects of aging. In Rossman, I., ed. *Clinical Geriatrics.* Philadelphia: J. B. Lippencott. 86–109.

Jenson, O. M., and A. M. Bolander. 1980. Trends in malignant melanoma of the skin. *World Health Stat Quarterly* 33:2–26.

Jeste, D. V., and R. J. Wyatt. 1981. Changing epidemiology in tardive dyskinesia: An overview. *Am J Psychiatry* 138:297–309.

Kaplan, N. M. 1983. Therapy of mild hypertension—toward a more balanced view. *JAMA* 249(3):365–67.

Kart, C. S., E. S. Metress, and J. F. Metress. 1978. *Aging and health: Biological and social perspectives.* Menlo Park, Calif.: Addison-Wesley.

Kegel, A. H. 1948. Progressive resistance exercises in the functional restoration of the perineal muscles. *Am J Obstet Gynecol* 56:238–48.

Kiesling, S. 1983. The trials of everyday tension. *American Health* Jan.–Feb.: 50.

Knudsen, F. S. 1984. Gastrointestinal and metabolic problems in older adults. In Steffl, B. M., ed. *Handbook of gerontological nursing.* New York: Van Nostrand Reinhold. 234–50.

Leeming, J. T., and I. W. Dymock. 1978. The upper gastrointestinal tract. In Brocklehurst, J. C., ed. *Textbook of geriatric medicine and gerontology.* New York: Churchill Livingstone 344–57.

Linos, A., J. W. Worthington, W. M. O'Fallon, and L. T. Kurtland. 1980. The epidemiology of rheumatoid arthritis in Rochester, Minn: A study of incidence, prevalence and mortality. *Am J Epidemiol* 111:87–98.

MacDonald, J. B., J. Baille, B. D. Williams, and D. Ballantyne. 1983. Coronary care in the elderly. *Age Ageing* 12:17–20.

Mahboubi, E., and G. M. Sayed. 1982. Oral cavity and pharynx. In Schottenfeld, D., and J. F. Fraumeni, eds. *Cancer epidemiology and prevention.* Philadelphia: W. B. Saunders. 583–95.

Mancia, G., F. Bertinieri, G. Grassi, et al. 1983. Effects of blood pressure measurement by patients' blood pressure and heart rate. *Lancet* 8352:695–97.

Maxwell, F. S. 1968. *The measure of my days.* New York: Penguin Books.

McAlister, N. H. 1983. Should we treat "mild" hypertension? *JAMA* 249(3):379–82.

Mechanic, D. 1966. Response factors in illness: The study of illness behavior. *Soc Psychiatry* 1:11–20.

Moe, R. E. 1985. Breast disease in elderly women. In R. Andres, E. L. Bierman, and W. R. Hazzard, eds. *Principles of geriatric medicine.* San Francisco: McGraw-Hill. 636–46.

Monto, A. S., M. W. Higgine, and H. W. Ross. 1975. The Tecumseh study of respiratory illness: VIII. Acute infection in chronic respiratory disease and comparison groups. *Am Rev Respir Dis* 111:27–36.

Moore, G. 1977. Influenza and Parkinson's disease. *Public Health Reports* 92 (1):79–80.

Murray, R., N. M. Huelskoetter, and D. O'Driscoll. 1980. *The nursing process in later maturity.* Englewood Cliffs, NJ: Prentice-Hall.

National Cancer Institute. 1985. *Cancer rates and risks.* NIH Publication No. 85–691 Washington, D.C.: National Institutes of Health.

National Diabetics Advisory Board. 1983. The prevention and treatment of five complications of diabetes. Publ. No. HHS 83–8392. Atlanta: Center for Disease Control.

Ouslander, J. G., R. L. Kane, and I. B. Abrass. 1982. Urinary incontinence in elderly nursing home patients. *JAMA* 248:1194–98.

Ouslander, J., R. Kane, S. Vollmer, and M. Menezes. 1985. Technologies for managing urinary incontinence. Health Technology Case Study 33, OTA-HCS-33, Washington, D.C.: U.S. Congress Office of Technology Assessment, July.

Painter, N. S., and D. P. Burkitt. 1971. Diverticular disease of the colon: A deficiency disease of Western civilization. *Br J Med* 2:450–54.

Palmer, J., and F. J. Myers. 1984. Benign prostatic hypertrophy and carcinoma of the prostate. Paper presented at the California Conference on Applied Clinical Geriatrics. University of California, Davis and Veteran's Home of California, Yountville. Oct. 11, 1984.

Parsons, T. 1958. Definition of health and illness in the light of American values and social structure. In E. G. Jaco, ed. *Patients, physicians, and illness.* Glenco, Ill.: Free Press. 165–87.

Podolsky, S., and B. El-Beheri. 1980. The principles of a diabetic diet. *Geriatrics* 35 (12):73–78.

Reichel, J. 1978. Pulmonary problems in the elderly. In Reichel, W. ed. *Clinical aspects of aging.* Baltimore: Williams and Wilkins. 85–90.

Rogot, E. 1978. Smoking and life expectancy among U.S. veterans. *Am J Public Health* 68:1023–25.

Rullis, I., J. A. Schaeffer, and O. M. Lillien. 1975. Incidence of prostate carcinoma in the elderly. *Urology* 6:295–97.

Samet, J., W. C. Hunt, and C. Key et al. 1986. Choice of cancer therapy varies with age of patient. *JAMA* 255:3385–3390.

Sklar, M. 1978. Gastrointestinal diseases in the aged. In Reichel, W., ed. *Clinical aspects of aging.* Baltimore: Williams and Wilkins. 173–82.

Speizer, F. E., and I. B. Tager. 1979. Epidemiology of chronic mucous hypersecretion and obstructive airway disease. *Epidemiol Rev* 1:124–42.

Spencer, H., and M. Lender. 1979. The skeletal system. In Rossman, I., ed. *Clinical geriatrics.* Philadelphia: J. B. Lippencott. 460–76.

Strauss, A. L. 1975. *Chronic illness and the quality of life.* St. Louis: C. V. Mosby Co.

Thornberry, O. T., M. A. Wilson, and P.M. Golden. 1986. Health promotion data for the 1990 objectives. *Advance Data from Vital and Health Statistics.* National Center for Health Statistics. Number 126. Sept. 19.

Tunbridge, W. M. G. 1981. Is hyperthyroidism causing your patient's lethargy? *Geriatrics* 36(5): 79–80, 82, 87–88.

U.S. Surgeon General's Report. 1982. *The health consequences of smoking* USDHHS Publ. No. 82–50179. Washington, D.C.: U.S. Govt. Printing Office.

U.S. Surgeon General's Report. 1986. *The health consequences of involuntary smoking.* USDHHS Pub No. 87-8398. Washington D.C.: U.S. Govt. Printing Office.

Urbach, F. 1983. Prevention and treatment of skin cancer in the elderly patient. In Yancik, R. et al. eds. *Perspectives on prevention and treatment of cancer in the elderly.* New York: Raven Press. 181–85.

Vaughn, C. C. 1976. Rehabilitation in post-menopausal osteoporosis. *Israel J Med Sci* 12(7):652–57.

Walsh, P. C., H. Lepor, and J. C. Eggleston. 1983. Radical prostatectomy with preservation of sexual function: Anatomical and pathological considerations. *Prostate* 4:473–85.

Weiss, S. T. 1984. Chronic bronchitis, asthma and obstructive airways disease: Age, smoking and other risk factors. In Bosse, R., and C. L. Rose, eds. *Smoking and aging.* Lexington, Mass.: DC Heath. 73–94.

White, J. R., and H. F. Froeb. 1980. Small airways dysfunction in nonsmokers chronically exposed to cigarette smoke. *N Engl J Med* 302:720–23.

Wolanin, M. O., and B. M. Steffl. 1984. Neurological disorders of the elderly. In Steffl, B. M., ed. *Handbook of gerontological nursing.* New York: Van Nostrand Reinhold. 303–17.

Wynder, E. L., and D. Hoffman. 1982. Tobacco. In Schottenfeld, D. and J. F. Fraumini, eds. *Cancer epidemiology and prevention.* Philadelphia: W. B. Saunders. 277–92.

Yeates, W. K. 1976. Normal and abnormal bladder function in incontinence of urine. In Willington, F. L., ed. *Incontinence and the elderly.* New York: Academic Press.

Acute Illnesses and Accidents

6

Flu

Oh, wow Lord
This flu bug, this virus
has hit me hard,
laid me low.
Scares me, too
Because at my age when you get knocked down,
You don't know if you'll ever get up.
Well, nobody ever knows that
Or knows for sure anything's going to happen
All we do know is that a lot of the happening is up to us.

Take my friend Wilhemina Gray,
Broke her hip at eighty, and they say
When you break a hip,
That's I. T. It.
But Billy's up and around walking without a limp.

Introduction

Long-standing chronic illnesses account for the largest proportion of death and disability of elders. However, acute illnesses (primarily influenza and pneumonia), and accidents are also significant. For a number of reasons elders are more likely to suffer severe consequences from accidents and infections than other age groups. Acute illnesses and accidents are also major causes of admissions to hospitals and consequently comprise a high proportion of the health care expenditures for those over sixty-five.

This chapter will address acute illnesses common among older adults, both those that are caused by infection and those that are environmentally-induced (hypothermia and hyperthermia). The chapter will also discuss the common types of accidents among elders, factors that increase accident susceptibility, and accident prevention.

San Francisco police, on duty, during the 1918 influenza epidemic.

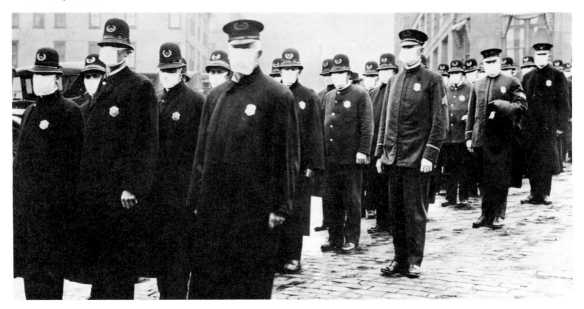

Common Acute Illnesses Among Elders

Elders are generally no more susceptible than younger groups to infections, but they have a higher incidence of sickness and death from several infectious diseases (Yoshikawa 1981). Mortality from pneumonia and influenza are particularly high in the older population and, when taken together, are the fifth leading cause of death in that group. Elders are at triple the risk of nosocomial (hospital-acquired) infection as compared with the general population—12 percent vs. 4 percent (Freeman and McGowan 1978).

A number of factors place older people at a higher risk of debilitation from common infections. Age-associated physiological decrements increase susceptibility to viral or bacterial invasion. For instance, diminished pulmonary function, especially the ability of the lung to clear foreign matter, increases the likelihood of pneumonia and other respiratory tract infections. Changes in the skin, such as decreased vascularization, less subcutaneous fat, and thinning of the skin make elders susceptible to skin and wound infections.

The high prevalence of chronic illness among elders plays a role in their high rate of acute illnesses and accidents. A number of chronic diseases predispose elders to infections. For example, chronic bronchitis increases susceptibility to pneumonia and other respiratory infections. Those with diabetes are more likely to develop infected foot ulcers. Urogenital disorders make one more susceptible to urinary infections. Chronic disease may also indirectly increase the presence of infection. Some instruments used to treat chronic illnesses (e.g., catheters, intravenous equipment) predispose the user to infections. Some drugs lower resistance to infection. The immobility caused by some chronic illnesses can predispose individuals to urinary tract infections, pneumonia, and decubitus ulcers. Finally, if a chronic disease is present, the ill person is likely to become more debilitated and take longer to get well than those others who do not have chronic diseases.

Certain environmental factors increase the opportunity for acute illnesses. A hospital or nursing home setting encourages infection because confining many ill people in a small area increases their chances of contracting an infection. It is estimated that at any one point, 20 percent of nursing home residents have an infection acquired within the home. The most common are urinary tract infections and decubitus ulcers (Cohen et al. 1979; Garibaldi et al. 1981). Malnutrition is also thought to lower resistance to infections in all age groups. Extremes of environmental temperatures may cause hypothermia or hyperthermia, especially among those who are frail.

Elders have a higher rate of latent infections. Some types of bacteria or viruses, which have been residing in the body in a latent state for years, suddenly reappear. Tuberculosis and Herpes zoster (shingles) are the most common latent infections among those over fifty.

Diagnosis of acute illnesses is more difficult in elders than other age groups because important warning signs of infection, especially fever and elevated white blood cell count, may be atypical or absent. Those with congestive heart failure and those who take drugs such as aspirin, corticosteroids, or other anti-inflammatory agents are even less likely to develop a fever. In older people, nonspecific symptoms often accompany an infection: confusion, change in mental status, fatigue, appetite loss, decline in performance, or lack of interest in environment. A physician may either misdiagnose or ignore these symptoms, attributing them to age-related decline, drug side effect, or a pre-existing chronic illness. Finally, elders themselves are less likely to report symptoms to their physician, especially if they are vague and not extreme.

Respiratory Infections

Acute respiratory illnesses are more common in elders than the general population. If an elder smokes or is around those who do, the likelihood of contracting a respiratory infection is significantly greater. Those with chronic bronchitis and emphysema are also at increased risk of respiratory infections. Increased susceptibility to respiratory infection is related to age-associated pulmonary conditions that lower pulmonary reserves and increase the impact of disease: less elastic airways and tissues, reduced chest cavity size, and reduced capacity of respiratory muscles. The most obvious mechanism to prevent occurence of respiratory infection is to stop smoking or to reduce the amount of exposure to cigarette smoke. A healthy diet, exercise, sufficient sleep, indoor humidifiers, drinking plenty of fluids, and avoiding those with a respiratory infection are other mechanisms to prevent these illnesses.

Common Cold

The common cold is responsible for over half the acute illnesses in the general population in the United States. Since over two hundred types of viruses have been identified to cause the common cold, it is difficult to develop a vaccine to prevent it. Even though there is no cure for the common cold, more than a billion dollars is spent annually on cold remedies to relieve its symptoms.

The common cold is a viral infection of the cells that line the nose and throat. In response to the virus, the mucous membranes lining the respiratory passages secrete large amounts of fluids. The most common symptoms of a cold are nasal congestion, runny nose, scratchy or sore throat, sneezing and coughing.

Symptoms of a cold develop from one to three days after infection occurs. Stress, poor general health, lack of sleep, and smoking predispose one to a cold. After infection, one is immune to that particular rhinovirus for three to four months, but another cold can develop from a different virus. Rest, drinking plenty of fluids, and drugs for symptom relief are generally recommended to treat a cold. Aspirin is no longer recommended because it reduces the fever, which may serve a part in the body's defense against the virus. Although controversial, some studies indicate that vitamin C as a preventive reduces both the duration and symptoms of the common cold (for a review, see Pauling 1986). Zinc gluconate lozenges have been reported to significantly reduce the duration of the common cold (Eby et al. 1984).

In the adult years, the likelihood of contracting a cold is reduced and they become milder in nature due to increased immunity (Lamy 1980). However, in elders, a cold is more likely to lead to more serious complications, such as sinusitis, ear infections, acute bronchitis, and pneumonia. Signs of secondary infection that require physician care are an extended fever, a bloody discharge from the nose or mouth, recurring chest pains, persistent cough, earache, sinus congestion, or sore throat.

Influenza

Influenza, commonly called the flu, is a viral infection of the respiratory tract. Three types have been identified: A, B, and C. Type A influenza, generally the most severe and debilitating, was responsible for five world-wide epidemics. The largest, in 1918, killed about 65,000 people (mostly the very old and very young) from pneumonia, a chief complication. Type B causes symptoms similar to Type A, but they are usually less severe. Type C is very similar in symptoms and treatment to the common cold.

Although elders are less likely to contract influenza than younger people, the mortality among those over age sixty-five is much higher. This increased mortality is attributed to the fact that the flu lowers elders' resistance to more serious infections, usually pneumonia. Elders are more likely to have heart disease, emphysema, bronchitis, kidney disease, and diabetes than younger groups, so they are at high risk of developing secondary infections after a bout with influenza. Symptoms are sudden onset of high fever, headache, severe muscle aches, chills, loss of appetite, and total prostration for several days.

The symptoms of influenza are generally treated similarly to the common cold. In addition, Symmetral (amantodine) is a safe, powerful and useful drug to prevent and treat all influenza infections. It can be taken in small doses to prevent the flu when it is known to be in the community, or a larger dose may be taken to reduce the duration and intensity of the flu once the symptoms are noticed (Graedon and Graedon 1986). Because of the high death rate of Type A influenza, those over sixty-five, those with chronic illness, and the institutionalized are advised to be vaccinated annually during the fall. The immunity lasts for a year and the vaccine seldom causes side effects.

Pneumonia

Both the incidence and mortality from pneumonia increase with advancing age. Together pneumonia and influenza are the fifth leading cause of death among those over sixty-five. Although the advent of antibiotics has significantly decreased the death rate from pneumonia among the young, it has not in elders.

Pneumonia is an infection of the lung alveoli and in older people is generally caused by a bacteria. Pneumonia usually begins with a colonization of bacteria in the back of the throat that is not cleared by normal respiratory mechanisms. Immobile individuals are at particularly high risk for this reason. Other reasons for reduced pulmonary defenses may be smoking, chronic illnesses (especially respiratory), and malnutrition. Pneumonia is frequently a complication of heart failure, stroke, and surgery. Hospitalization itself places one at higher risk because of increased exposure to bacteria.

The usual symptoms of pneumonia include fever, chills, productive cough, and chest pain. However, older people may not exhibit respiratory symptoms, only mental confusion, weakness, or congestive heart failure. Antibiotic therapy is used to treat pneumonia after determining the type of bacteria from blood, lung fluid, or lung tissue. As noted by the mortality incidence, drugs are not always effective. A vaccine to protect against pneumonia is available, but has been more successful in the young and middle aged than the elderly. It used to be recommended only for elders at high risk for pneumonia complications (those with kidney, lung, or heart disease, diabetics, and alcoholics). However, a recent study of high risk individuals over fifty showed that those given the vaccine were no more protected from pneumonia than those given a placebo (inert substance) (Simberkoff 1986).

A particular threat to elders is aspiration pneumonia, which develops when oral secretions, gastric contents, or food is aspirated into the lungs. This type of pneumonia is more likely to occur among the bedridden, those with chronic illnesses (e.g., Parkinson's disease, stroke, and Alzheimer's disease), the semiconscious or sedated, and those fed with a nasogastric tube. The seriousness of aspiration pneumonia depends on what is aspirated, but can result in lesions on the lungs, bacterial infection, or suffocation. As a preventive measure, those who are bed-bound should be positioned to avoid aspiration of secretions and should not be prescribed drugs that depress respiration or produce sedation.

Gastrointestinal Illnesses

Gastrointestinal symptoms such as indigestion, abdominal pain, heartburn, and gas are very common in older adults. Eating highly processed foods, overeating, sedentary life-style, drug use, emotional upset, and tooth loss are major causes or contributing factors to the common digestive complaints. Identifying their source and embarking on a cure is usually not easy. Some common symptoms can be addressed with over-the-counter medications. Other symptoms may be serious (cancer or appendicitis). All symptoms should be assessed before they are dismissed as insignificant. The most common acute illnesses of the gastrointestinal system are periodontal disease, appendicitis, and diverticulitis.

Periodontal Disease

Periodontal (gum) disease is a common, nonfatal disease that affects all age groups, but predominantly elders. It has been estimated that about 15 percent of elders in the United States require treatment for periodontal disease (Pearlman 1981). Periodontal disease is the primary cause of tooth loss among middle-age and older adults. In the United States, almost half the population over age sixty-five have lost all their teeth (Baum 1985). Periodontal disease is a chronic bacterial infection of the gum tissue that can eventually destroy the roots of the teeth and even the supporting jawbone. Bacteria collect at the meeting of the tooth and gum or other locations and form plaque, a sticky substance composed of food debris and bacteria. If not removed daily, the plaque hardens into calculus and can only be removed by a dental professional. The gum tissue reacts to the calculus with swelling and tenderness.

There are two forms of periodontal disease: gingivitis and periodontitis. The former is a mild, easily reversible inflammation, swelling, and sometimes bleeding of gum tissue around one or more teeth. In contrast, periodontitis is more destructive. The gums gradually become detached from the teeth, and pockets develop. As the gums recede, some of the roots of the teeth are exposed. Eventually the connective tissue fibers that fasten the teeth to bone are destroyed. Much of the bone socket disintegrates, loosening and eventually destroying the tooth. Those who smoke are at increased risk of periodontal disease.

It is now believed that gingivitis does not always lead to periodontitis. It is estimated that most people have gingivitis, but only about 20 percent of the population gets periodontitis. However, early stage periodontitis is hard to diagnose. One expert recommends that scrapings from the bacterial pockets be placed under the microscope to determine the extent of infection. The treatment for periodontitis is the removal of calculus and irrigation of the infected pockets with antibiotics. Although not a proven preventive against periodontitis, dentists recommend regular removal of calculus by a dental professional, flossing, and tooth-brushing to prevent gum disease. Keyes, a dental researcher, recommends brushing with baking soda and rinsing between the teeth with an irrigating device. (Napoli 1986). However, many elders are unable to brush their own teeth or are unconvinced of its value. Institutionalized elders may not have assistance with daily dental hygiene or access to a dentist. Dental professionals seldom make home or institutional visits for preventive dental care.

The condition of the oral cavity is vital to physical and mental health as it affects appearance, the ability to communicate, and the ability to chew. The number of elders retaining their natural teeth is likely to increase in the future because of water fluoridation, improvement in oral hygiene, health education, and improvement in dental procedures. If Medicare included dental coverage, the number might increase further. Currently, many elders do not seek professional dental care because of lack of funds.

Appendicitis

Appendicitis is caused by a bacterial infection within the appendix, a small pouch located at the beginning of the large intestine. The disease usually progresses rapidly. If surgery is not accomplished promptly, the appendix may rupture, causing life-threatening complications. Although elders are less likely to have appendicitis than younger age groups, they have a higher mortality and complication rate (Rosenthal and Andersen 1985).

Appendicitis may be more dangerous in elders, not because of age, but because of delay in diagnosis and treatment. Researchers differ regarding the usual signs of appendicitis among elders. Some believe that fever and abdominal pain are less likely to be present while others find no difference in symptoms with age (Ryden et al. 1983; Villaverde and MacMillan 1980).

Complications are relatively common in the older population. A perforated appendix may occur in as many as 60 percent of appendicitis cases, prolonging the hospital stay. One report found one-third of those over sixty-five had postoperative wound infections. Other complications noted were increased incidence of blood clots, pneumonia, and heart attack (Ryden et al. 1983).

Diverticulitis

Diverticulitis is characterized by an inflammation of the diverticuli, small indentations in the mucous membrane in the wall of the colon. Elders often develop these diverticuli with age; however, they cause no problems until they become infected. About one-fourth of those who have diverticuli will develop diverticulitis at some time (Burakoff 1981). The diverticuli become inflamed when they fill with fecal material, irritating the mucous lining. Symptoms include abdominal pain or tenderness, diarrhea followed by constipation, and sometimes fever. The usual treatment for mild cases is a liquid diet and stool softeners. When there is marked abdominal pain and fever, antibiotics are indicated. When the inflammation is controlled, fiber is added to the diet to prevent further recurrence.

Urinary Tract Infections

The prevalence of urinary tract infections increases with age and is widespread in some older populations, especially among women. In general, about 10 percent of elder men and 20 percent of elder women living at home have a urinary tract infection. In institutionalized elders, the incidence rises sharply. Depending on the setting, 20 to 35 percent of older men and 25 to 40 percent of older women have urinary tract infections (Kaye 1980), making urinary tract infections the most common hospital-acquired infections (Lye 1978). Elders are at higher risk because they are more likely to have health conditions that predispose them to urinary infections, such as incomplete emptying of the bladder, contamination from fecal incontinence, enlarged prostate, and diabetes. Those who are immobile and who use catheters are at significantly greater risk, which partially explains the high incidence of urinary infections among the institutionalized.

The most common infecting organisms are *E. coli,* bacteria normally residing in the intestinal tract. Most elders exhibit no symptoms with the infection and when they do, they include increased frequency and urgency of urination, pain or burning upon urination, lower abdominal discomfort, and sometimes fever. However, elders may not exhibit these symptoms. Usual drug therapy includes antibiotics or sulfa drugs. A high fluid intake may help to prevent and treat urinary tract infections because it relieves symptoms by diluting the urine and increasing urine flow. However, excessive amounts of water taken with drugs may lower the effectiveness of drug therapy.

Pressure Sores

Decubitus ulcers, also called bedsores or pressure sores, are areas of the skin where soft tissues are progressively destroyed. This tissue destruction is caused by unrelieved pressure that interferes with the blood supply to the skin. If left untreated, bedsores progress rapidly into ulcers that spread into underlying tissues, eventually invading the bone. Pressure sores occur predominantly among those who are immobilized in bed or a wheelchair. The amount of pressure and time needed to produce an ulcer depends on the condition of the individual. Changes in the skin can occur from as little as two hours of pressure on an area. It may begin with a reddened area of the skin, and, if not attended, can progress to a deep cavity of dead tissue that is highly susceptible to infection and ultimately gangrene.

It is generally agreed that the presence of decubitus ulcers in a facility indicates poor care. Nevertheless, incidence is high among immobile, frail elders, despite intensive effort (Rowell and Steffl 1984). Those who are obese, underweight, malnourished, incontinent, diabetic, confused, or highly sedated are also at high risk for bedsores. In the obese, fat tissue does not have many blood vessels, making the skin more susceptible to blood loss. On the other hand, those who are very underweight do not have sufficient fat or muscle to cushion bony protuberances. The localization of bedsores is dependent on whether the person is sitting or lying. The most likely locations for bedsores are on the heel, lower back, knee, pelvis, hip, or buttocks.

A bedsore must be regularly cleaned and given protection so it does not worsen. Antibiotics are usually administered to reduce infection of the sores. A number of types of topical preparations have been used with varying degrees of success. Patients recovering from decubitus ulcers need a high protein diet to supply the body with nutrients to build antibodies and repair tissues.

The best prevention for decubitus ulcers is attentive nursing care. Some institutions determine patients at high risk for decubitus ulcers upon admission and give special attention throughout their stay. The diet should be high in proteins, calories and fluids. The patient should be kept as active as possible, including a walking program, if possible, and range-of-motion exercises. For the bedfast, turning the patient every two hours is imperative. Some experts believe every half hour is needed in some cases (Taylor 1980). Devices to relieve pressure such as sheepskin pads, waterbeds, and foam padding are helpful. Good skin care, including body oils and massages, increase blood flow to the skin.

Latent Infections

A latent infection is one in which bacteria or viruses appear earlier in life, and, after the initial outbreak, remain dormant in the body until stress, trauma, or lowered immunity reactivate the microorganisms. Two latent infections, *Herpes zoster* and tuberculosis, are most common in the older population.

Herpes Zoster (Shingles)

Herpes zoster, or shingles, is a painful viral disease caused by the same virus as chickenpox and only occurs in those who have had chickenpox earlier in life. Shingles may occur among all age groups but most commonly appears in those age fifty and older. Even though most adults carry the latent virus, not everyone gets shingles. It is hypothesized that disease, stress, or lowered immunity may trigger an attack although the majority of affected persons are apparently healthy. The virus remains dormant in the spinal nerves and travels from the nerve to the skin, triggering pain under the skin accompanied by a fever. After four or five days, a rash of small blisters appears, usually on a band clustered on one side of the trunk or face. The blisters last about two weeks, but the pain may remain for months, even years after the outbreak, especially in older people.

For those with mild shingles, talcum powder, calamine lotion, and analgesics are the common treatment. Wet compresses with an aluminum acetate solution several times daily soothe the pain (Fretwell and Lipsky 1985). Elders are often given cortisone to prevent the complication of long-lasting pain after the shingles attack. However, cortisone depresses the immune system and may cause the shingles to spread to other parts of the body. Preliminary studies with the drug acyclovir show it to shorten the period of pain and improve the rate of healing (Fretwell and Lipsky 1985).

Tuberculosis

Tuberculosis is a communicable disease that commonly occurs in the lungs that is caused by a tubercle bacteria. The bacteria is found in the sputum of infected persons and is spread when the bacteria becomes airborne by coughing and sneezing. Tuberculosis is now considered a disease of the elderly because they were initially infected when they were young and the disease was more prevalent.

In those over sixty-five, tuberculosis usually occurs as a reactivation of the primary disease acquired many years earlier. Many elders are likely to have been exposed to the bacteria and developed immunity earlier in life, even though they may not have exhibited symptoms. It is estimated that from 10 to 40 percent of elders have been exposed to the bacteria (Kasik and Schuldt 1977). These tubercle bacteria can remain dormant for many years, reappearing when the individual has decreased resistance.

Symptoms of tuberculosis include fatigue, evening fever, sweating, cough, weight loss, and, in the later stages, chest pain. Although the symptoms of tuberculosis are flu-like, they persist and increase in severity with time. Tuberculosis patients are treated with several drugs that eliminate the bacteria from respiratory secretions and reduce the infectiousness of the disease. Treatment may take from nine to thirty-six months. It is important that infected individuals continue the prescribed drug regimen and have periodic medical evaluations so they can be monitored for treatment effectiveness, drug toxicity, and development of drug-resistant bacteria (Bergersen 1979). Elders can be treated in their own homes as long as family members are under surveillance because the disease is highly infectious.

Environmentally-Induced Acute Illnesses

Body temperature is carefully regulated by a complex mechanism that enables the body to maintain a constant body temperature even when the environment is warm or cold. The normal body temperature fluctuates about two degrees Fahrenheit within a 24-hour period, generally decreasing at night and increasing during daylight hours. This section will discuss hyperthermia (raised body temperature) and hypothermia (lowered body temperature), two emergencies that result when the body temperature lies outside the normal range. Both hyperthermia and hypothermia are more common and more serious in the elder population.

Hyperthermia

Hyperthermia occurs when the body temperature is one-hundred degrees Fahrenheit or more because of infection or high environmental temperatures. Normally, the body cools itself by dilating the surface blood vessels in the skin to increase heat loss and by increasing production of sweat to enable the body to lose heat by its evaporation on the skin. With advancing age, however, the body becomes less able to respond to extended heat exposure. Elders require a higher core body temperature to initiate sweating and less sweat is produced per gland (Fennel and Moore 1973). This may be due to age-related changes in the cardiovascular system or shrinkage of the sweat glands themselves.

The summer of 1980 in the United States was a particularly hot year. Heat stroke rates for those sixty-five and older were reported to be twelve to thirteen times that of the general population (U.S. Dept of Health and Human Services 1981). At highest risk are the frail, chronically ill, users of certain prescription drugs, alcoholics, and those who cannot afford air-conditioning. Deaths from diabetes, respiratory illness, and hypertension have been reported to increase significantly during heat waves, reflecting the stressful effect of high environmental temperature upon those who are already impaired (Schuman 1972). Similarly, an increased rate of hospital admission has been recorded among elders during heat waves (Fish et al. 1985).

The most common heat-related illnesses among elders, especially the frail, are heat stroke and heat exhaustion. *Heat stroke,* a life-threatening emergency, is due to a high internal body temperature caused by the inability to perspire sufficiently. The symptoms are hot, dry, flushed skin, faintness, dizziness, headache, rapid pulse, and body temperature over 104 degrees Fahrenheit. Treatment includes cooling the body by removing outer clothing, using a fan, cool baths, and ice washes. Since the individual needs to be closely monitored during this process, medical personnel should be contacted as soon as possible.

Heat exhaustion is slower in onset and is not life-threatening. It is a result of the pooling of the blood near the skin surface as the body attempts to cool itself. There is a loss of body fluids and salts due to heavy sweating. Weakness, disorientation, lightheadedness, and nausea are common symptoms. Treatment for heat exhaustion includes lowering the body temperature if it is elevated, giving liquids, and encouraging the person to rest away from heat.

To prevent heat-related conditions in hot weather, elders should keep themselves cool, avoid heavy exertion, and get adequate rest. Those who are unable to afford air-conditioning should go to a public place that is air-conditioned to spend the hottest hours of the day. Cool baths, increased ventilation, electric fans, staying out of direct sunlight, drinking plenty of fluids, and dressing in lightweight, breathable clothing will reduce the effects of the heat. Elders need to be aware of the symptoms of heat-related conditions since heat stroke may be fatal.

Hypothermia

The body has two mechanisms to preserve body heat in a cold environment: shivering, and constriction of surface blood vessels. Shivering constricts the muscles to warm the blood that circulates to the internal core to protect vital organs. The constriction of surface blood vessels conserves heat loss at the body surface. With advancing age, these mechanisms are less efficient; many elders lose their sensitivity to cold or become less able to respond to the stress of extreme cold. Accidental hypothermia occurs when the body temperature drops below 95 degrees Fahrenheit because of exposure to environmental cold without sufficient protection. Hypothermia may occur after exposure to even mildly cool temperatures. For elders, hypothermia may occur indoors at temperatures between fifty and sixty-five degrees Fahrenheit over an extended period of time (Besdine and Harris 1985).

While a cold environment can be harmful at any age, it is especially hazardous for the old: nearly half the victims of hypothermia are elderly. For all ages, the death rate of hypothermia is 40 percent, but those age seventy-five and older are five times more likely to die than those who are younger (Rango 1980). Elders who live alone, are frail, are too poor to afford heat, and are taking drugs that interfere with thermoregulation are at highest risk of hypothermia. Experts believe the incidence of hypothermia is underreported. Its symptoms mimic those of other disorders and elders who die of hypothermia often manifest a number of other chronic conditions that are more likely to be listed as the cause of death.

Hypothermia takes a few days to develop. When body temperature is reduced, the metabolic rate decreases, heart rate slows, pulse weakens, there is decreased blood flow to the brain, reflexes are slowed, and elders may become confused, feel drowsy, or fall into a coma. Those with hypothermia often shiver uncontrollably, have a slow, irregular heartbeat, slurred speech, slow shallow breathing, and lack of coordination. The victim may not complain about feeling cold. The signs of hypothermia can be confused with those of a stroke, diabetic coma, heart attack, or other conditions.

Treatment of victims of accidental hypothermia involves warming their core body temperature with hot water bottles, electric blankets, or another's body heat. If conscious, warm fluids should be administered. If unconscious, the head should be lowered and feet raised to prevent shock. Upon hospitalization, sometimes transfusions of warm blood are administered. The most serious problem during hypothermia and rewarming of the body is ventricular fibrillation, a form of irregular heartbeat that can lead to death. The chances of recovery depend on the severity and length of exposure and previous general health. Hypothermia can worsen pre-existing chronic conditions such as heart disease and diabetes. Serious hypothermia can cause kidney, liver, and pancreas damage or death.

Hypothermia can be prevented by keeping the house warm, using an electric blanket, practicing good nutrition, and keeping active. Elders should be encouraged to dress warmly in cold weather, even if they don't feel cold, and to wear a hat outdoors. For the poor, financial support for home weatherization programs and fuel costs would likely reduce the incidence of hypothermia.

Accidents

Accidents are the seventh leading cause of death among elders. Even though elders constitute 12 percent of the total population, they comprise 36 percent of all accidental deaths (National Center for Health Statistics 1986). Elders are more apt to become injured during an accident, their injuries are more apt to be serious, and they take longer to heal than younger groups. Older accident victims remain in the hospital significantly longer than their younger counterparts. Many elders are repeatedly admitted to hospitals after the first accident (Catchen 1983). Accidents are responsible for a significant proportion of hospital care expenses. The average length of hospital stay for accident victims over age sixty-five is longer than for most diseases. The consequences of accidents may be increased dependence, permanent physical damage, institutionalization, and death. In some cases, there may be no physical effect, but self confidence is reduced, causing excessive cautiousness because of the fear of a future accident.

Even though the risk of injury or death due to accidents increases with advanced age, chronological age itself is not the cause. Age-associated physiological deficits in vision, hearing, muscular strength, and coordination play a role, as do drug side effects, symptoms of some chronic health problems, and psychological factors. The following pages will explore the multiple factors that make elders susceptible to accidents and the types of accidents most common in elders. As accidents are often a signal of a more serious problem, appropriate assessment after an accident to determine an underlying cause will also be discussed. Finally, methods to reduce accidents will be addressed.

Factors Increasing Accident Susceptibility

Contrary to popular opinion, an accident is not due to fate, chance, or luck, but a combination of individual susceptibility and environmental hazards that predispose one to an accident. The following paragraphs will describe the multiplicity of factors that promote accidents in elders.

Although the effects of aging vary considerably among elders, there is a general decline in the neurosensory system that reduces awareness of environmental hazards. Age- and disease-associated visual decrements increase accident susceptibility. One small study compared a group of elders living at home who fell with a similar group who did not fall. The group of elders who fell were reported to have significantly poorer visual acuity (Wilder-Smith and Thorpe 1981). Auditory deficits, commonly experienced among elders, may result in failure to recognize signs of an impending accident. Temperature and pain receptors in the skin are not as efficient in many elders, increasing the possibility of scalding and hypothermia.

Circulatory disorders among elders can temporarily impair blood flow to the brain causing transient lightheadedness, which increases accident susceptibility. Orthostatic hypotension results from a temporary loss of blood flow to the brain as the blood pools in the lower extremities when one moves rapidly from a supine or sitting position to an upright position. It is believed that orthostatic hypotension occurs in 20–30 percent of elders living at home. This dizziness is compounded in some elders who have inner ear disturbances or problems in visual perception that reduce the ability to maintain balance. Fainting is also common among elders with metabolic problems, such as diabetes. Small strokes and abnormal cardiac rhythms also affect circulation of blood to the brain, increasing the risk of falls and other accidents. Because diabetics have reduced blood flow to their extremities, they have reduced pain and pressure sensation in their feet which increases accident susceptibility.

Diseases of the central nervous system also increase accident risk. For instance, those with organic brain disorders may experience disorientation, memory loss, poor judgement, poor comprehension, or emotional imbalances that affect awareness and appropriate response to the environment.

Musculoskeletal diseases and disorders increase accident susceptibility. For instance, a seemingly minor fall can result in a major fracture because of the excessive bone loss of osteoporosis. Arthritis can reduce joint flexibility so

that when balance is lost, it is difficult to recover quickly enough to avert a fall. Many elders complain of drop attacks—a sudden weakness in the legs without specific cause—that precedes a fall. Consciousness is not lost with a drop attack, but it may take some time for the muscles to regain their power. Drop attacks may be associated with anemia, postural hypotension, irregular heartbeat, or small strokes. One report estimated that drop attacks accounted for one-fourth of all falls among elders (Sheldon 1960).

Individuals with gait disturbances are more susceptible to accidents, especially falls. The usual gait of some elders—stooped posture and shuffling walk—makes them more susceptible to tripping and falls and decreases their ability to catch themselves when they begin to fall. One report measured the gait of a group of elders admitted to the hospital after a fall and reported it to be more abnormal than other groups (Guimaraes and Isaacs 1980). Many elders have an increased body sway, further increasing the tendency to fall. Not surprisingly, these limitations are most common in the very old and frail. Many musculoskeletal diseases cause gait disturbances that increase the likelihood of accidents (e.g., arthritis, Parkinson's disease). Those relying on walking aids, such as canes and walkers, are even more susceptible to accidents (Sobel and McCart 1983).

Problems in walking may be due to foot problems. The American Podiatry Association estimates that about 80 percent of the population over fifty has at least one foot condition, occurring more commonly in women than men (89 percent vs. 61 percent). Only one-third of those with problems seek medical care (Schank 1977). Those with sore or deformed feet are more likely to wear loose-fitting shoes or floppy slippers that create an added risk. Poorly fitting shoes can unbalance an elder and also cause gait disturbances. Some with aching feet may go barefoot, encouraging cuts, bruises, and broken toes.

Drug side effects increase the likelihood of accidents. Psychotropic drugs, such as phenothiazine and other tranquilizers, produce drowsiness, lethargy, and reduce awareness of

Proper foot care may make the difference between dependence and independence.

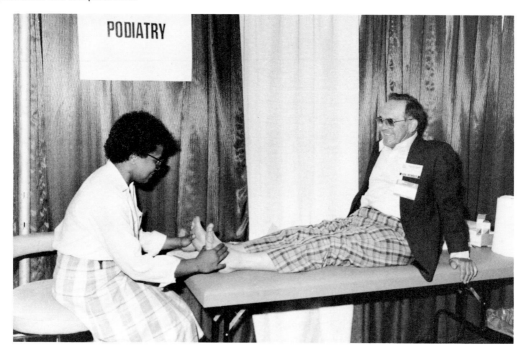

environmental hazards. Antidepressants have a sedative effect, decreasing reaction time and awareness of surroundings. One large controlled study of elders indicated that long-acting antianxiety, antidepressant, and antipsychotic medications increased risk of falls and hip fractures in that population. The risk increased with higher dosages. Although the results do not prove that such drugs directly cause falls and hip fractures, the sedative effect of confusion, drowsiness, loss of muscle coordination can be dangerous (Ray et al. 1987). Both barbiturates and alcohol are an important cause of falls at night and in the hangover period the following morning because they commonly produce drowsiness, and distortion of judgement and motor skill. A number of drugs may induce postural hypotension and consequent dizziness and possible falls: diuretics, sedatives, antidepressants, and hypoglycemics. Feist (1978)

investigated falls in one nursing home and reported that 80 percent of those who fell were undergoing drug therapy.

Undernutrition may also be a factor increasing accident susceptibility. Bastow and colleagues (1983) studied 744 elderly women admitted to the hospital in midwinter with a fractured hip. Those who were very thin had seven times the risk of fractures than those who were well-nourished. Further, 70 percent of the accidents among the well-nourished occurred outside in mid-winter while outdoor accidents were not an important variable in the very thin (only 19 percent of these cases occurred outside). The core body temperature upon hospital admission was significantly lower in those who were very thin as compared with the well-nourished. The researchers hypothesized that thinness or undernutrition itself impairs thermoregulation, increasing the risk of hypothermia, lack of co-ordination, and accidents. The study also reported that thinness increased death rate after an accident; those who were very thin had a mortality rate during the hospital stay of 18 percent as compared with 8 percent who were thin and 4.4 percent who were well-nourished.

Psychological status affects accident susceptibility; transient or chronic emotional illness can place a person at risk. Any illness, regardless of symptoms, tends to cause apathy and a detachment from the environment. Preoccupation with illness reduces alertness and decreases self-care, which increases accident susceptibility. Depression retards psychomotor function so that the ability to think and react to the environment are too slow to enable the depressed or apathetic person to avoid danger. Some mental illnesses make an individual oblivious to the reality of the surroundings, resulting in poor judgement.

Accidents are more likely to occur during or after periods of transient emotional stress. When individuals are temporarily tense, angry, anxious, frightened, or disappointed, they are preoccupied with emotions and less alert to danger. Further, in an intense emotional state, the ability to respond to danger is temporarily impaired. An elder who is usually cautious may become accident-prone under the stress of loss and grief. Repeated falls, scalds, or other accidents may be indicative of psychological distress.

Some experts believe that unconscious motivation plays a significant role in some accidents. Lawton (1967) sees some accidents as indifferent suicides—self-destructive events that may result after would-be victims place themselves in hazardous situations beyond their ability to control. Individuals may provoke accidents to satisfy unconscious needs for punishment or sacrifice, or to make restitution for previous acts or wishes. The sense of helplessness in those who are dependent can produce unconscious feelings of rage and fear. These individuals take risks because of the absence of goals and a removal of a strong impulse to live. In less extreme cases, a disabled elder may

not accept the limitations of ability to perform everyday activities and refuse needed assistance, increasing accident risk.

In some cases, a loss of confidence can follow a fall, leading to increased cautiousness and decreased mobility. An elder may restrict activity to the point of social isolation because of fear of accidents. The combination of decreased activity, social isolation, and lack of confidence in personal capabilities lead to a downward spiral of dependency. Many elders who complain of dizziness are often describing the fear of falling and a loss of confidence in walking safely (Overstall 1980). Ironically, overcaution and fear may make elders even more susceptible to accidents.

Some contributors to accident susceptibility can be reduced or eliminated by changing drug dosage or types, correcting vision and hearing impairments, and reducing the symptoms of chronic illness. However, some impairments cannot be corrected and the individual must learn to live with them. In these cases, elders can decrease the number and severity of falls by monitoring and treating medical conditions and learning to adapt to those impairments that cannot be corrected.

Some experts estimate that the number of accidents could be reduced significantly if environmental hazards were eliminated. Unlike the individual factors that increase susceptibility to accidents, environmental hazards are simple to detect and remedy. It is incumbent on those who live and work with elders to perceive those hazards and to correct them to reduce accident risks.

The environmental hazards that account for almost half the falls among elders relate to floors and flooring materials, and stairs (Czaja et al. 1984). The most common floor-related hazards include tripping over the edge of a rug, failure to notice the rug, slipping on scatter rugs and highly waxed floors, and moving from one flooring type to another. Staircases are hazardous because elders often miss the first and last step. This factor, combined with poor lighting, improper handrails and inadequate marking of top and bottom steps make stairs particularly dangerous for elders. However, environmental dangers are rarely a problem for elders who are healthy and active; accidents are usually a combination of individual susceptibility and environmental hazards.

Common Types of Accidents

The majority of accidental deaths among elders occur in the home as falls and on the streets as vehicular and pedestrian accidents, although some occur in hospitals and long-term care settings. From ages sixty-five to seventy-four, accidental deaths are most commonly due to motor vehicles, but among those seventy-five and older, falls are the most common. When both elder groups are combined, falls are the most common and are responsible for three-fourths of all accidental deaths. Vehicular or pedestrian accidents, fires and burns, and choking are responsible for most of the remainder of the accidental deaths among that age group. This section will describe the fre-

quency of each type, and ways to reduce their risk. Table 6.1 summarizes the accident types and frequencies among various age groups.

Falls

Although the incidence of falls among the elderly is high, the majority of falls result in only minor injury and loss of confidence. It is estimated that from one-third to one-half of those elders living at home will fall each year (Perry 1982). However, only one fracture occurs for every one-thousand falls (Nickens 1985). Serious injuries, such as a fracture, usually occur after a series of falls in which the fear of falling and tendency to fall has already been noted. Seldom do falls result in an injury among those who are otherwise healthy; usually the individual is already ill. Still, some falls are very serious. The rate of death and severe injury after a fall increases dramatically after age seventy-five. Falls and fractures among older people tend to be followed by declining

---

Table 6.1	Accidental deaths by age, sex, and type, 1983									
Age and Sex	All Types	Motor-vehicle	Falls	Drown-ing	Fires, Burns	Ingest. of Food, Object	Fire-arms	Poison (Solid, Liquid)	Poison by Gas	% Male All Types
All Ages	**92,488**	**44,452**	**12,024**	**6,353**	**5,028**	**3,387**	**1,695**	**3,382**	**1,251**	**69%**
Under 5	3,999	1,233	162	750	752	301	40	55	33	60%
5 to 14	4,321	2,241	70	711	422	54	203	22	34	68%
15 to 24	19,756	14,289	406	1,661	410	100	544	438	285	78%
25 to 44	24,996	14,323	1,021	1,897	987	358	562	1,743	425	79%
45 to 64	15,444	6,690	1,708	826	974	693	229	654	262	72%
65 to 74	8,336	2,287	1,656	264	603	609	69	205	98	61%
75 & over	15,636	2,849	7,001	244	880	1,272	48	265	114	46%
Male	**63,902**	**31,907**	**6,279**	**5,342**	**3,066**	**1,931**	**1,465**	**2,193**	**895**	
Female	**28,586**	**12,545**	**5,745**	**1,011**	**1,962**	**1,456**	**230**	**1,189**	**356**	
Per cent male	69%	72%	52%	84%	61%	57%	86%	65%	72%	

Figures from National Center for Health Statistics and National Safety Council. Table reproduced from *Accident Facts, 1986 Edition* from National Safety Council. Reprinted by permission.

health, decreased mobility, and in some cases, by bedrest, sedation, restraint, further dependency, and immobility.

Factors other than the trauma of the fall itself may debilitate elders. The psychological aftermath of a fall can alter behavior and lengthen recovery time. Murphey and Isaacs (1982) evaluated elder patients after a fall and recorded a post-fall syndrome that was correlated with a higher rate of re-hospitalization and mortality. This syndrome included a tendency to clutch and grasp and an inability to walk unsupported. It is unclear whether these behaviors are physiological disturbances in gait or balance or a psychological reaction to falling. Another study followed a sample of elders living in the community who fell. Although most elders who fell had only trivial injuries, some of those elders had a mortality rate five times higher than the general elder population. Of those who lay on the floor for more than an hour before being found, half died, even though their injuries were no worse than the others (Wild et al. 1981). Again, it is unclear whether these increased mortality rates are due to disease or psychological reaction to the fall. Repeated falls, whether or not accompanied by injury, are a common reason for admission into long-term care facilities (Rubenstein 1983).

Institutionalization does not decrease the risk of falling. In fact, severe falls are much more common among the institutionalized than those living at home. Those who are institutionalized are at higher risk because they are likely to have mobility problems, underlying illness, drug use, and confusion and disorientation due to an unfamiliar setting (Snipes 1982). The use of restraints to protect elders from harm may be counterproductive. They may create accidents because they are improperly fitted or the act of restraining itself may cause agitation of the patient.

Berry and colleagues (1981) reported that most accidents in nursing homes occurred during waking hours, and the activity promoting the most accidents was getting in and out of a bed or

Accidents among the institutionalized are most likely to occur when residents attempt to get in and out of wheelchairs.

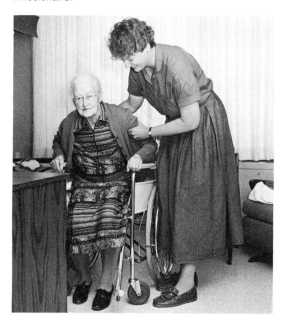

wheelchair or getting on or off the toilet. The authors stressed that the indiscriminate use of wheelchairs as a convenience for caretakers should be discouraged and staff and patients should be trained in the use of all assistive devices to ensure maximal safety.

Perhaps the best way to reduce accidents among institutionalized elders is to restore their function and release them as fast as possible. Minimizing drug dosages, using night lights, and orienting the newly admitted patient to the hospital environment are also helpful. Even though those who fall in institutions have a low death and injury rate, there is often significant immobility, prolonged institutional stay, and the patient and family may be demoralized by the event.

The Public Health Service estimates that two-thirds of all deaths due to falls are preventable. There are many ways that older people, their families and professionals can reduce falls in the home.

Steps to Reduce Falls in the Home

1. Illuminate all stairways and other danger areas inside and outside the home.

2. Provide convenient light switches at each end of the hall, by the bed, and at the top and bottom of stairs. Use nightlights in bedrooms, halls, and bathrooms.

3. Install handrails on stairs and place non-slip treads or carpeting on all stairways.

4. Carry only small loads on stairs to keep one hand free for handrail.

5. Keep stairways, halls, and traffic paths through rooms clear of obstacles such as lamp cords, low furniture, and clutter.

6. Use tape or paint to mark one step elevations, high thresholds at doorways, and top and bottom stair steps.

7. Do not use throw rugs unless they are firmly tacked down or have non-skid backing. Repair frayed, worn, or loose edges on carpet and other floor coverings. If the ends curl, fasten down with carpet tape or tacks. Eliminate torn carpet, broken linoleum, and loose stair treads.

8. Use no wax or non-skid wax on floors.

9. Wipe up all spills immediately.

10. Don't wear trailing bathrobes or loose-fitting slippers and shoes. Wearing socks or stockings without shoes also increases susceptibility to falls.

11. Install grab bars and hand grips in shower, bath, and near toilets. Use adhesive strips or rubber mats in shower and bath. If needed, use a bench or stool with rubberized seat for bathing.

12. Adjust height of beds and chairs to ease entry and exit.

13. Use only step stools or ladders in good repair. Reach no more than 12 inches from the ladder. Do not use a makeshift substitute, such as a chair.

14. Fill holes in yard and patch cracks and holes in outdoor walkways. Use non-skid paint or carpeting on outdoor steps. If rainy and snowy, remove wet leaves, snow, and ice from steps and walk.

Motor Vehicle Accidents

Motor vehicle accidents are the primary cause of accidents of elders from sixty-five to seventy-four (National Safety Council 1986). The major cause of vehicular accidents among elders is due to error in perception, judgement, and response time. Further, overcautiousness, not speeding, is more apt to be a cause among this age group.

A number of physiological factors can predispose older people to vehicular accidents. Arthritis and osteoporosis make it more difficult to turn the head to directly note traffic patterns. The effects of prescription drugs may cause confusion, drowsiness, and impaired reflexes, consequently reducing driving skill. Vision deficits—susceptibility to glare, poorer adaptation to dark, and blurred vision—also affect driving capability.

Motor vehicle accidents can be reduced in the older population if elders learn to compensate for those decrements by driving fewer miles, using public transportation, and driving less during bad weather, rush hour, and in the dark. It is also important to refrain from driving when under the influence of drugs that interfere with perception and reaction time. Updating knowledge on the current driving rules might also increase confidence and reduce accidents. The American Association for Retired Persons (AARP) distributes an educational program for drivers over fifty-five (1909 K Street, N.W., Washington, DC 20049).

A physician may have to recommend driving limitations to protect the elder as well as other drivers and pedestrians. Limitations such as driving only in town, during non-rush hours, and during the day may be a reasonable compromise for many. This issue is very touchy because serious psycho-social consequences may result when an individual is no longer able to drive.

Pedestrian Accidents

Death rates for pedestrians struck by vehicles increase after middle age. Elders account for one-fifth of all pedestrian fatalities. Not only are elder pedestrians more likely to be involved in a pedestrian accident, but they also run a greater risk

---

Driving

I'm not as young as I'd like to be but
I've got my health
My eyesight
Most of my marbles
and an old rattletrap of a car.
I'm so glad I can still drive.
Days on end, the old jalopy sits in the driveway
And I don't go anywhere,
But just knowing I could
Feels good . . .

---

of dying from it. Their injuries are more serious because the bones of an elder are more likely to break and their wounds take longer to heal than their younger counterparts. The death rates for pedestrians living in downtown areas are greatest and progressively lessen in less populated living environments (Allard 1982).

Although older pedestrians are generally more cautious than younger groups, hearing and vision impairments, gait problems, and other disabilities increase their susceptibility to pedestrian accidents. For example, they are less able to recognize the speed and distance of oncoming vehicles. Seventy percent of elder pedestrian accidents occur at an intersection in a crosswalk. The brief duration of the green light often deters the ability of slow-moving elders to safely cross the street. Difficulty in ascending and descending street curbs also increases pedestrian accident risk. The lack of extra energy to run out of harm's way increases with those who are old. Most fatal pedestrian accidents among older people happen in early evening. Whether it is because the driver is unable to see the older pedestrian or vice versa is not clear. However, the pedestrian may be at

Those who are disabled are at higher risk for pedestrian accidents.

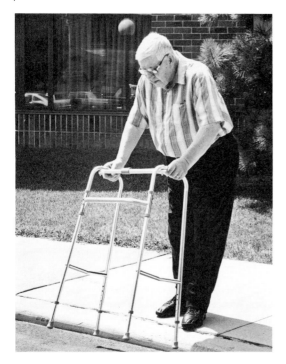

fault in some cases. A significant number of elder pedestrian deaths and injuries occur after the pedestrian has violated a traffic law or done something unsafe. There are many ways to reduce pedestrian accidents.

Communities can reduce the incidence of pedestrian accidents by lengthening the walk phase of signals at crosswalks, especially in areas heavily used by elders. Eliminating curbs at crosswalks by installing ramps would eliminate a common pedestrian hazard. Further, when streets have safety islands in the middle of the road, especially on a multi-lane road, pedestrians can cross the street in two stops instead of one.

Fires and Burns

Accidents due to fire and burns are not nearly as common as falls among elders, but when they occur, they are more likely to cause serious injury or death. Most deaths from fire are caused indirectly: about four-fifths are due to smoke and gas inhalation and one-fifth are due to panic and burns. Careless personal behaviors (e.g., leaving lighted cigarettes untended) are the primary causes of fire accidents. Cooking accidents are the second most common cause of fire-related accidents.

When a fire occurs, elders, especially those who are frail, may not be able to respond quickly and with agility. Often they are living alone and have no assistance in perceiving danger or getting to safety. Sometimes, elders are trapped in their homes because they have installed multiple locks that are difficult to open when an emergency arises. The risk of accidents from fires and burns can be reduced by installing smoke detectors and devising a fire escape plan.

Although not as serious, burn injuries due to hot liquids (scalding) are much more common than burns due to fire (Katcher 1981). They account for 40 percent of all cases of hospitalized burn patients (Feck and Baptiste 1979). Elders are particularly vulnerable to scald burns because of their decreased pain and temperature sensation. Many elders, especially those with diabetes or other health problems, soak their feet in warm water then later realize they have severely burned themselves. Water temperature and duration of exposure affect severity of burn. Tap water at 140 degrees Fahrenheit will cause a serious burn after only a few seconds whereas water at 120 degrees will cause the same burn in ten minutes. Almost all scald injuries could be prevented by keeping the temperature of household water between 120–125 degrees Fahrenheit (Katcher 1981).

Respiratory Obstruction

Elders suffer a higher death rate due to breathing obstruction than any other age group. An obstruction (food, vomited matter, mucus, or even water) enters the windpipe instead of the esophagus, subsequently blocking air passages or causing reflex closing of the epiglottis. Perhaps the most common respiratory obstruction among elders is a piece of food that partially or completely blocks air intake. Choking is more likely

Chapter 6

Strategies to Reduce Pedestrian Accidents

1. Wait for a new green light before starting across the street to guarantee plenty of crossing time.

2. Whenever possible, wait to cross with other pedestrians.

3. Look both ways before stepping into a crosswalk, even when the light indicates you may walk.

4. Be alert for drivers who are turning. Before crossing the street, gain their attention by making eye contact.

5. Cross only at intersections. Do not jaywalk and do not walk between parked cars or in front of or behind a stopped bus or truck.

6. Wear reflective or white clothing or reflector patches if out at night, or carry a flashlight.

7. Stand on the curb, not on the street, while waiting to cross.

8. Whenever possible, walk on sidewalks, not on the road. If you must walk on the road, use the left side facing the oncoming traffic.

9. Concentrate on the traffic around you as well as what you are doing and where you are going.

10. If you are on medication or have used alcohol, be wary of their side effects.

11. Do not carry umbrellas or packages in a way that blocks vision or hampers mobility.

among frail elders since difficulty in swallowing is more common among that group. Other factors that contribute to unintentional aspiration of food or fluid into the lungs are overmedication, alcohol intoxication, inappropriate positioning during feeding, poorly fitting dentures, many missing teeth, and emotional excitement.

Typical signs of choking are: victim is unable to speak, grasps the throat, turns pale, then blue. Sometimes people who are choking may show no evidence of distress except they suddenly stop eating and talking, followed by collapse. The act may be misinterpreted as a heart attack. In any case, a choking person will sustain permanent brain damage from lack of oxygen unless the object is removed within four minutes. The safest and easiest first aid procedure for choking is the Heimlich maneuver (Heimlich 1975).

Medical Assessment after an Accident

The first concern of medical personnel after an accident is to look for signs of treatable injury. As soon as the acute problems from the accident are stabilized, it is the responsibility of the physician to explore the circumstances surrounding the accident. Unfortunately, physicians too often make the assumption that accidents are due to old age and merely examine elders for injuries instead of delving into the reasons. As mentioned earlier, accidents often indicate the presence of disease, drug side effects, or other serious conditions. Unfortunately, elders tend to underreport their accidents, especially falls, to physicians and family members, assuming they are due to old age.

The Heimlich Maneuver and Other Means to Assist a Choking Victim.

The most effective first aid for a choking victim is the Heimlich maneuver. The rescuer grasps the choking victim from behind, making a fist with one hand and clasping it with the other hand so that the fist lies thumb side against the victim's upper abdomen. The fist is then pressed sharply into the abdomen just below the sternum with a quick upward thrust. This maneuver can be repeated several times if necessary.

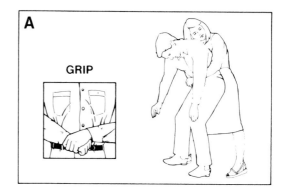

When the respiratory distress is not due to food and the Heimlich maneuver does not work, the rescuer should extend the jaw to partially relieve the obstruction. At the same time the mouth should be freed of mucus or other secretions. If the obstruction still persists, mouth aspiration, in which the rescuer strongly sucks in with direct mouth contact may create a suction sufficient to dislodge the obstruction.

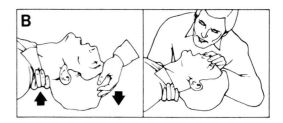

If mouth aspiration is not effective, the person should be placed face down on a table or bed, with the entire body above the waist hanging over the side and should be struck sharply between the shoulder blades.

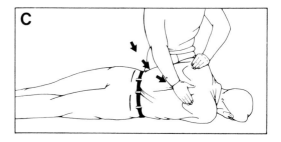

If the victim is sitting, the rescuer simply stands or kneels behind the chair and follows the same procedure. If the victim is found lying on his/her back, the rescuer faces the victim astride the hips, and follows the same procedure outlined above. The rescuer presses with a quick upward thrust on the upper part of the abdomen with the heel of one hand, instead of a fist, but using both hands to exert adequate pressure. This position is good for small or weak rescuers who can use the weight of their own body to apply the thrust of the Heimlich maneuver. This maneuver should not be used if the victim can breathe (Henderson 1978). When one is choking while eating alone, it is necessary to apply force below the diaphragm by pressing against a table, chair, or using the fist.

Although this may possibly move the object further into the windpipe, it is a drastic step that may succeed when other steps failed. If the object is still not dislodged, mouth to mouth respiration should begin, making sure the jaw and head are maximally extended to permit some air past the obstruction. Finally, if these measures fail, a tracheotomy (cutting a temporary opening in the windpipe) is necessary (Henderson 1978).

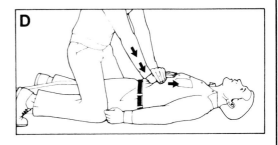

Box Fig. 6.1 Choking strategies. (Source: Fireman's Fund American Life Insurance Company, reprinted with permission).

A careful history of the circumstances surrounding the accident should be taken: What was the person doing at the time? Were physical symptoms present before the accident? What symptoms occurred at the time of the accident? It is seldom easy to determine the circumstances leading up to an accident because elders may be very vague about how it happened, or they may not remember any physical symptoms preceeding it. In falls, many are not willing to disclose how they fell as they may have been doing something dangerous or foolish. If witnesses were present during the episode, they may be questioned so the cause of the accident can be better determined. Questions regarding the presence of environmental hazards should also be asked (Gordon 1982).

A comprehensive physical assessment should be part of the evaluation after an accident. Disorders of vision, hearing, and balance are common correlates of accidents and should be checked. Many chronic and acute illnesses predispose one to falls, so both a physical examination and medical history are necessary. Circulatory problems affecting blood to the brain (hypotension, small stroke, cardiac arrhythmia) are often responsible for a fall. One survey found that 32 percent of institutionalized elders who fell had a cardiac arrhythmia as the primary cause of their falls (Gordon et al. 1982). This is understandable because they commonly cause confusional states, dizzy spells, fainting, and brief neurological disorders. Drug history and current drug regimen should be assessed since drug side effects causing sleepiness, dizziness, weakness, and confusion can increase accident susceptibility.

A home visit can shed light on whether an environmental hazard contributed to the accident. A checklist will enable the assessor to determine the safety of the environment and suggest improvements that reduce accident risks. This is especially important for those who are already frail. If available, family members may be instructed on safety practices, especially if the elder has a history of falls.

Personal susceptibility may be reduced under the guidance of health professionals. Disorders of vision and hearing can be corrected, acute illnesses can be diagnosed and brought under control, the symptoms of chronic illnesses can be reduced, and drug dosages can be altered. Those with balance problems may be directed to exercises that increase balance and instill confidence. Those with gait problems may be prescribed a cane, walker, or wheelchair. Since those who use mobility aids are more susceptible to falls, elders should be instructed in their proper use. The health professional needs to be aware of personality traits, emotional reactions, or periods of emotional disturbance that may lead to accidents and to treat them.

Sometimes the factors that predispose one to future accidents cannot be treated medically. The client and family may need counseling to restore confidence and to reduce the fear of another accident. When a physical limitation cannot be reduced, it is important that the limitation be explained and counseling be initiated to enable the elder to accept the disability and to learn to accomodate to it. Rehabilitation therapists are especially helpful in this regard.

Accident Prevention

There is a great need for both professionals and elders themselves to learn how to prevent accidents. Not only do accidents cause unnecessary deaths, but also those who survive may have serious disabilities and be dependent for the remainder of their lives. Estimates vary, but as many as two-thirds of the accidents occuring among elders may be prevented by treating underlying medical conditions and reducing environmental hazards.

Safety programs for elders and their families and friends need to be implemented to reduce the environmental hazards associated with many accidents. Education is also important for health and social service providers to enable them to recognize environmental hazards and reduce their risks when they visit elders in their homes. The National Safety Council (444 N. Michigan Avenue, Chicago, Ill. 60611) has a number of materials to assist providers in educating elders regarding accident prevention, including a home-safety checklist.

Chapter 6

Family and friends of elders, especially of those living alone, are rightly concerned about safety. However, overprotectiveness can undermine self-confidence and increase overcautiousness which may promote accident susceptibility. Family and friends can assist in accident prevention by eliminating environmental hazards, making daily phone calls or visits, and monitoring drug intake, among others. Some communities have services that make a daily visit or phone call that serves to reduce an elder's fear of falling and not being found for days.

Summary

Although chronic conditions account for the majority of death and disability among elders, acute conditions and accidents remain an important cause of death. For a number of reasons, older people are more likely to suffer severe consequences from accidents and infections than other age groups. A number of factors place elders at higher risk of disability from accident or infection including age-associated physiological decrements, drug side-effects and existing chronic illness. Acute illnesses may be more difficult to diagnose in elders because symptoms may be vague and warning symptoms may be absent. Acute illnesses of elders include respiratory infections (cold, influenza, pneumonia), gastrointestinal conditions (periodontal disease, appendicitis, diverticulitis), urinary tract infection, latent infections (herpes zoster and tuberculosis), and environmentally-induced illnesses (hypothermia and hyperthermia).

Even though elders comprise only 12 percent of the population, they comprise 36 percent of all accidental deaths. Common accidents among elders include falls, vehicular and pedestrian accidents, fires and burns, and respiratory obstruction. Because so many factors can contribute to an accident, it is important that a thorough assessment be conducted to prevent further accidents and to treat underlying conditions. Accident prevention programs may be effective in reducing accident susceptibility among elders.

Activities

1. Last year what was the death rate from accidents among persons sixty-five and older in your state? What about specific accident types? How do death rates among elders differ from those eighteen–sixty-four?
2. What programs in your community reduce accidents among elders (e.g., driver education for those over sixty-five, safety checks of homes)? Compile a list of ways your community could further decrease accidents among elders.
3. Interview a group of elders and a group of younger people about their fear of accidents and how they consciously prevent accidents. Do elders seem to be more preoccupied with avoiding activities that may cause accidents? In your estimation, are some too cautious?
4. Question elders on their knowledge of prevention and treatment of acute illnesses. How do they know whether their condition is severe enough to see a doctor? What methods do they use to prevent or treat minor acute illnesses?
5. Attend a senior nutrition site, senior center, or other places where elders congregate, and look for environmental hazards that may cause falls. Write a letter to the director outlining the problems and suggestions to reduce them.
6. Using a checklist for home safety, assess the safety of your home or that of an older friend (ask permission). Discuss your findings with the occupant.
7. Consider an accident you were involved in within the past two years. What was the cause? How might it have been prevented? Discuss this accident in terms of individual susceptibility and environmental factors.
8. Simulating some of the age changes outlined in the chronic illness chapter (such as putting petroleum jelly over eyeglasses, or using a walker or wheelchair), attempt to cross the street, manipulate curbs, enter

and leave the car and go up or down stairs. Discuss how accidents may happen. When you do this, pair up with a friend to reduce your risk of accidents.

9. Find out how nursing homes cope with patients with colds, flu, or other infectious diseases. How is disease contagion prevented?

10. Find data on severe climatic changes occuring in the United States. What age group suffered the most severely from these temperature extremes? Were all elders at risk or just those with pre-existing health problems?

11. Research the years of major epidemics of influenza and tuberculosis. What age groups were affected most severely? What age-groups of elders still living survived those epidemics?

Bibliography

Allard, R. 1982. Excess mortality from traffic accidents among elderly pedestrians living in the inner city. *Am J Public Health* 72(8):853–54.

Bastow, M. D., J. Rawlings, and S. P. Allison. 1983. Undernutrition, hypothermia and injury in elderly with fractured femur: An injury response to altered metabolism? *Lancet* 8317:143–46.

Baum, B. J. 1985. Alterations in oral function. In R. Andres, E. L. Bierman, and W. R. Hazzard eds. *Principles of geriatric medicine.* San Francisco: McGraw-Hill Book Company. 288–96.

Bergersen, B. S. 1979. *Pharmacology in nursing.* St. Louis: C. V. Mosby.

Berry, G., R. H. Fisher, and S. Lang. 1981. Detrimental incidents, including falls, in an elderly institutional population. *J Am Geriatr Soc* 29(7):273–75.

Besdine, R. W. and T. B. Harris. 1985. Alterations in body temperature (hypothermia and hyperthermia). In R. Andres, E. L. Bierman, W. R. Hazzard, eds. *Principles of geriatric medicine.* San Francisco: McGraw-Hill Book Company. 209–17.

Burakoff, R. 1981. An updated look at diverticular disease. *Geriatrics* 36:83–91.

Catchen, H. 1983. Repeaters: Inpatient accidents among the hospitalized elderly. *Gerontologist* 23(3):273–76.

Cohen, E. D., W. J. Hierholzer, C. R. Schilling, et al. 1979. Nosocomial infection in skilled nursing facilities: A preliminary survey. *Public Health Reports* 94:162–65.

Czaja, S. J., K. Hammond, and C. C. Drury. 1984. A major research project about: Accidents and aging (executive summary). BOSTI, Buffalo, N.Y.

Eby, G. A., D. R. Davis, and W. W. Halcomb. Reduction in duration of common colds by zinc gluconate lozenges in a double-blind study. 1984. *Antimicrob Agents: Chemother* 25(1):20–24.

Feck, G., and M. S. Baptiste. 1979. The epidemiology of burn injury in New York. *Public Health Reports* 94:312–15.

Feist, R. R. 1978. A survey of accidental falls in a small home for the aged. *Gerontol Nurs* 3(6):10–13.

Fennel, W., and R. Moore. 1973. Responses of aged men to passive heating. *J Physiol* 231:18–19.

Fish, P. D., G. C. Bennet, and P. H. Millard. 1985. Heatwave morbidity and mortality in old age. *Age Ageing* 14:243–45.

Freeman, J., and J. E. McGowan. 1978. Risk factors for nosocomial infection. *J Infect Dis* 138:811–19.

Fretwell, M., and B. A. Lipsky. 1985. Infectious agents: The compromised host. In Andres, R., E. L. Bierman, and W. R. Hazzard, eds. *Principles of geriatric medicine.* San Francisco: MacGraw-Hill. 477–506.

Garibaldi, R. A., S. Brodine, S. Matsumiyo. 1981. Infections among patients in nursing homes. *N Engl J Med* 305:731–5.

Gordon, M. 1982. Falls in the elderly: More common, more dangerous. *Geriatrics* 37(4):117–20.

Gordon, M., M. Huang, and C. I. Gryfe. 1982. An evaluation of falls, syncope and dizziness by prolonged ambulatory cardiographic monitoring in a geriatric institutional setting. *J Am Geriatr Soc* 30:6–12.

Graedon, J., and T. Graedon. 1986. Symmetrel for the flu. *Medical Self-Care* 22:15–16.

Guimaraes, R. M., and B. Isaacs. 1980. Characteristics of the gait in old people who fall. *Int Rehabil Med* 2:177–80.

Heimlich, H. J. 1975. A life-saving maneuver to prevent food-choking. *JAMA* 234:398–401.

Henderson, J. 1978. *Emergency medical guide.* San Francisco: McGraw-Hill Book Co.

Kasik, J. E., and S. Schuldt. 1977. Why tuberculosis is still a health problem in the aged. *Geriatrics* 31(3):63–72.

Katcher, M. L. 1981. Scald burns from hot tap water. *JAMA* 246(11):1219–22.

Kaye, D. 1980. Urinary tract infections in the elderly. *Bull NY Acad Med* 56:209–20.

Lamy, P. 1980. *Prescribing for the elderly.* Boston: PSG Pub. Co.

Lawton, A. H. 1967. Accidental injuries to the aged and their psychological impact. *Mayo Clin Proc* 42:685–99.

Lye, M. 1978. Defining and treating urinary infections. *Geriatrics* 33(3):71.

Murphy, J., and B. Isaacs. 1982. The post-fall syndrome. A study of 36 elderly patients. *J Gerontol* 28:265–70.

Napoli, M. 1986. Peridontal disease—a challenge to the standard advice and treatment. *Health Facts* 11(83):1–6.

National Center for Health Statistics. 1986. Advance report of final mortality statistics. *NCHS Monthly Vital Statistics Report* 35(6) Suppl 2, Sept. 26, 1986. 18–19.

National Safety Council. 1986. *Accident Facts,* 444 N. Michigan Dr., Chicago.

Nickens, H. 1985. Intrinsic factors in falling among the elderly. *Arch Intern Med* 145:1089–93.

Overstall, P. W. 1980. Prevention of falls in the elderly. *J Amer Geriatr Soc* 11(28):481–84.

Pauling, L. 1986. *How to live longer and feel better.* New York: W. H. Freeman and Co.

Pearlman, S. 1981. Oral health needs of the elderly: Manpower training and health care delivery system. Prepared for the White House Conference on Aging.

Perry, B. C. 1982. Falls among the elderly: A review of the methods and conclusions of epidemiologic studies. *J Amer Geriatr Soc* 30(6):367–71.

Rango, N. 1980. Old and cold: Hypothermia in the elderly. *Geriatrics* 35(11):93,96.

Ray, W. A., N. P. Griffen, W. Schaffner, et al. 1987. Psychotropic drug use and the risk of hip fracture. *New Engl J Med* 316(7):363–369.

Rosenthal, R. A., and D. K. Anderson. 1985. Surgery in the elderly. In R. Andres, E. L. Bierman, and W. R. Hazzard, eds. *Principles of geriatric medicine.* San Francisco: McGraw-Hill Book Co. 909–32.

Rowell, G. and B. M. Steffl. 1984. Pressure ulcers: prevention and treatment. In Steffl, B. M. ed. *Handbook of gerontological nursing.*

Rubenstein, L. Z. 1983. Falls in the elderly: A clinical approach. *West J Med* 138(2):273–75.

Ryden, C. I., T. Grunditz, and L. Janzon. 1983. Acute appendicitis in patients above and below 60 years of age. *Acta Chir Scand* 149:165–70.

Schank, M. J. 1977. A survey of the well-elderly: Their food problems, practices and needs. *Jour of Ger Nurs* 3(6):10–13.

Schuman, S. 1972. Patterns of urban heat wave deaths and implications for prevention: Data from New York and St. Louis during July 1966. *Environ Res* 5:59–75.

Sheldon, J. H. 1960. On the natural history of falls in old age. *Br Med J* 5214:1685–90.

Simberkoff, M. S., A. P. Cross, M. Al-Ibrahim, et al. 1986. Efficacy of pneumococcal vaccine in high-risk patients. *N Engl J Med* 315(21):1318–27.

Snipes, G. E. 1982. Accidents in the elderly. *Am Fam Physician* 26(1):117–22.

Sobel, K. G. and G. M. McCart. 1983. Drug use and accidental falls in an intermediate care facility. *Drug Intell Clin Pharm* 17:539–42.

Taylor, V. 1980. Decubitus prevention through early assessment. *J Gerontol Nurs* 6(7):389–91.

U.S. Department of Health and Human Services. 1981. Heat stroke—United States, 1980. *Morbidity and Mortality Weekly Report,* Center for Disease Control, Public Health Service, 30:277.

Villaverde, M. M., and C. W. MacMillan. 1980. *Ailments of aging: From symptom to treatment.* New York: Van Nostrand Reinhold.

Wild, D., U. S. L. Nayak, and B. Isaacs. 1981. How dangerous are falls in old people at home? *Br Med J* 282(24 Jan):266–68.

Wilder-Smith, O. H. G., and T. A. S. Thorpe. 1981. Letter in response to "How dangerous are falls in old people at home?" *Br Med J* 282 (27 Jun):2132–33.

Yoshikawa, T. T. 1981. Important infections in elderly persons. *West J Med* 135(6):441–45.

7

Medication Use

This small white pill is what I munch
at breakfast and right after lunch.
I take the pill that's kelly green
before each meal and in between.
Those loganberry-colored pills
I take for early morning chills.
I take the pill with zebra stripes
to cure my early evening gripes.
These orange-tinted ones, of course,
I take to cure my Charley horse.
I take three blues at half past eight
to slow my exhalation rate.
On alternate nights at nine p.m.
I swallow pinkies. Four of them.
The reds, which make my eyebrows strong,
I eat like popcorn all day long.
The speckled browns are what I keep
beside my bed to help me sleep.
This long flat one is what I take
if I should die before I wake.

Dr. Theodore Seuss Giesel (1986)
You're Only Old Once!
Reprinted with permission

Introduction

Many advances of modern medicine have been brought about by the use of drugs to prevent and treat disease. The development of antibiotics to control bacterial infection, vaccines to prevent communicable disease, and drugs to treat the symptoms of chronic illnesses have improved the quality of life for many who would have suffered or died without them. Drugs also rid us of small irritants, such as headaches, itching, minor aches and pains, and constipation. Despite their many benefits, drugs may exacerbate illness or even cause death.

Because they have a high prevalence of chronic illnesses, those over sixty-five consume more medications than any other age group. Both prescription and over-the-counter (OTC) drugs are used and these drugs often must be taken over a period of many years. Drug therapy provides significant benefits in managing chronic illness symptoms that would otherwise impair the quality of life. However, elders are at higher risk of adverse drug reactions than other age groups because of age-related changes in physiology, disease characteristics, and patient factors, and inadequate assessment, education, and supervision of drug therapy by the physician. These issues, as well as a description of common OTC and prescription drugs, adverse drug reactions, and guidelines for promoting rational drug use will be discussed in the following sections.

Older people are more likely to use prescription drugs than any other age group.

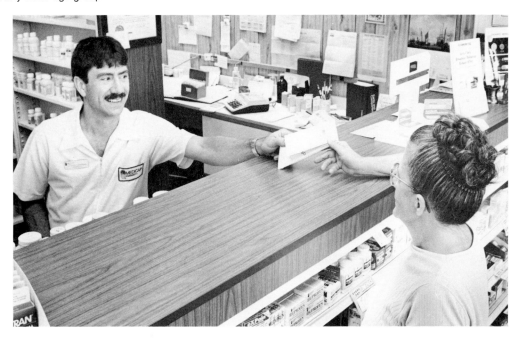

Elder Medication Consumption and Expenditures

Elders in the United States are prescribed more medication than any other age group (Koch and Knapp 1987). Although survey results vary, it is estimated that 57–81 percent of elders living at home take at least one prescription drug (Kasper 1982; Health Care Financing Administration 1982). Because institutionalized elders have more chronic illnesses than those living in the community, their average medication use ranges from three to seven prescriptions taken daily (Kalchthaler et al. 1977). However, institutionalized patients are often prescribed drugs that others purchase over the counter; thus, aspirin, laxatives, and antacids are often counted as part of the total, inflating the figure.

Those sixty-five and over comprise 12 percent of the total United States population, but account for 30 percent of the total drug expenditures. Because Medicare does not cover prescription or OTC drugs purchased by outpatients, elders pay most of the cost from their personal funds (Health Care Financing Administration 1982). Not all elders use medications. Some elders spend very little on medications, while others spend a significant proportion of their income on medicine. For impoverished elders that need them, the high costs of pharmaceuticals may mean a choice between living expenses or needed medication.

Polypharmacy

A medical consumption pattern sometimes seen in elders is polypharmacy, the practice of using medications excessively and unnecessarily. Polypharmacy is common among elders who are taking a number of medications to treat multiple illnesses and encompasses a number of drug-taking behaviors. A person might take the medicine even though there is no health problem. For instance, a medication may be continued for years after the health problem has gone. Duplicate medications may be used simultaneously, creating excessive drug concentrations in the body. Polypharmacy also includes the use of medications that interact with one another, creating either a heightened or reduced drug effect. Those who use drugs to reduce the adverse effects of other drugs, rather than adjusting the dosage or changing the original drug, are practicing polypharmacy. Polypharmacy predisposes an individual to a greater chance of adverse reactions, more health problems, and increased expense of drugs and physicians visits.

Polypharmacy is often instigated by a physician. However, the consumer may also be responsible. Some consumers visit more than one physician without telling one about the drugs prescribed by the others. They may borrow prescriptions from others, hoping to cure themselves without an expensive doctor's visit or pharmacy bill. Or, they may use a number of OTC drugs in addition to their prescribed medication in order to deal with a health problem.

Factors Affecting Medication Use

Our country is afflicted with widespread chemophilia, a love of chemicals. Many people are less concerned with modifying behaviors to prevent disease than with finding a miracle pill to make them feel better. The overflowing medicine cabinets of most households is an example of our country's obsession with drug cure-alls.

Pharmaceutical companies are primarily responsible for this attitude because they successfully promote the idea that there is a 'pill for every ill,' a chemical solution to every physical, emotional, or social problem. Drug companies invest a significant proportion of their profits on advertising to encourage the use of both OTC and prescription drugs. One pharmacist writes that he was able to predict what had been advertised on television the hour before because people came into his store requesting those products. The elderly were prominent among them (Lofholm 1978).

Since pharmaceutical companies must rely on physicians to sell their prescription products, their goal is to maximize their profits by encouraging physicians to write as many prescriptions as possible. The companies advertise heavily in professional journals and send salespeople to inform physicians of their latest products. This is counterproductive to good patient care; a good physician should minimize prescriptions, prescribe non-drug alternatives and, if drugs are necessary, keep the costs as low as possible.

The physician is the primary factor influencing prescription medication use. Elders visit physicians more often than younger groups because they have more health problems. Almost seventy percent of all elders' visits to a physician are associated with the initiation or continuation of at least one prescribed medication, and in 40 percent of all visits, two or more drugs are prescribed or continued (Koch and Knapp 1987). It is logical to infer that the more one visits a physician, the greater the chance of obtaining a prescription.

Physicians vary in their propensity to prescribe drugs, but it is apparent that a few physicians prescribe a large proportion of the drugs. A Drug Enforcement Agency study of 200 physicians found that 25 of them over-prescribed (Jernigan et al. 1980). Another study of 770 general practitioners found that 16 percent of the physicians wrote nearly 75 percent of the prescriptions. Over one-thousand prescriptions were written by 3.5 percent of the physicians, while only two hundred were written by 80 percent of the physicians (Maryland Department of Health and Mental Hygiene 1977).

Physicians' drug-prescribing practices are influenced by past training, attitudes toward elders, and pressure received from patients. Some physicians prescribe the minimum amount of drugs possible and explore alternative treatments—such as lifestyle modification—before prescribing drugs. However, others prescribe drugs as an easy way to conclude a visit when the cause of vague complaints cannot be easily determined. Further, the physician may write a

Impact of Medical Advertising on Prescribing Practices

Scientific papers delivered at physicians' conferences or published in medical journals should determine the physician's drug choices; yet many studies have shown that salespeople and advertising have a greater impact. One such study conducted at Harvard in 1982 had an interesting twist (*Medical World News* 13, September, 1982). Of the primary care physicians polled, 62 percent believed that scientific papers had the strongest influence on their prescribing practices. Yet this survey contained catch questions that enabled investigators to ascertain the differences between the sources physicians *think* determine their drug choices and the sources that *do* determine them.

The two drugs used as markers were Darvon and cerebral vasodilators. The former is a painkiller that has been promoted extensively for fractures and major surgery. However, it was shown in controlled studies to be less effective than a placebo and was highly toxic. The cerebral vasodilators, drugs that dilate the blood vessels to the brain, are advertised to physicians to treat senile dementia, despite the fact that studies show they have no value for this condition.

Although 68 percent of the physicians believed that drug ads had minimal influence on their prescribing habits, results showed otherwise. Half the physicians polled believed that Darvon was a more potent painkiller than aspirin. As for cerebral vasodilators, 32 percent found them "useful in managing confused geriatric patients" and 71 percent incorrectly believed that "impaired cerebral blood flow is a major cause of senile dementia."

Reprinted with permission from *Health Facts,* the monthly newsletter published by the Center for Medical Consumers in New York City, (September, 1985).

Over the counter drugs are commonly used by older people to reduce symptoms of many illnesses.

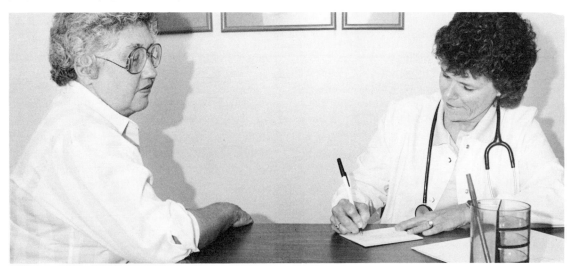

prescription in response to a patient's expectations. Prescriptions are a sign to many that their pain is real and can be helped. Without a prescription, patients may feel the problem is untreatable or their complaints were not taken seriously.

Pharmacokinetics

Pharmacokinetics is the study of what happens to a drug after it enters the body: how it is absorbed into the bloodstream, distributed throughout the body, metabolized, and finally excreted by the kidneys. These pharmacokinetic processes are important in determining optimum drug dosage to maximize benefits and minimize risks. The effectiveness and toxicity of many medications are related to their concentration in the blood. Ideally the amount of drug to be administered is the minimum blood levels to cause a therapeutic effect and subsequent dosages to maintain that effect. However, a number of physiological variables can affect the pharmacokinetics of a drug: age, body weight, kidney function, and presence of disease. Temporary alterations in physiology such as dehydration, vitamin deficiencies, presence of other drugs in the bloodstream, and immobility can also affect drug response.

The high frequency of adverse drug reactions and drug sensitivity in elders has stimulated research on the effects of physiological aging on pharmacokinetics. It has been postulated that the medication dosage needed for a therapeutic effect changes as a person ages because age-associated changes in physiology alter the action of the drug in the body. A simplified overview of the effects of age on drug absorption, distribution, metabolism, and excretion can assist those who work with elders to understand why older people may respond differently to drugs than younger adults.

Age-Changes in Drug Absorption

After ingestion, most drugs are absorbed into the bloodstream from the stomach or small intestine. Injected drugs enter the bloodstream directly. Although a number of changes in the digestive system may accompany aging, pharmacokineticists do not believe significant alterations in the rate and extent of drug absorption occur with age. Digestive diseases or food and other drugs taken at the same time are more likely to affect drug absorption than age changes alone (Vestal 1985).

Age-Changes in Drug Distribution

After medication is absorbed into the bloodstream, it is distributed to body tissues. Cells at the site of action have receptors on their surface that bind chemically with the drug. To be effective, an adequate amount of the drug must be made available at the various sites. This process is complicated by differences in the way the body distributes various drugs. Some drugs dissolve in the blood and are carried that way. However, the majority of drugs are attached to carrier proteins in the blood. Drugs may also be stored in fat or muscle to be released when the blood concentration of the drug declines.

A number of age-related changes cause elders to distribute drugs differently, which ultimately affects the needed dose. Elders generally weigh less than younger adults so appropriate dosages for younger adults may be excessive for elders. In addition, elders generally have more body fat and less body fluid than younger adults. Because many medications are distributed in body fat or body water, changes in these constituents may significantly affect drug distribution. For instance, drugs distributed in body water are more concentrated in elders because they have less body water. Conversely, drugs stored in fatty tissues may last longer in elders because they have more fatty tissue.

Another factor affecting the distribution of medication within the body is the degree to which the drug attaches itself to the carrier protein (albumin) in the bloodstream. Most drugs can bind or unbind with this protein and thus can be carried throughout the body. When a drug is bound to albumin, it is inactive; only the unbound drug has a pharmaceutical effect. Since the percentage of the unbound drug is an important determinant of drug distribution, change in the level of albumin in the blood will affect drug action.

Blood levels of albumin are reduced significantly in elders, especially those who are malnourished, severely debilitated, or have advanced illness (MacLennan et al. 1977). Low albumin levels may result in a decreased proportion of bound (inactive) drug and an increased proportion of the unbound (active) drug. Consequently, more of the drug will be distributed to action sites, perhaps to a toxic level. If a drug is 90 percent bound in young adults, a 10 percent decrease in binding capacity in elders would nearly double the blood concentration of the active drug. Further, with age, each albumin molecule becomes less able to temporarily inactivate drug molecules. Thus, if an elder is taking many drugs that bind to albumin in the bloodstream, the active drug concentrations will increase. Low albumin levels have been shown to be directly related to a number of adverse drug reactions in elders.

Age-Changes in Drug Metabolism

The liver metabolizes (breaks down) many medications before they are removed from the body. It has been hypothesized that decline in liver function due to the age-associated changes could cause an increased life of the medications within the body. However, it appears that any age-related decrements in the liver have minimal effects on liver function and consequent drug metabolism.

Age-Changes in Drug Excretion

Kidney excretion is the major route of elimination for many medications. Not only do the kidneys excrete some drugs in unchanged form, they also excrete drug products broken down by the liver. Studies conflict regarding the decrease in kidney function with advanced age. One study estimated kidney function was reduced more than one-third between the ages of twenty and ninety (Rowe et al. 1976). However, one longitudinal study showed no difference in kidney excretion rate due to age itself and reduced function was more likely due to disease and other factors (Shock et al. 1978). For whatever reason, a decrease in kidney function allows a drug to circulate longer in the body, thus increasing its effect.

Laboratory tests can measure kidney function to determine if medication dosages should be altered.

Conclusion

Many drugs on the market have not been tested on elders. Only 17 percent of the two hundred most commonly prescribed drugs include recommendations for geriatric dosages (Simonson 1984). Because of the great variability of age changes, disease states, and other drugs used concurrently by elders, physicians should carefully monitor blood levels of the drug, observe the patient's response, and adjust dosage to prevent adverse reactions. Standard pharmacology textbooks, drug company information, and articles in medical and pharmacological journals contain some information to assist a physician in adapting dosages for elders. It is often recommended that physicians reduce normal adult dosages of many medications by one-third to one-half for elders. Although this method is imprecise, it is a step in the right direction. For the reader who desires more detail on this subject, including specific drugs that are altered pharmacokinetically with age, refer to Lamy (1980), Bender (1980), and Ritschel (1983).

Drug Interactions

The effect of a drug upon the body can be influenced by other drugs and food taken at the same time. A drug-drug interaction occurs when the action of one drug in the body is altered as a result of the administration of another drug. The more drugs consumed, the greater the probability of a drug-drug interaction. Drug-drug interactions are more likely to occur in elders because of their higher than average drug consumption. Further, elders are high users of a number of medications frequently implicated in drug interactions, especially antihistamines, tranquilizers, and antidepressants. Other behaviors that contribute to drug-drug interactions are inappropriate drug dosages or schedules or ingesting alcohol with

Table 7.1 Foods that foil drugs

If Your Patient Takes:	And Eats or Drinks:	The Combination May:	So Intervene to:
Acetaminophen	Carbohydrates	Retard the absorption rate of the drug, though not the total amount absorbed	Explain that the therapeutic effect will be delayed
Anticoagulants (Coumadin and others)	Food high in vitamin K: citrus fruits, egg yolks, large amounts of fish, fish oil, potato chips, vegetable oil, leafy green vegetables	Decrease prothrombin time	Watch for changes in prothrombin time, limit intake of foods high in vitamin K
Bisacodyl tablets	Milk or alkalinizing food	Disintegrate the enteric coating prematurely in the stomach or intestine	Give the medication with water or another beverage. Watch for gastric irritation or lack of therapeutic effect if the patient did take milk
Cardiac glycosides	Milk or other food high in calcium	Diminish the therapeutic effect and lead to arrhythmia	Withhold milk; give the drug after meals to lessen gastric irritation
Erythromycin stearate	Acidic fruit or juice, carbonated beverages	Decompose the drug prematurely	Give the drug 1 hour before or 3 hours after meals
Griseofulvin	Very little fat	Cause incomplete absorption of the drug	Serve butter or margarine at each meal
Iron salts	Cereal, eggs, milk	Form insoluble chelates	Withhold these foods

medications. For an extensive list of drug-drug interactions refer to Block (1983), and Gomolin and Chapron (1983).

Study of drug-drug interactions can be very complex as thousands of drugs may be ingested in millions of different combinations. One person's response to a drug interaction may be life-threatening, while another may exhibit little or no effect. Because drug companies are not required to determine drug interactions and there is not yet an organized way for physicians to report observations of drug-drug interactions in their patients to other physicians, data on this subject are scarce. Information is spread slowly by physicians who send letters concerning individual cases to scientific journals.

Drug-food interactions include both the effect of food on drug action and how drug intake influences nutritional status. This section will address how food affects drug action. How drugs affect the absorption of nutrients in the body will be discussed in Chapter 9.

The presence of food in the stomach may impede or enhance the absorption of a drug into the bloodstream. For example, acetominophen

Iron salts	Citrus fruit juice	Hasten absorption and cause toxic reactions: nausea, vomiting, peripheral vascular collapse, anaphylaxis	Withhold these juices
Levodopa (Larodopa, Sinemet)	Foods high in vitamin B_6— yeast, liver, muscle meat, whole grain cereals, fish, vegetables, molasses	Interfere with the therapeutic effect	Limit intake of these foods
Lincomycin (Lincocin)	Any food or beverage	Interfere with absorption of the drug	Allow only water for 1–2 hours before and after administration of the drug
Lithium	Insufficient salt and water	Cause lithium toxicity: diarrhea, vomiting, drowsiness, muscular weakness, lack of coordination	Insure adequate salt and fluid intake; watch for toxicity
MAO inhibitors	Foods high in pressor amines: aged cheese, processed cheese, beer, wine (especially Chianti), chocolate, yeast extract, avocado, pickled herring, chicken liver, broad bean pods	Cause possibly fatal hypertensive crisis or intracranial bleeding	Warn patients of the danger; watch for signs of crisis: severe headache, chest pain, profuse sweating, palpitation, fast or slow pulse, visual disturbances, stertorous breathing, coma

(e.g., Tylenol) is absorbed faster in fasting subjects than in those consuming a high carbohydrate meal. Tetracycline, when ingested with dairy products, impairs calcium absorption. In contrast, the absorption of griseofulvin, a medication that combats fungus infections, is enhanced when one eats fatty foods before taking the drug.

The most hazardous drug-food interactions are those that increase the toxicity of the medication. For instance, when a monoamine oxidase (MAO) inhibitor (prescribed for depression or hypertension) is consumed with foods that contain tyramine (a protein found in aged cheese, red wines, and other foods), blood pressure increases causing severe hypertension in individuals who already have elevated blood pressure (Horwitz et al. 1964). Even though this interaction has been cited in the literature more than any other drug-food interaction, reports of toxic reactions still occur. Physicians and pharmacists need to educate patients who use MAO inhibitors of the danger. In contrast, some foods taken with drugs decrease the toxicity of the medication. Some medications (aspirin, for example) should be taken with food to reduce gastrointestinal irritation commonly associated with them. Table 7.1 indicates the more common drug-food interactions.

Physicians should prescribe drugs for older clients only after exploring less-invasive alternatives.

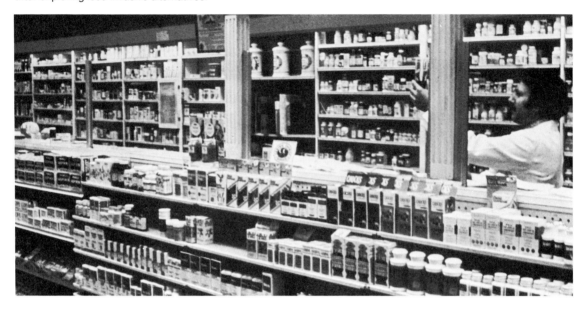

Non-Prescription (OTC) Drugs Commonly Used by Elders

When consumers select and use non-prescription or over-the-counter (OTC) drugs, they take complete charge of reducing symptoms or curing a health problem. It has been estimated that almost all elders use OTC drugs, either as a substitute for medical care or as a supplement to it. Elders may use such drugs because they cannot see a physician as soon as needed, may not want to bother a physician with a minor condition, or cannot afford to pay for a physician's visit and a prescription.

Over-the-counter drugs should not be underrated. They are a quick and inexpensive drug therapy for temporary, minor conditions. Most OTCs are effective. In fact, some are the same compound as a prescription drug, but with different packaging. If consumers had to go to a physician for every small ailment, not only would it cost them more, but it would create a tremendous overload on the medical care system. Further, many problems that are self-medicated are

limited minor conditions that go away whether treated or not, such as the common cold, constipation, or transient headaches.

On the negative side, many laypeople are not adequately informed to diagnose their own health problems and to choose an appropriate drug. They may select a drug because of its packaging or advertising. The drug may have no effect, or worse, delay needed care for serious problems. For instance, what may be interpreted as heartburn, may, in fact, be angina. Use of self-prescribed medications might confuse a physician's diagnosis if the physician is not told of its use. Further, because nonprescription drugs are thought by most laypersons to be less potent than prescription drugs, consumers may over-medicate. Finally, there is a potential for drug interactions when some OTCs are taken with prescription drugs. For instance, taking over-the-counter antihistamines can cause severe reactions when used with valium or other antianxiety agents.

Despite the disadvantages, nonprescription drugs can contribute to good health if used for the right problem and if label directions are followed. The most common OTC drug families will be discussed in the following section. When indicated, the brand names begin with capital letters while the generic equivalents are in lower case letters.

Analgesics

Analgesics, or pain relievers, are the most commonly used OTC drugs. Two main types are sold over the counter: those with aspirin (salicylates) and those without aspirin (acetaminophen and ibuprofen). Aspirin is the most widely used analgesic. Daily consumption in our country is estimated at twenty tons (Taylor 1980–81). Not only is it sold as a single product, but it is an active ingredient in over two hundred different over-the-counter products. It effectively reduces pain, fever, and inflammation. It is inexpensive, less toxic than other analgesics, does not lead to physical dependence, and the body does not build up tolerance for the drug. Aspirin is considered to be the most effective drug for arthritis because it reduces pain and swelling in joint tissues. To be effective in reducing inflammation, a large amount of aspirin must be taken regularly over a long period of time. It is also recommended for those susceptible to blood clots because it acts as an anticoagulant (Flower et al. 1980). There is also evidence that aspirin reduces cardiac death and nonfatal heart attacks in those with angina (*FDA Drug Bulletin* 1985).

Aspirin is not without its disadvantages. In high doses, it irritates the stomach and promotes blood loss from the stomach lining, sometimes causing anemia. High doses of aspirin may cause nausea, hearing and vision disturbances, abdominal pain, confusion, or dizziness in elders (Vivian and Goldberg 1982). Because aspirin reduces fever, it can cause subnormal temperature in elders; those on long-term aspirin therapy frequently complain of being cold (Lamy 1980). The fever-reducing property of aspirin may interfere with the body's own healing mechanisms (see box on right). Aspirin also interacts with a number of prescription drugs and may affect the results of kidney function tests. Because aspirin reduces the ability of the blood to clot, it can be detrimental if taken before surgery.

Aspirin, Fever, and Infection

The earlier belief that fever is harmful and should be reduced is erroneous. Although an extremely high fever can damage body organs, especially in small children, a moderate fever is one way the body defends itself against infection. It is believed that invader microorganisms alert the immune system to produce a substance that activates the hypothalamus in the brain to elevate the body temperature. High body temperature not only creates a hostile environment to inhibit the growth of bacteria and viruses, but also enhances some immune functions by speeding chemical reactions in the body.

Aspirin used to be commonly prescribed to reduce fever. However, it is now believed that aspirin may interfere with the body's fight against infection. Aspirin not only reduces the natural mechanisms of the body to fight invading organisms, but also blocks the output of prostaglandins. Although many of the benefits of prostaglandins are unknown, it is agreed that they stimulate the production of interferon—a known fighter of viruses.

A fever is most often a sign of infection, but it can also occur in those with inflammatory conditions (e.g., gout, rheumatoid arthritis), circulatory problems (e.g., heart attack), metabolic conditions (e.g., heat stroke), and some cancers (Glew 1985). It may also be a reaction to some medications. Because body temperature in elders tends to be lower and less likely to respond to infection with a fever, even a moderate fever in that group may indicate severe illness.

The most popular analgesic without aspirin is acetaminophen (Tylenol, Datril). It relieves minor pain and fever, but does not reduce inflammation and for that reason is not used for rheumatoid arthritis. Acetaminophen is less irritating to the stomach than aspirin and can be used by those allergic to aspirin. It does not affect blood clotting or renal function laboratory tests as aspirin does. However, an overdose of acetaminophen may cause permanent liver damage, which occurs without any warning symptoms. It is not as effective in treating severe pain as aspirin and it costs more.

Another nonaspirin painkiller that reduces fever, inflammation, and pain is ibuprofen. It used to be sold as a prescription drug (Motrin and Rufen), but in 1984 was approved as an OTC drug (Advil and Nuprin). It has less potential to cause gastrointestinal effects than aspirin. Ibuprofen can be used to treat rheumatoid and osteoarthritis and other forms of mild to moderate pain. Davison (1978) suggests elders, especially those with hypertension, avoid ibuprofen because the drug causes fluid retention.

Antacids

Antacids relieve symptoms of upset stomach, heartburn, and acid indigestion by neutralizing excess stomach acid. There are over six hundred different antacid products on the market in many forms: pills, lozenges, gum, powder, and liquids. Popular brand names are Alka Seltzer, Tums, Milk of Magnesia, and Maalox. Antacids generally begin acting in minutes and may be effective for up to forty minutes. All contain one or more of thirteen active ingredients, many of which have side effects. Aluminum hydroxide has a constipating effect; magnesium salts have a diarrheal effect. Antacids with high sodium content can cause fluid retention. Antacids may also decrease the absorption of some drugs, aggravate symptoms of upset stomach, or mask symptoms of an ulcer.

Laxatives

Laxatives—agents to promote bowel movement or soften the stools—are the most frequently used drug in nursing homes. One study reports almost 60 percent of all patients in such facilities receive at least one laxative daily (U.S. Dept. of HEW 1976). Among elders living in the community, it is estimated that one third to one half use laxatives at least occasionally (Cummings 1974).

A number of factors can predispose an elder to constipation: poor nutritional intake, lack of teeth, inadequate fluid intake, insufficient exercise, and drug side effects. In most cases, constipation may be reversed by nondrug alternatives: increasing dietary fiber and fluids, exercising more, and consuming foods with natural laxative properties. However, laxative use is indicated in those with weakened abdominal muscles, inadequate food intake, partial or complete loss of rectal reflex, and altered bowel motility caused by drug therapy (American Medical Association 1977).

There are many types of laxatives and each works differently. *Bulk laxatives* (e.g., Metamucil) increase volume and water content of stools. They are used when a low fiber diet cannot be corrected and should be taken with a lot of water to avoid intestinal obstruction. Bulk laxatives are the least likely to be abused and do not seem to interfere with intestinal absorption of essential nutrients. However, in elders, bulk-forming laxatives can reduce appetite because the individual feels full. *Saline laxatives* (e.g., Milk of Magnesia) attract water to the intestinal tract where it is retained, creating intestinal motility. They should not be taken with a low salt diet because they can cause dehydration and fluid-salt imbalances. *Stool softeners* promote defecation by allowing water to penetrate the fecal mass, thus softening the stool. They work for people who have normal intestinal tone but dry, hard stools. Mineral oil, though an effective stool softener,

Chapter 7

prevents absorption of fat-soluble vitamins and may leak from the rectum. *Stimulant laxatives* (e.g., Ex-Lax) increase intestinal activity by directly irritating nerves and muscles of the intestine. Prolonged use can lead to laxative dependency, fluid-salt balance disturbances, severe cramps, diarrhea, and dehydration.

Cough and Cold Preparations

One of the most common self-limiting illnesses is the common cold, a viral infection of the upper respiratory tract. Antibiotics are ineffective against viruses, so the only therapy is to reduce the symptoms while the cold runs its course.

Currently there are thousands of remedies on the market to temporarily relieve one or more of its symptoms. While some cold remedies contain only one ingredient, the majority contain a combination of ingredients. However, these "shotgun approach" products are undesirable because many of their ingredients are unnecessary. All individuals who have a cold do not have the same symptoms or require the same dosages. Many combination products have insufficient dosages of each ingredient to give relief. They cause needless drug exposure and increase the possibility of drug interactions and adverse side effects. Further, combination products may interfere with the healing process. For example, most cold preparations contain an analgesic, that reduces the fever that stimulates the body's immune system to fight the infection. Finally, combination products cost more money than single ingredient medications. Physicians recommend that single drugs in appropriate dosages be used to reduce particular symptoms.

Combination cough and cold remedies contain two or more of the following major ingredients:

1. *Cough suppressants* control coughs that cause chest pain or interfere with sleep or breathing. Most combination products do not contain high enough quantities to suppress coughing. Further, cough suppressants may be harmful because coughs may be important in clearing the respiratory passage by bringing up phlegm.

2. *Expectorants* thin and loosen the thick mucus common in the airways of a cold sufferer. Although desirable, the FDA review panel concluded that the common expectorants are ineffective.

3. *Bronchodilators* enlarge the bronchial passageways and promote easier breathing. They also relax bronchial muscle spasms that occur in asthma attacks.

4. *Decongestants* unclog blocked nasal passages and sinuses and prevent postnasal drip in the throat by constricting blood vessels in the nasal passages. Nearly all cold preparations contain a decongestant or bronchodilator. Some may cause nervousness, dizziness, or insomnia.

5. *Analgesics* reduce the aching feeling that may accompany a cold. However, they also reduce fever, which may not be desirable.

6. *Antihistamines* block the effects of the allergy-producing chemical, histamine, to relieve allergic reactions such as sneezing, watery eyes, runny nose, and itchy nose, or throat. However, these do not relieve the sinus or nasal congestion of a cold and also tend to thicken bronchial secretions in the airway, counteracting the effect of an expectorant.

7. *Alcohol* is a common ingredient in liquid cold and cough remedies: some products contain as much as 40 percent. There is no evidence that alcohol relieves the symptoms of colds or coughs. When the combination medication contains an antihistamine, the alcohol heightens its effect and produces drowsiness.

8. *Sugar* is present in large amounts in some liquid cough and cold preparations, which may harm diabetics.

Prescription Drugs Commonly Used by Elders

Prescription medications can only be procured under the direction of a physician and dispensed by a pharmacist. They are used to treat more serious disease conditions and are more likely to cause unexpected and adverse side effects. Over five-thousand prescription drugs are available and are classified into major drug families or groups that share important chemical characteristics and intended action within the body. Each family has several medications marketed under different brand names, but all contain the same or similar basic drug ingredients. The following provides an overview of the medication families commonly used by elders. See Sheridan (1984), Conrad and Bressler (1982), and Lamy (1980) for detail on prescription drugs used by elders.

Analgesics

Although some analgesics can be procured over the counter, others are available only by prescription. Prescription analgesics are narcotics that may either be naturally derived from opium (heroin, morphine, codeine), or contain a non-opiate, synthetic narcotic, such as methadone (Dolophine) and meperidine (Demerol). Low doses of narcotic agents in elders provide effective pain relief. However, they may promote physical or psychological addiction, constipation, respiratory depression, and urinary retention. Chronic narcotic use can lead to major cognitive deficits in elders (Lamy 1980). For the intense pain of terminally ill patients, special narcotic mixtures containing different combinations of heroin or morphine, cocaine, ethyl alcohol, and chloroform are used. Although such drugs are addictive and the patient may need a increasingly greater dosage to achieve the same results, this is not an important consideration in a terminally ill patient (Lamy 1980).

Antiarthritics

This group includes the analgesics just described as well as other drug types. Antiarthritics reduce joint swelling, morning stiffness, inflammation, and pain so that immobility associated with rheumatoid arthritis and osteoarthritis can be minimized. As mentioned earlier, the most widely used and effective drug for arthritis is aspirin. Other antiarthritic drugs are useful for both long- and short-term treatment when aspirin cannot be used (e.g., ibuprofen, naproxen, fenoprofen). Although these drugs have fewer gastrointestinal side effects than aspirin, they cause fluid retention and should not be used by those with hypertension or congestive heart failure. These drugs are no more effective than aspirin and are more expensive.

Gold salts are sometimes injected or taken orally to treat rheumatoid arthritis. However, it may be several months before improvement is noted. Gold salts may also adversely affect the skin, blood, and kidneys.

Steroids (e.g., cortisone) reduce the inflammation of rheumatoid arthritis quickly, but should only be prescribed after other treatments have failed. In elders, these drugs should be used sparingly because they increase bone loss and consequent risk of fractures. They also depress serum albumin levels, alter glucose metabolism, increase fluid retention, aggravate glaucoma and cataracts, and increase risk of infections by depressing the immune system.

Antibiotics

Antibiotics destroy or inhibit the multiplication of disease-producing bacteria that invade the body. Some antibiotics attack only certain types of bacteria. Others are broad spectrum, because they inactivate many bacteria types. Broad spectrum antibiotics alter the normal bacterial population within the body, leading to gastrointestinal upset and/or yeast overgrowth in the vagina. Tetracycline also causes the skin to sunburn more easily.

Kidney function plays a major role in the choice of antibiotics and dosage since reduced kidney function leads to increased drug levels in the blood, and possible toxicity. For most infections in elders (except urinary tract) Penicillin G is preferred because it has a wide margin of safety in dosage.

Antidiabetics (Hypoglycemic Agents)

Two major drug types help the body maintain blood sugar at a nearly normal level: oral hypoglycemics for those with diabetes who still produce insulin and insulin for those who cannot produce it. Oral hypoglycemics (Orinase, Dymelor, Tolinase, Diabinese) stimulate insulin production. The use of oral hypoglycemics is controversial; some health professionals worry they may not only be ineffective, but harmful (University Group Diabetes Program 1970). Elders using long-acting oral hypoglycemic agents should be closely monitored since some can cause excessively low blood sugar.

For diabetics who do not produce insulin, daily insulin injections are necessary. Insulin injections may also be used for adult-onset diabetics who do not respond to behavioral modification or oral hypoglycemic drugs. Appropriate dosage and careful monitoring is important as too much or too little can be harmful.

Antiparkinsonism Agents

The goal of drug therapy for patients with Parkinson's disease is to increase the dopamine levels in the brain. Because direct administration of dopamine cannot cross the blood-brain barrier, precursors of dopamine have been developed (levodopa and combinations). These precursors can cross the barrier and enter the brain where they are then converted into dopamine. Although these drugs do not reduce the progression of the disease, they do reduce symptoms. However, the drug may cause a number of adverse effects with prolonged use. Anticholinerginic drugs and antihistamines may be used in combination with levodopa for symptoms of Parkinson's disease. They are sometimes used alone if levodopa therapy is not tolerated, but are generally less effective.

Antianginal Agents

There are currently three types of antianginal drugs: nitrates, calcium blockers, and beta blockers. The *nitrates* (isosorbide dinitrate, nitroglycerine) relax the smooth muscles of the arteries and veins that increase circulation to the heart and decrease anginal pain. Nitrates may be used in a fast-acting form when an attack is imminent. The slow-acting form to prevents further attacks. They may be swallowed like a pill, dissolved under the tongue, rubbed on the chest in ointment form, or diffused slowly into the bloodstream through a small patch on the chest. Adverse effects include low blood pressure that can lead to weakness, dizziness, and fainting. Severe headaches are also common with high dosages.

Calcium blockers (nifedipine, verapamil) inhibit calcium from entering cardiac and smooth muscles. Since calcium is necessary for muscle contraction, this reduces heart contraction and constricts small arteries, causing a decreased blood flow to the heart. These actions decrease the frequency and intensity of anginal pain. However, the drug is associated with lightheadedness or dizziness because low blood pressure is a common side effect.

Beta blockers slow breathing and heart rate by inhibiting nerve impulses to the heart and lungs. Propanolol (inderol) is the most commonly prescribed beta blocker. Abrupt withdrawal of the drug may cause anginal pain or even a heart attack, so it must be gradually reduced when therapy is terminated.

Diuretics

Diuretics rid the body of excess water and salt. They are the most common treatment for congestive heart failure and mild to moderate hypertension. Diuretics are one of the most commonly prescribed drugs in the United States. Two types of diuretics are commonly used: potassium depleting (thiazide diruretics) and potassium sparing (nonthiazide or kidney loop diuretics).

Thiazide diuretics reduce fluid outside the cells by increasing output of water and electrolytes, mainly sodium, chloride, and potassium. Adverse effects in elders include excessive potassium loss, impaired glucose tolerance, and increased uric acid level in the blood, which may cause gout. Potassium and chloride supplements or potassium-rich foods are often prescribed with thiazides to counteract the problem.

Potassium-sparing diuretics rid the body of water without eliminating potassium. In addition, they do not seem to disturb glucose or uric acid metabolism like the potassium depleting diuretics. However, in elders, the drug often causes too much potassium to be retained, especially in those with decreased kidney function, and may result in heart failure. Patients on potassium sparing diuretics should avoid foods high in potassium (such as bananas). Both types may also cause excessive fluid loss that leads to dehydration and to postural hypotension (a drop in blood pressure when rising), causing dizziness and fainting.

Antihypertensive Drugs

When diuretics are ineffective in reducing high blood pressure, a hypertensive drug is usually added. There are many types and they affect the body in many different and complex ways. The most commonly prescribed antihypertensive drugs are inderal (a beta blocking agent), and methyldopa (Koch 1983). All hypertensive drugs commonly have side effects, many of which are severe and affect psychological state, cognitive function, sexual functioning, and other body systems. Sometimes the side effects of these drugs are more difficult to cope with than hypertension itself. Various antihypertensive agents have been documented to significantly decrease quality of life of those who take them (Croog et al. 1986). Refer to Sheridan (1984) for more detail on specific antihypertensive medications and their side effects.

Antiarrhythmics

Antiarrhythmic drugs restore heart rhythm and increase the strength of heart contractions. They are commonly used for elders with congestive heart failure. The most commonly prescribed antiarrhythmic is digoxin (lanoxin), an extract from the foxglove plant. Although widely used, digitalis preparations frequently cause adverse drug reactions that often require hospitalization. Perhaps this is because the therapeutic dose is very close to the toxic dose. Digitalis is eliminated more slowly in elders, so the potential for adverse affects (e.g., appetite loss, weakness, confusion, depression, and abnormal heart rhythms) is increased. Many experts believe this drug is overused in elders.

Inderal, a beta blocker mentioned earlier as a hypertensive drug, is also considered an antiarrhythmic and is commonly prescribed to restore heart rhythms. Like digoxin, inderal is metabolized more slowly in elders, resulting in higher blood concentrations of the drug and a greater potential for low blood pressure that could cause weakness, dizziness, and fainting. Those with congestive heart failure should not use inderal. In addition, the drug masks symptoms of low blood sugar, so diabetics taking hypoglycemic drugs should avoid it.

Anticoagulants

Anticoagulants reduce blood clotting by decreasing the production of clotting factors by the liver. These drugs reduce the incidence of stroke and mortality in patients with cerebrovascular disease. The most commonly prescribed anticoagulant drug is warfarin. Elders are more sensitive to anticoagulants than younger groups so the dosage should be closely monitored. The effectiveness of warfarin is altered if it is taken with vitamin K or aspirin. Vitamin K, which increases blood clotting, will work against the drug, while aspirin, also an anticoagulant, increases the action of warfarin. Anticoagulants have a high rate of adverse reactions. Up to one-third of elders taking anticoagulants may suffer cerebral hemorrhages because of this drug and one-fifth may experience gastrointestinal hemorrhage (May et al. 1977). One of the biggest risks of anticoagulants is the large number of drugs that can interact with them.

Sedative/Hypnotics

Sedative/hypnotics induce drowsiness or sleep and are suitable for temporary use during acute, stressful incidents. There are two types of sedative/hypnotics: barbiturates (phenobarbital, atropine), and nonbarbiturates (chloral hydrate). Barbiturates are used extensively in the elder population, despite their well-documented paradoxical effects of agitation, insomnia, and nocturnal restlessness in that group. These drugs also suppress rapid eye movement sleep (REM) patterns, the necessary dream sleep. Further, barbiturates have a high rate of drug interactions. For instance, their effect is significantly increased with alcohol use. They also have a hangover effect, evidenced by impaired judgement and motor coordination. Barbiturates should be used no longer than a few days because long-term use causes drug dependency, intellectual impairment, slurred speech, and an unsteady gait (Davison 1978).

Chloral hydrate, a nonbarbiturate, is one of the oldest, and perhaps most effective, hypnotic drugs for elders. It does not appear to modify rapid eye movement sleep patterns, stay in the body as long as barbiturates, or cause a hangover effect. However, tolerance and dependence are possible.

Other nonbarbiturates used as hypnotics are in the benzodiazepine group (Valium, Librium, Dalmane). Although they are antianxiety agents, if used as a short-term hypnotic, they act as a barbiturate, with a much lower addiction potential. Many professionals recommend cautious use of these drugs because their activity is prolonged in elders and dosage must be reduced. Adverse effects include excessive sedation and drowsiness, dizziness, weakness, and confusion (Sheridan 1984).

Antipsychotics

Antipsychotics, or major tranquilizers, are used to treat major mental disorders: psychosis, organic mental disorders, personality disorders, or agitated, disruptive behavior. There are many different kinds of antipsychotics, each with different chemical structure, site of action, and side effects. However, all inhibit certain sites in the nervous system that create mental symptoms. Elders require reduced doses of these drugs because they are excreted more slowly. Authorities question the use of antipsychotics for long-term therapy. One investigator reports that the difference between those treated with antipsychotics and those who were not decreases with time (Crane 1973).

Side effects of many antipsychotics are postural hypotension, abnormal heart rhythms, dry mouth, blurred vision, constipation, urinary retention, and unsteadiness. Drowsiness, lethargy, weakness, and fatigue are common side effects in elders (Ziance 1979). Motor function may be affected and excessive dosages for a long period of time may cause a serious side effect called tardive dyskinesia.

Tardive dyskinesia is an inability to control movement of various body parts, especially in the lower face, causing rapid involuntary muscle twitches and difficulty in speaking or swallowing (Sheridan 1984). These symptoms often develop after six months of treatment with antipsychotic drugs and may first appear when the antipsychotic drug is reduced or withdrawn. At present, this side effect cannot be reversed, but lower dosages can reduce the possibility of these effects. Specifics of drug management are complicated and must be carefully monitored; often other drugs must be given to counteract side effects.

Antianxiety Agents

Antianxiety agents are prescribed to reduce anxiety and tension, relax skeletal muscles, and facilitate alcohol withdrawal. Major drugs in this group are the benzodiazepines (e.g. Librium and Valium). These drugs should only be prescribed for temporary episodes of anxiety and should be taken for a week or less. Tolerance and dependence occur with prolonged use. Many patients habitually take these drugs when no longer indicated. The misuse of benzodiazepines is considered to be the largest drug abuse problem in the United States.

Antianxiety drugs are eliminated more slowly as one ages, placing elders at higher risk. One researcher estimates elimination time at twenty hours for twenty-year-olds and ninety hours for eighty-year-olds (Rosenberg et al. 1976). Because of this, physicians should initially prescribe

Shown above are three name-brand drugs and their generic equivalents.

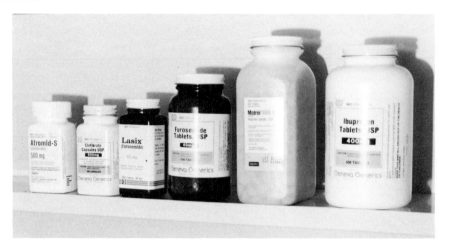

very small doses and increase as needed. Common adverse effects for elders are drowsiness, sedation, confusion, dizziness, and fatigue and these effects increase when dosage is high. Unfortunately, the side effects are often attributed to old age and the prescription is not altered. Antianxiety agents have less potential for drug interactions than most drugs; however, they should not be taken with alcohol.

Before antianxiety drugs are prescribed, other alternatives should be explored: stress reduction, meditation, counseling, physical activity, among others. One study compared the value of benzodiazepines with several minutes of "listening, explanation, advice, and reassurance by the physician during the office visit. The drugs and interaction were equally effective in reducing anxiety and those in the interaction group were more satisfied with their care than the drug group (reported in *Health Letter* 1987).

Antidepressants

Antidepressants are prescribed to relieve abrupt-onset depression, reduce anxiety, or produce a sedative effect. There are two main types of antidepressants: tricyclic antidepressants and monoamine oxidase (MAO) inhibitors. Tricyclic

compounds have a mood-elevating action in depressed patients. They are most effective for those with severe, abrupt-onset depression and least effective in patients with long-standing, chronic depression (Lamy 1980). When first administered, these drugs exert a sedative effect that may worsen depression for a few days; often mood elevation is not evident for two to three weeks. Adverse side effects are dry mouth, constipation, blurred vision, postural hypotension, dizziness, rapid heartbeat, and urinary retention. As depressive symptoms disappear, the antidepressant should be gradually withdrawn and psychotherapy initiated to forestall another episode. Even though the MAO inhibitor antidepressants are effective, they are particularly hazardous to older people and should not be used unless other treatments have failed. The drug is inherently toxic and predisposes them to a host of both drug-drug and drug-food interactions (Lamy 1980).

Generic Vs. Brand-Name Drugs

When a drug company develops a new drug, it is patented and sold under a single brand name. After seventeen years, the patent runs out and any drug company can manufacture the drug using

Chapter 7

another brand name or its generic name. A generic drug has the same ingredients as the original patent but has no fancy labeling and advertising. The name of a generic drug is a simplified version of its chemical name.

Many people erroneously believe brand name drugs to be better than generic drugs. A number of pharmaceutical companies encourage that belief by directing misleading advertising towards physicians and laypeople that portray generic drugs as ineffective and unsafe. Both the FDA and consumer groups are taking action against such unethical advertising (*AARP Bulletin* 1987). Both brand name and generic versions must meet the same FDA standards of quality. About 90 percent of the generic drugs are produced by the major drug firms who also produce brand name drugs. The FDA is responsible for assessing whether a generic drug is therapeutically equivalent (absorbed by the body at the same rate as the brand name). Thus far, of more than 5,000 approved prescription drugs on the market, one-third are still under patent and cannot be sold generically, but about 2,400 brand name products have generic drugs that have been tested and approved to be therapeutically equivalent.

A generic drug is significantly lower in cost, sometimes as much as 50 percent. This is a considerable savings, especially if the drug must be taken over an extended period. Even though in the last three decades, the generic prescribing rates have more than doubled, brand name prescribing still occurs about 80 percent of the time (Koch and Knapp 1987). Unfortunately, those found to be the least likely to use generic drugs are the elderly poor. (Lambert et al. 1980).

Physicians generally prescribe brand name drugs because they are familiar with the brand name. This behavior is mainly due to the influence of medical journal advertising and drug sales representatives. Generic drugs are not advertised or otherwise promoted by the drug companies. Physicians may also have more confidence in the brand name. Finally, a number of brand name drugs do not yet have generic equivalents so the physician must prescribe a brand name in some cases.

The patient may not trust a generic drug, believing it to be inferior because it is less expensive. Many elders have the attitude, "I want the best possible medication and I'm willing to pay the price." Generic drugs may arouse suspicion because they differ in shape and color than the brand elders may previously have taken. Educating elders that generic drugs are safe, effective, and less expensive would counteract negative attitudes towards these drugs. Elders need to learn to ask the pharmacist or physician to prescribe the generic equivalent. Most states now permit the pharmacist to substitute a generic equivalent unless the physician specifically expresses that the substitution would not be in the patient's best interest (Food and Drug Administration 1982).

Table 7.2 illustrates the generic equivalent of many commonly used brand name medications—both prescription and non-prescription.

Adverse Effects of Medications in Elders

An adverse drug reaction is any undesirable and unexpected response to a medication that occurs when a drug is used routinely and appropriately to prevent, diagnose, or treat a disease state. Gastrointestinal disturbances are the most common adverse effect. Others are confusion, depression, loss of appetite, weakness, lethargy, unsteady gait, forgetfulness, tremor, or constipation (Karch and Lasagna 1975). Note that these symptoms are the stereotypical view of old age. In elders, many adverse drug reactions are ignored because they are unfairly viewed as part of the aging process.

Table 7.2 Generic equivalents to common drugs

Brand Name	Generic Name	Uses
Amcill, Omnipen	Ampicillin	Antibiotic
Bayer	Aspirin	Analgesic
Lanoxin	Digoxin	Regulates heartbeat
Valium	Diazepam	Relieves anxiety
Inderal	Propanolol hydrachloride	Hypertension, Angina
Motrin, Rufin	Ibuprofen	Antiarthritic, Analgesic
Achromycin V	Tetracycline	Antibiotic
Tagamet	Cimetidine	Duodendal ulcer
Esidrix, Oretic HydroDIURIL	Hydrochlorothiazide	Hypertension, Diuretic
Aldomet	Methyldopa	Hypertension, Diuretic
Veetids, Pen Vee K, V-Cillin K	Penicillin	Antibiotic
Thorazine	Chlorpromazine	Antipsychotic
Cort-Dome	Hydrocortisone	Anti-inflammatory

Studies indicate that about one-fourth of older people living in the community report undesirable effects from the drugs they use (Klein et al. 1981; Eberhardt and Robinson, 1979). Drug-induced illness is an important reason for hospitalization among elders. Williamson (1980) reported that of two-thousand admissions to a geriatric ward in the United Kingdom, about one in eight were admitted because of adverse drug reactions. Elders also represent the largest proportion of patients who develop an adverse reaction while hospitalized. One study indicated as many as one third of those from ages sixty-six to seventy-five had an adverse drug reaction while in the hospital, and only one-half of the reactions were minor (Miller 1973).

Although almost all prescription and OTC drugs can cause adverse effects, some medications elders commonly use are responsible for a large percentage of the adverse drug reactions.

Table 7.3 (Simonson 1984) lists those prescription and nonprescription drugs that commonly cause adverse reaction in elders. For a more complete listing of medications and adverse effects, see Friesen (1983).

Compliance

Even if the physician accurately diagnoses a disease or disorder and prescribes the appropriate drug, the problem cannot be cured or controlled unless the patient complies with the therapy. Compliance is defined as adherence to a prescribed medical regimen. Although elders differ little from other populations in compliance rates, compliance is especially important for elders because they are prescribed more drugs and are more susceptible to drug interactions and adverse effects.

Senility Caused by Medication

My father suffered a heart attack on December 26, 1980. He was 76 years old. Two days after he was hospitalized, he began to show symptoms of confusion, agitation and restlessness after he was given several drugs to tranquilize him. But as his agitation and confusion increased, the medication was increased. After three weeks of hospitalization, he came home and did not recognize his surroundings. He would not stay there, he said, all the time insisting he wanted to go home. He could not sleep and my mother was desperately trying to calm him and keep him in the apartment.

In desperation, we had him readmitted to another hospital for further testing to see if perhaps he had suffered a stroke. Results of the testing were negative, but he continued to be agitated and violent. He was switched from drug to drug, all of which seemed to feed his agitation and feelings of paranoia, so that he had to be restrained. At this point he was too physically weak to walk without assistance and could hardly open his mouth to speak audibly.

The doctors involved were a cardiologist, a neurologist and a psychiatrist. Their joint diagnosis was organic brain syndrome and irreversible dementia. A nursing home was their recommendation for his future care. Although we suggested many times that he be taken off medication, the doctors would not listen.

It was hard for us to believe that my father had turned senile overnight, especially since he had been working five days a week and driving a car up until his heart attack. . . .

We were very fortunate to get my dad admitted to a hospital where, under medical supervision, he was gradually taken off all medication. About a week after the last medication was withdrawn, my dad returned to complete normalcy. He returned home with my mother and is a whole person once again. He has no memory of the past three months from the time of his heart attack to the time he was off all medication. . . .

Table 7.3 Significant adverse reactions to medications in elderly patients

Type of Drug	Generic Name	Brand Name Example	Adverse Effect(s)
Prescription drugs Cardiac	Digoxin	Lanoxin®	Loss of appetite, vision disturbances, depression, confusion, breast enlargement in males, abnormal heart rhythm
	Propranolol	Inderal®	Slow pulse, low blood pressure, complicates diabetic monitoring
Diuretic	Hydrochlorothiazide Chlorothiazide Furosemide	HydroDIURIL® Diuril® Lasix®	Potassium loss, dehydration, low blood pressure, diabetes, gout
	Spironolactone	Aldactone®	Excess potassium levels, breast enlargement in males
Antihypertensive	Methyldopa	Aldomet®	Drowsiness
	Reserpine	Serpasil®	Depression, sedation, gastrointestinal distress, abnormal heart rhythm
Antiarthritic	Phenylbutazone	Butazolidin®	Gastrointestinal irritation, fluid retention, serious blood disorders
	Indomethacin	Indocin®	Headache, gastrointestinal irritation, dizziness, mental confusion, ringing in ears
Anticoagulant	Warfarin	Coumadin®	Bleeding problems
Corticosteroids	Prednisone	Deltasone®	Fluid retention, diabetes, decreased immunity, ulcers, softening of bones, glaucoma, cataracts, confusion, psychosis
Bronchodilator	Theophylline	Elixophyllin®	Nausea, seizures, abnormal heart rhythm
Gastrointestinal	Cimetidine	Tagamet®	Confusion, disorientation
	Atropine	Donnatal®*	Dry mouth, blurred vision, constipation, urinary retention, confusion, psychosis
Narcotic Analgesic	Codeine	Empirin® with Codeine* Tylenol® with Codeine*	Constipation, sedation

Sedative-Hypnotic	Pentobarbital	Nembutal®	Confusion, residual drowsiness, agitation, psychosis
	Flurazepam	Dalmane®	Drowsiness, confusion, unsteady walking
Antianxiety	Diazepam	Valium®	Drowsiness, sedation, confusion, dizziness
Antidepressant	Amitriptyline	Elavil®	Dry mouth, confusion, low blood pressure, constipation, increased pulse, heart rhythm disorders, glaucoma
Antipsychotic	Chlorpromazine	Thorazine®	Sedation, low blood pressure, dry mouth, blurred vision, constipation, urinary retention, extrapyramidal effects, including: restlessness, exaggerated facial movements, and symptoms of Parkinson's disease
	Haloperidol	Haldol®	Less toxicity than chlorpromazine but increased extrapyramidal effects
Nonprescription medication			
Analgesic	Aspirin	Bayer Aspirin®	Nausea, gastrointestinal irritation, ulcers, confusion, drowsiness, metabolic disturbances
Antacids	Magnesium hydroxide Aluminum hydroxide Calcium carbonate		Diarrhea Constipation
	Sodium bicarbonate		Can worsen high blood pressure, congestive heart failure, kidney disease
Saline and stimulant Laxatives		Ex-Lax, Milk of Magnesia	Dehydration, electrolyte loss

From Simonson, W. 1984. *Medication and the elderly*, pp. 133–134. Reprinted with permission of Aspen Publishers, Inc. Copyright © 1984.

*contains more than one active ingredient

Note: This table does not include all important adverse drug effects that occur in the elderly nor does it list all drugs capable of causing adverse effects.

Causes of Noncompliance Among Elders

I. Patient Factors
  1. Never start the drug therapy
  2. Forgetfulness
  3. Lack of knowledge
    a. Does not understand disease or importance of therapy
    b. Does not know how to take medication properly
    c. Visual or hearing decrements that preclude knowledge of medication use
  4. Intentionally altering medication schedule
    a. Fear of dependence on medication.
    b. Lack of trust in physician
    c. Dissatisfaction with results of medication

II. Nature of Disease and/or Therapy
  1. High number of medications and dosage frequency
  2. Long treatment time
  3. Medication causes unacceptable side effects
  4. High cost of medication
  5. Disease has no symptoms
  6. Unacceptable dosage forms (bad-taste, can't swallow pills)
  7. Low potential for therapy to cure disease or relieve symptoms

III. Physician Inadequacies
  1. Lack of explicit written and oral instructions
  2. Poor relationship with patient
  3. Phyusician's lack of confidence in treatment
  4. Complicated drug regimen prescribed
  5. Lack of specific instructions on medication label

Noncompliant Behaviors

A number of behaviors can be classified as non-compliant. An individual may never begin a drug therapy, forget to take the drug, or take the drug improperly because of lack of education. One study found that elders usually remember less than one-half the instructions concerning the proposed regimen and one-third of the explanation about the illness to be treated (Lamy 1980). Patients may take drugs at the wrong times and in the wrong dosages, or they may discontinue the drug therapy before it is appropriate. Noncompliance may be caused by the patient, the nature of the disease or therapy, and physician inadequacies. The reported incidence of drug noncompliance among adults ranges from 25–50 percent, depending on the defining criteria for noncompliance. Noncompliance extends the recovery rate, consequently increasing the costs of drugs, physicians, and hospitalization.

Education to Increase Compliance

Effective education increases the success of drug therapy. Although education does not guarantee compliance, it is a necessary prerequisite. Patient education should include an understandable description of the disease and its progression, treatment goals, and details about the drug therapy. Elders generally need more time to learn about the drugs they are prescribed than other populations. Many elders are hearing or vision impaired, and some speak little English or have had little formal education. To compensate for these difficulties, information should be relayed in a personal, easily understood manner, free from technical jargon.

The health professional should ensure that the patient understands the specifics of the drug therapy and is able to carry out the instructions. It is important to determine whether the client can administer the medication (e.g., swallow large pills, put drops in own eyes). The client should be questioned about the regimen to evaluate what information has been learned. Also, elders need time to ask questions about their health problem and treatment plan. Finally, if possible, someone close to the patient should be involved in drug education, especially if she or he will be responsible for the supervision or administration of the medication.

One of the most important, and neglected, means of patient education to increase compliance is clear instructions on drug labels and provision of supplemental materials. Boyd (1974) found that the more information put on the drug label, the better the client understood the drug directions and the higher the compliance rate. Whenever possible, verbal information regarding drugs or disease should be supplemented with large-print, readable, written materials that the client can refer to later.

Another aspect of drug education that is seldom addressed concerns childproof containers. The Federal Poison Prevention Act requires childproof containers be used for both OTC and prescription medication. Medication packaged in this way has reduced the incidence of poisoning in children by 75 percent (Breault 1974). However, it is estimated that one-fourth of elders living in the community cannot open such containers (Robbins and Jahnigen 1984), usually because of impaired eyesight, manual dexterity, or strength.

The most obvious consequence of the inability to open a childproof container is that elders will not take the medication. Another problem is that elders may break the container to open it, possibly destroying the medication and accompanying instructions. Many elders injure themselves as they try to force the cap open with a screwdriver or knife. Once the lid is off, elders may leave the cap off, predisposing the contents to deterioration. In addition, many elders transfer the medications to an unmarked container. This can decrease compliance because the labels or directions are seldom transferred. It is the responsibility of the physician and pharmacist to ensure medication prescribed to older people is in a container they can open. If the patient requests or receives a cap that is not childproof, drug storage away from children should be discussed.

The following information should be discussed when any prescription is given:

Name of medication (both generic and brand name)
How much medication is in each dose
Appearance of the medication
What the drug is for (why prescribed)
Expected outcome (what will it do)
Major benefits and risks of medication
Quantity to be taken
Dosage frequency
Method of administration
Duration of therapy
Precautions when using
Special instructions
What to do if dose is missed
Prescription refill information
Storage requirements
Knowledge of adverse effects to report
Interactions with food, other medications or alcohol
When effects of medication should be noticed
When to stop taking a drug
How long prescription should last
What to expect if medication is not taken

The Noncompliant Patient: Disobedient or Self-Reliant?

The word *noncompliant* describes a patient who does not conform to a physician's instructions. Noncompliance may be an unintentional act (lack of knowledge or forgetfulness) or intentional (a deliberate choice not to comply). Noncompliance does not always result in negative consequences. Some patients may make a necessary drug dosage

Memory Aids to Increase Compliance

Because elders often undergo multiple drug therapies simultaneously, keeping track of which medications to take when can be a major impediment to compliance. There are many techniques to help people remember medication schedules. Medication-taking may be incorporated with an activity that is done every day, such as breakfast or toothbrushing. In this way, medication can be placed in an obvious place (beside the coffee, toothbrush, or razor) to jog the memory. A different type of technique is to have older people divide all pills to be taken at a particular time in labeled containers. For instance, once weekly, medication is compartmentalized by day or hour of ingestion in a labeled compartmentalized pill box, egg carton, or set of envelopes. A more expensive, but effective, use of this method is to request the pharmacist to consolidate all daily medication by day in a sterile

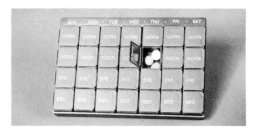

bubble package on a chart that is labeled clearly with days of the week. If there are many pills to be taken at various times, the package may be labeled with times of day. A third way to keep track of medication intake is to purchase or make a medication calendar and have the client check off boxes when drugs have been taken. Finally, a timer may be purchased to remind the client to take drugs. An electronic pill cap has been developed with a flashing red light and a seventy-five decibel sound that goes off a pre-set number of times a day.

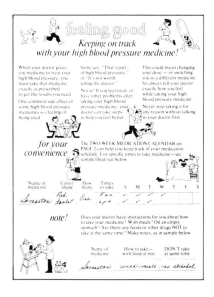

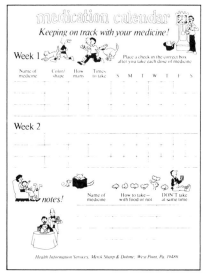

adjustment to minimize adverse effects or discontinue unnecessary medication without the physician's consent. In one study, 10 percent of patients on drug therapy were judged to be intelligent noncompliers (Weintraub 1981).

Until the consumer health movement of the early 1970s, physicians and pharmacists were instructed to withhold information on what medication patients were prescribed. Now, the majority believe patients have a right to know about their health status and all aspects of their medications—benefits, side effects, and alternatives. Further, consumers have the right to decide whether or not to agree to a prescribed regimen. It is the physician's responsibility to give clients appropriate information to allow them to make these decisions rationally.

Role of Professionals in Promoting Rational Drug Use

A number of health professionals should be involved in effective drug therapy. Many have the potential to minimize adverse drug effects and provide helpful drug information to elders. In a team approach, the physician, nurse, pharmacist, social worker, family members, and the individual cooperate to maximize benefits and minimize problems with drug therapy. The following paragraphs discuss the role of each team member in promoting rational drug use. Unfortunately, the team approach is seldom used—especially in community settings.

Role of the Physician

Physicians have the primary responsibility for drug therapy. They must accurately assess the health problem, prescribe the correct type and dosage of medication, and supervise drug therapy. In addition, the physician is responsible to educate the patient about the disease and drug therapy. In some cases, these responsibilities are delegated to a nurse, educator, or pharmacist. Because their responsibility in drug therapy is so

great, there are many areas where physicians may fall short. Lamy (1983) asserts that physicians may contribute to drug misuse by:

Failure to obtain a complete drug history
Inaccurate diagnosis of the health problem
Failure to consider drug interactions
Failure to consider nondrug alternatives
Inappropriate drug treatment (e.g., wrong drug, wrong dose)
Overmedication (prescribing unneeded or ineffective drugs or for an excessive length of time)
Failure to prescribe most inexpensive drug
Failure to consider drug side effects
Failure to consider effects of age and disease on drug
Failure to consider patient's lifestyle
Failure to give clear instructions regarding medication
Inadequate supervision of long-term medication
Failure to periodically review need for all medications

Perhaps the two areas in which physicians are most inadequate is knowledge of drug side effects and appropriate dosages for elders. Side effects of a drug may be misinterpreted as another disease or a worsening of the existing condition. More drugs may be prescribed to treat the negative effects of the first instead of reducing the original dosage or prescribing a different drug or other therapy. One survey of physicians found that only 27 percent felt qualified to recognize and treat drug side effects in older patients (U.S. Senate 1983). In addition, physicians often prescribe drugs for elders in higher dosages than are necessary because age and lower weight were not considered. One study of thirty-three elder heart patients in a teaching hospital showed most prescriptions were administered in dosages higher than recommended for elders by the drug company (reported in Lamy and Vestal 1976). Much of physician's lack of knowledge in this area is attributed to a dearth of geriatric focus and pharmacology content in most medical schools and limited opportunities for continuing drug education for practicing physicians.

Role of the Pharmacist

The traditional role of the pharmacist was to procure, store, prepare, and dispense drugs. However, with increased awareness of adverse drug reactions and other problems associated with drug use, pharmacists have expanded their role to prevent, recognize, and intervene in drug-associated problems.

Most community pharmacists now serve a number of important roles. Many of their services augment the work of the physician. Pharmacists serve as a resource for both clients and physicians as they provide information on proper drug use and adverse effects of both prescription and OTC drugs. Pharmacists are experts in drug and food interactions and symptoms of adverse drug effects. Further, pharmacists provide a confidential record-keeping service for their customers. This includes drug history, drug allergies, and medical history. They consult with the physician periodically to assure the client is using the drug properly and alert the physician of potential drug interactions, adverse drug effects, and the negative impact of prescriptions ordered by other physicians. They can identify symptoms of serious diseases in their clients and refer them to their physician when necessary. Pharmacists provide information on generic drugs and can assist the patient with medication scheduling and memory aids. Pharmacists can instruct clients on the use of childproof containers and assess need for easy-open containers. Finally, many pharmacies provide emergency service, delivery, charge accounts, and insurance billing service.

Despite the potential of pharmacists, many physicians and clients do not utilize their expertise. Smith and Sharpe (1984) studied a group of community elders and found that even though most used one pharmacy for all their drug needs, little medical information was exchanged between the elder and pharmacist. It is unclear whether clients are unaware of the services provided or pharmacists volunteer little information. The authors suggest pharmacists hold group information sessions and encourage clients with prescriptions to ask questions. Another researcher suggests pharmacists should enter in the field of home health care by visiting clients in their homes to assess medication use (Lamy 1983).

Low utilization of pharmacists' expertise may be due to the relatively recent expansion of the role of the pharmacist. With time, it is expected that both physicians and clients will rely increasingly on the pharmacist to educate clients about drugs. Many long-term care institutions and hospitals have already instituted clinical pharmacy services to dispense and administer drugs, review drug utilization, and educate patients. When such services are implemented in an institutional setting, drug misuse drops significantly.

Role of the Nurse

The nurse's responsibility in drug therapy depends on the work setting. In a physician's office, nurses commonly provide drug education. In hospitals, long-term care institutions, or home health care, nurses are fully responsible to carry out the plan of care devised by the physician. They administer medications and monitor drug reactions and report them to the physician. Nurses also need to intervene when the physicians over- or underprescribe, question the advisability of an order if it interferes with other drugs, and suggest medication to help the patient.

Nurses carry out the Five Rights of medication administration: administering the right drug, in the right dose, through the right route, at the right time, to the right patient. Although this seems a straightforward task, data from a number of studies indicate a high degree of error in the administration of medications in hospitals. A report from the U.S. Senate Subcommittee on Long Term Care (1975) reported that those who administer drugs to elders in long-term care facilities make medication errors about 30 percent of the time.

In institutional settings, nurses are responsible to give the right drug in the right dose through the right route at the right time to the right patient. Unfortunately, many mistakes are made.

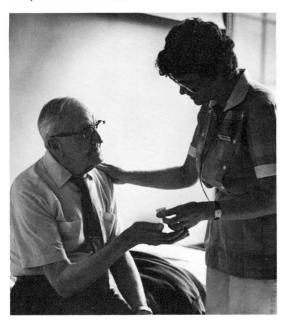

Role of the Social Worker

Social workers in both institutional and community settings should have a basic knowledge of medication-related problems and be able to refer clients with those problems to appropriate health care professionals. Social workers in community settings generally have closer contact with elders than the physician, so they are in a good position to monitor medication consumption and adverse effects. Social workers might also discuss problems with compliance or medication complications with their client's physician. Unfortunately, few social workers are educated to deal with health concerns of elders in general and have little knowledge of drug issues.

Perhaps the primary role of social workers in the care of older people is to serve as health advocates by recognizing medication-related problems, helping to resolve them, and encouraging health practices that could reduce drug use. The advocate is in a position to inform the elder about

generic drugs and assist in developing memory aids to increase compliance. The advocate can encourage the elder to keep a medication record and discuss all drugs with a pharmacist or physician. The social worker's role as an advocate becomes more important for those elders living alone because they may be their only professional contact (Giannetti 1983).

The Responsibility of the Drug Consumer

Consumers must take responsibility for their medication use. To do this, they need to actively seek drug information from their physician and pharmacist, make decisions about the treatment plan, and monitor their own drug therapy program. Elders are less apt to initiate discussion with their physician than other adults, perhaps because they do not want to waste the physician's valuable time or be labeled as a complainer. Those working with older people should impress upon them that the physician is responsible to discuss health problems and medications in as much detail as needed. Also elders should be aware that questions related to drug use can be answered by their pharmacist in person or by phone. Box 7.4 suggests a number of ways older consumers may take more responsibility for drug therapy.

If the individual cannot be responsible for personal medication use, family and friends can reduce the risks of misuse by supervising or assisting with drug administration (Simonson 1984). A family member or friend can also monitor the elder's reaction to the drug, determine if symptom relief is sufficient, keep drug intake records, and serve as a health advocate. In addition, the helper should be alert to potential adverse drug reactions and should contact the physician when they occur.

Alternatives to Drugs

Many health complaints and disease states should not be answered by a prescription or a trip to the OTC drug counter. In some cases, drug treatment causes more damage than no treatment at

How the Consumer Can be Responsible for Drug Therapy

1. Tell the physician all physical complaints; lack of complete data can lead to inappropriate drug use. It might help to bring a written list to the doctor's office.

2. Be aware that a physical problem may be caused by adverse drug effects or drug-drug/drug-food interaction and report it to the physician.

3. Keep a personal medication record, including both prescription and OTC drugs. Share this record when you visit each physician.

4. Tell the physician of any allergic reactions experienced previously with drugs.

5. Question the physician about alternatives to drug therapy.

6. Know when, how, and with what to take drugs as well as which foods to avoid. Read all drug inserts and consult your pharmacist or physician with unanswered questions.

7. Follow medication instructions exactly. If in doubt, contact your physician or pharmacist.

8. Don't mix medications without permission from your physician.

9. If the drug schedule interferes with your lifestyle, tell your doctor immediately.

10. Do not share prescription medication with others.

11. Do not mix similar looking medications in a pill box.

12. Do not take medications in the dark or when not fully awake.

13. Do not drink alcohol when taking drugs.

14. Keep medications away from children.

15. Destroy all outdated medication.

16. Ask that childproof containers not be used if they are a problem for you.

17. Ask for a generic substitution, if available.

18. Ask for large-print prescription labels if you have vision problems.

all. For instance, those with moderate hypertension may be at greater risk from the adverse effects of antihypertensive medication than from the high blood pressure itself (Briant 1977). Some diseases can be treated more effectively by nondrug means (such as exercise, change of diet, and other life-style modifications). For instance, many times insomnia can be controlled without side effects by behavioral modifications such as reading in bed, eliminating daytime naps, or drinking a glass of warm milk. Patients who are constipated might increase dietary fiber and exercise. In many cases, exercises for lower back pain might be more helpful than muscle relaxants and pain-killers. Drugs should only be used when less risky treatment alternatives have failed.

This is not to say that drug therapy is never necessary. However, when initiating drug therapy, the long- and short-term benefits and risks need to be assessed. Will the side effects be worse than the disease symptoms? Does the complaint justify a medication or could it be the result of malnutrition, inadequate exercise, or psychosocial problems? Studies show that the more time a physician spends with a patient, the fewer drugs prescribed (Lamy and Vestal 1976). This makes sense since the longer a physician spends with a client, the more the psychosocial issues surrounding the symptoms can be examined.

Summary

Elders use more medications then any other age group because of their high prevalence of chronic conditions. Advances in drug technology have revolutionized the management of symptoms of chronic illnesses in elders. However, with their benefits come several risks. Elders are especially susceptible to adverse drug effects, drug-drug, and drug-food interactions because of the high number of OTC and prescription drugs they take. Effective patient education can increase compliance with drug regimens and reduce the risk of adverse drug effects. Nurses, pharmacists, physicians, social workers, and the consumer can work together to maximize rational drug use. Finally, nondrug alternatives should be tried before drug therapy is initiated as all drugs are accompanied by risks.

Activities

1. Ask an older relative or friend to show you the OTC and prescription drugs available in the home. Find out the level of knowledge of their use, side effects, directions for administration, and shelf life. Ask what drugs are currently being used. From your reading, do you note any drug misuse?
2. Observe individuals buying over the counter drugs at the drug store for a half-hour period. Compare the purchases of elder and younger people. Keep a record and compare your results with those of other students in the class.
3. Collect as many types of childproof containers as you can from pharmacists and other class members. Have a container-opening session in class and assess which would be most difficult to open for elders with decreased visual and touch sensitivity and reduced physical strength. Interview five elders regarding their opinion of childproof caps. Are they aware they can request a regular container?
4. Ask ten people (any age) if they know what generic drugs are and if they request them. Be prepared to educate them on the difference between generic and brand name drugs. What laws in your state encourage the use of generic drugs?
5. View "It's Up to You," a free film used to educate elders on prescription drugs (National Pharmaceutical Council, 1030 15th St., NW, Washington, D.C. 20005). Critique the usefulness of this film as part of a drug educational effort for elders. What issues were covered well? Which

were overlooked? Collect other relevant educational materials from pharmacists, the city or county health department, drug centers, mental health departments, and hospitals that can be used to educate elders on drug use.

6. Collect all the OTC and prescription drugs in your home. Is the name and label clear on the prescription drugs? Do you know why it was purchased? Is the medicine still usable (look at the expiration date)? Is it being properly stored? Concerning the OTCs, are they needed? Have you tried alternative behaviors for headache, insomnia, constipation, acid indigestion?

7. Collect and analyze drug adverisements in medical journals and regular magazine publications. How many are geared to older people? How many purport to give scientific information in the advertisement?

8. Each student is requested to bring an OTC medication to class. Without reading the label information, the rest of the class discusses what they believe the medication is used for and how they know about the product. Then the label is read. Any surprises? Discuss nondrug alternatives to each product.

Bibliography

AARP News Bulletin 1977. Generic drug wars: consumer activists challenge industry whispering campaign against generics. October, 11.

American Medical Association, 1977. *Drug evaluations.* Littleton, Mass: PSG Publ. Co.

Bauwens, E., and C. Clemmons. 1980. Foods that foil drugs. In Medical Economics Co., ed. *Practical guide to medications.* Oradell, N.J.: Medical Economics 96–98.

Bender, A.D. 1980. Therapeutic drug monitoring in the elderly. In A. A. Dietz, ed. *Aging—its chemistry.* Washington, D.C.: Amer. Assoc. for Clin. Chemistry. 394–416.

Block, L. H. 1983. Drug interactions in the geriatric client. In Pagliaro, L. A., and A. M. Pagliaro, eds. *Pharmocologic aspects of aging.* St. Louis: C. V. Mosby. 140–91.

Boyd, J. R., T. R. Covington, W. F. Stanaszek, R. T. Coussons. 1974. Drug defaulting (two parts). *Am J Hosp Pharm* 31:362–67; 485–91.

Breault, H. J. 1974. Five years with five million child resistant containers. *Clin Toxicol* 7:91–95.

Briant, R. H. 1977. Drug treatment in the elderly: Problems and prescribing rules. *Drugs* 13: 225–9.

Conrad, K. A., and R. Bressler. 1982. *Drug therapy for the elderly.* St. Louis: C. V. Mosby.

Crane, G. E. 1973. Clinical pharmacology in its 20th year. *Science* 181:124–8.

Croog, S. H., S. Revine, M. A. Teslo, M. A., et al. 1986. The effects of antihypertensive therapy upon the quality of life. *N Engl J Med* 314 (26):1657–64.

Cummings, J. H. 1974. Progress report: laxative abuse. *Gut* 15:758–66.

Davison, W. 1978. The hazards of drug treatment in old age. In J. C. Brocklehurst, ed. *Textbook of geriatric medicine and gerontology.* New York: Churchill Livingstone. 651–69.

Eberhardt, R., and L. A. Robinson. 1979. Clinical pharmacy involvement in a geriatric health clinic at a high rise apartment center. *J Am Geriatr Soc* 27:514–17.

FDA Drug Bulletin. 1985. Aspirin for myocardial infarction. Vol. 15 (4). December, 35.

Flower, R., S. Moncada, and J. R. Vane. 1980. Analgesic-antipyretics and inflammatory agents. In A. G. Gillman et al., eds. *The pharmacological basis of therapeutics.* New York: Macmillan. 682–728.

Food and Drug Administration. 1982. Generic drugs: How good are they? *FDA Consumer.* HHS Publication No. (FDA) 80–3068. Washington, D.C.: U.S. Govt. Printing Office.

Friesen, A. J. 1983. Adverse drug reactions in the geriatric client. In Pagliaro, L. A., and A. M. Pagliaro, eds. *Pharmacologic aspects of aging.* St. Louis: C. V. Mosby. 257–93.

Giannetti, V. J. 1983. Medication utilization problems among the elderly. *Health Soc Work* 8(4):262–70.

Giesel, T. S. 1986. *You're only old once!* New York: Random House.

Glew, R. H. 1985. Fever and infection. In E. P. Hoffer, ed. *Emergency problems in the elderly.* Pradell, N.J.: Medical Economic Books, 175–96.

Gomolin, I. H., and D. J. Chapron. 1983. Rational drug therapy for the aged. *Compr Ther* 9(7):17–30.

Health Care Financing Administration. 1982. Reported in *Developments in Aging, 1982,* Volume 1. U.S. Senate Special Committee on Aging.

Health Facts, Sept. 1985. Impact of medical advertising on prescribing practices. p. 1.

Health Letter. 1987. Drug-induced tranquility. April, 6–8. Published by the Public Citizen Health Research Group.

Horwitz, D., W. Lovenby, K. Engelman, and A. Sjoerdsme. 1964. Monoamine-oxidase inhibitors, tyramine and cheese. *JAMA* 188:1108–10.

Jernigan, J. A., J. C. Gudat, J. L. Blake, et al. 1980. Reference values for blood findings in relatively fit elderly persons. *J Am Geriatr Soc* 28(7):308–14.

Kalchthaler, D. O., E. Coccaro, and S. Lichtiger. 1977. Incidences of polypharmacy in a long-term care facility. *J Am Geriatr Soc* 25:308–13.

Karch, F. E., and L. Lasagna. 1975. Adverse drug reactions. *JAMA* 234:1236–41.

Kasper, J. A. 1982. Prescribed medications: Use, expenditures and source of payment. (Data preview 9. National Health Care Expenditures Study, U.S. Dept. of HHS, Pub. No. (PHS) 82–3320), April.

Klein, L. E., P. S. German, and D. M. Levinew. 1981. Adverse reactions among elderly: A reassessment. *J Am Geriatr Soc* 29:525–30.

Koch, H. 1983. Drugs most frequently used in office practice: National Ambulatory Medical Care Survey, 1981. *NCHS Advance Data* 89:1–9.

Koch, H., and D. A. Knapp. 1977. Highlights of drug utilization in office practice: National Ambulatory Medical Care Survey, 1985. *Advance Data* from *Vital and Health Statistics.* No. 134, May 19, 1987. Hyattsville, MD: Public Health Service.

Lambert, Z. V., P. L. Doeving, E. Goldstein, and W. C. McCormick. 1980. Predisposition toward generic drug acceptance. *J of Consumer Research* 7:14–23.

Lamy, P. P. 1980. *Prescribing for the elderly.* Boston: John Wright.

Lamy, P. P. 1983. Drug abuse by older adults—who is responsible? *Drug Intell Clin Pharm* 18: 657–59.

Lamy, P. P., and R. E. Vestal. 1976. Drug prescribing for the elderly. *Hosp Prac* 11(1):111–18.

Lofholm, P. 1978. Self medication by the elderly. In Kayne, R. C., ed. *Drugs and the elderly.* Los Angeles: U. of Southern Cal. Press. 8–28.

MacLennan, W. J., P. Martin, and B. J. Mason. 1977. Protein intake and serum albumin levels in the elderly. *Gerontology* 23:360–67.

Maryland Department of Mental Hygiene. 1977. *Physician prescribing practices in the Maryland Medical Assistance Program.* Medical Care Programs Drug Utilization Review. Baltimore. State of Maryland.

May, F. E., R. B. Stewart, and L. E. Cluff. 1977. Drug interactions and multiple drug administration. *Clin. Pharmacol Ther* 22(3):322–8.

Miller, R. R. 1973. Drug surveillance utilizing epidemiologic methods: A report from the Boston Collaborative Drug Surveillance Program. *Am J Hosp Pharm* 30:584–92.

Ritschel, W. A. 1983. Pharmokinetics in the aged. In Pagliaro, L. A., and A. M. Pagliaro. eds. *Pharmacologic aspects of aging.* St. Louis: C. V. Mosby. 219–58.

Robbins, L. J., and D. W. Jahnigen. 1984. Child-resistant packaging and the geriatric patient. *J Amer Geriatr Soc* 32 (6):450–52.

Rosenberg, J. M., W. A. Simon, P. Sangkachand, et al. 1976. Benzodiazepines for the elderly. *Hosp Pharm* 11:308.

Rowe, J. W., R. Andres, J. D. Tobin, et al. 1976. The effect of age on creatinine clearance in man: A cross-section and longitudinal study. *J Gerontol* 31:155–63.

Sheridan, E. S. 1984. Drugs and the elderly. In Steffl, B. M., ed. *Handbook of gerontological nursing.* New York: Van Nostrand Reinhold. 394–424.

Shock, M. W., R. Andres, A. H. Morris, and J. H. Tobin. 1978. Patterns of longitudinal changes in renal function. Proceeding XII, International Congress of Gerontology, Tokyo, August 20–25. Amsterdam: Excerpta Medica. pp. 525–27.

Simonson, W. 1984. *Medications and the elderly.* Rockville, Md.: Aspen.

Smith, M. C., and T. R. Sharpe. 1984. A study of pharmacists' involvement in drug use by the elderly. *Drug Intell Clin Pharm* 18:525–29.

Taylor, F. 1980–1981. Aspirin: America's favorite drug. *FDA Consumer.* Dec. 1980–Jan. 1981. HHS Pub. No. (FDA) 81–3115,1.

University Group Diabetes Program. 1970. A study of the effects of hypoglycemic effects on vascular complexities in patients with adult onset diabetes. *Diabetes* 19 (2):474–830.

U.S. Dept. of HEW. 1976. Long term care facility improvement campaign, Monograph No. 2. *Physicians' drug prescribing patterns in skilled nursing facilities.* DHEW Publ. No. (OS) 76–50050. Washington, D.C.: U.S. Govt. Printing Office.

U.S. Senate. 1983. *Aging reports.* Drug misuse focus of joint hearing, Special Committee on Aging. Summer. Washington, D.C.: U.S. Govt. Printing Office.

U.S. Senate Subcommittee on Long-Term Care of the Special Committee on Aging. 1975. Nursing home care in the United States: Failure in public policy. Supporting Paper N. 2: *Drugs in nursing homes: Misuse, high costs, and kickbacks.* Washington, D.C.: U.S. Govt. Printing Office.

Vestal, R. E. 1985. Clinical pharmacology. In Andres, R., E. L. Bierman, and W. R. Hazzard, eds. *Principles of geriatric medicine.* San Francisco: McGraw-Hill.

Vivian, A. S., and I. B. Goldberg. 1982. Recognizing chronic intoxication in the elderly. *Geriatrics* 37 (11):91–97.

Weintraub, M. 1981. Intelligent non-compliance with special emphasis on the elderly. *Contem Pharm Pract* 4:8–11.

Williamson, J. 1980. Adverse reactions to prescribed drugs in the elderly: A multicenter investigation. *Age and Aging* 9:73–80.

Ziance, R. J. 1979. Side effects of drugs in the elderly. In Peterson, D. M., F. J. Whillington, and B. Payne, eds. *Drugs and the elderly: Social and pharmacological issues.* Springfield, Ill.: Charles C. Thomas. pp. 53–79.

Mental Health and Illness 8

Growing old in a youth-oriented society that places primary value on independence, competence, energy and productivity is not easy. It is the primary adaptive task of old age to find satisfaction and self-esteem when role loss, social status loss and physical ailments are more noticeable and decrements more likely than ever before.

Iris Winogrond (1982)

Introduction

Contrary to popular belief, most older people are not emotionally and physically debilitated, but continue to function well and lead meaningful lives. The ability of a person to adapt and grow in later life is related to a number of physical, psychological, and situational variables. A failure to adapt to change and loss can result in physical and emotional illness. Although most older people can adjust without help, a few cannot. Friends or relatives may offer help, while mental health services may provide more formal assistance.

This chapter will discuss the life transitions commonly faced in old age and the multiple factors that influence successful adjustment. The nature, prevalence, and treatment of common mental disorders will also be addressed. Finally, a summary of the types of mental health services, both community and institutional are included.

Mental Health Defined

There is no clear distinction between what is normal or abnormal behavior as it varies with age, situation, and societal norms. Behaviors accepted as normal for those of one age are often considered signs of mental illness when manifested by those in another age group. For example, dependent behavior in a middle-aged man may be abnormal, but dependence in a small child or a physically impaired older person is not. Whether a behavior is classified as abnormal or normal may also depend on the situation. Anxiety is considered normal before a test or job interview, but if it lasts for an extended period, it is considered abnormal. Finally, whether a behavior is classified as normal depends on cultural and societal norms. Suicide after the death of a spouse is considered the norm in some cultures, but in most, this behavior is an indication of a severe mental problem. What constitutes abnormal or normal behavior also depends on the individual's personality and past actions. For instance, lethargy may be normal in an elder who acted that way throughout life, but abnormal when suddenly appearing in another elder who usually is self-motivated and energetic.

Mental health is especially difficult to define for elders. The definition should not be based on stereotypes associated with how old people should behave, but must include special characteristics of elders. Too often, stereotypes of how elders should behave limit our view of elders' potential. We all believe there are appropriate ways for elders to respond to retirement, widowhood, poor health, or grandparenthood, and reinforce elders for meeting our expectations or "acting their age." However, this problem is not remedied by applying the same criteria for mental health to all individuals, regardless of their differences. For instance, defining mental health in terms of independence denies mental health to the elder who is physically debilitated and unable to care for some personal needs. Defining mental health in elders is further complicated by the heterogeneity of the elder population.

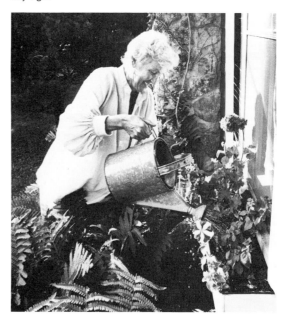

A positive outlook on life promotes mental health at any age.

Jahoda (1958) suggests six criteria for positive mental health: positive self attitudes, growth and self-actualization, integration of the personality, autonomy, reality perception, and mastery of environment. However, Birren and Renner (1979) suggest that these criteria cannot be easily applied to some older persons. For example, environmental mastery may be difficult or impossible for elders who are poor, handicapped, or institutionalized. Likewise, elders facing retirement, poor health, or widowhood may be forced to give up activities that formerly fulfilled their needs for autonomy or self-esteem and satisfy this need through a more restricted set of alternatives. Further, for elders, self-actualization may focus on living in the present and reviewing the past rather than setting goals and orienting toward the future. Birren and Renner (1980) state that mental health among elders entails maximizing individual potential in regard to changing abilities and resources.

Transitions in Later Life

Like any other period in life, old age is accompanied by transitions that require adaptation. However, the transitions faced by each age group differ. In general, the young are preparing for employment, finding a mate, setting up a home; the middle-aged are raising children, maintaining a job, and caring for aged parents. In the later years, the transitions are characterized by loss: loss of job, loss of spouse, loss of health, loss of youthful appearance, loss of income, loss of status, loss of residence, loss of independence.

One of the most profound transitions an elder commonly faces is *multiple losses of loved ones—* siblings, parents, friends, and spouse. The death of a spouse is considered to be one of the most traumatic of life experiences. In addition to grief itself, the individual must adapt to a new social role, increased responsibility, and, often for widows, financial hardship.

Retirement is often a severe life crisis, especially for men. Many have few other interests or social contacts outside their job, making adjustment to retirement very difficult. Common emotional reactions include depression, restlessness, boredom, and feelings of uselessness. Often social status, as seen by self and others, is connected to job performance. Women generally find the transition easier because they are used to domestic activity whether they work outside the home or not. Further, they are more likely to have social ties that extend beyond the workplace.

Marital transitions are also common in later life. After retirement, couples generally have more time to spend together. They may welcome the renewed time for intimacy or they may irritate each other by constant exposure. When one partner becomes ill, the other must adapt to more responsibility, altered relationship roles, and less personal time.

Elders, especially the very old, must often cope with *multiple physical illnesses* and *sensory* and *mobility decrements* that alter their mobility and daily routine and often force them to rely on others for basic care. Increased disabilities may require elders to move to a more sheltered living environment. This is not always negative; some welcome a change of residence.

Factors Affecting Adjustment

Despite the many transitions in later life, most older persons do adapt. Effective adjustment to these transitions is influenced by a number of factors: personality, health status, income, social supports, and coping skills.

Neugarten (1977) asserts that *personality* profoundly influences adaptation to the physical and social transitions that occur with advancing age. Personality characteristics are consistent throughout adulthood. A number of large scale longitudinal studies report little to no significant change in personality traits with age (Costa et al. 1980). When marked changes do occur, they are considered to be an indication of mental or physical illness.

The effect of *physical health* upon adaptation becomes more important with age because elders, especially the very old, have more chronic illnesses than other age groups. Multiple studies have shown physical health to be one of the strongest correlates with life satisfaction, adjustment, self esteem, and mental health. Both the symptoms of illness and the treatment regimen strain adaptive capacity. Illness, pain, debilitation, and dependence have a tremendous effect on life-style and emotional health. Because many chronic illnesses worsen over time, elders are fearful of progressive debilitation and dependence. Physical illnesses are often accompanied by mental distress, especially anxiety and depression. Further, the treatment of physical problems may cause mental symptoms (e.g., depression, insomnia, hallucinations). Decline in sensory abilities (especially vision and hearing) can result in withdrawal from social contacts, confusion, depression, and impairment of orientation and mobility.

Despite their physical decrements, the majority of elders rank themselves in better health than others their age. Thus, the perception of

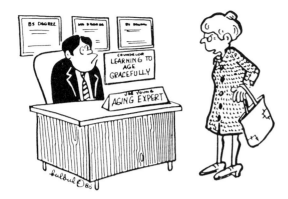

GOT ANY IDEAS ON AGING GRACEFULLY
WITH NO HOUSING, NO MEDICAL CARE
AND NO INCOME!

health or disability may be more important in determining successful adaptation than the actual extent of illness or decrement.

Financial situation can also affect mental health. Those with sufficient income are able to have their food, shelter, recreational, and health needs met. In contrast, those who are poor have the additional stress of maintaining their health with limited resources. As income generally declines after age sixty-five, many elders must deal with poverty and its concomitant problems for the first time. Poverty and the fear of poverty affect the sense of security and increase anxiety and depression at any age.

It is well established that the presence of *social support* promotes health. Isolated adults have a significantly higher death rate than those with social ties; the more ties, the lower the death rate (Berkman and Syme 1979). The presence of social supports not only buffers stress, but may reduce the symptoms of physical illness (Cohen et al. 1985).

The *ability to cope with stress* is an important factor in determining successful adaptation to old age. Stress is any physiological or psychological situation that challenges the individual's capacity to adapt. For instance, extreme temperatures, radiation, noise, and starvation are physical stressors, while life events such as death of a loved one, change in residence, and retirement are psychological stressors. Individual response to

stress is likely more important than the amount of stressors experienced. Certain personality types are able to adapt more easily to stress than others: some people are debilitated by it; others are challenged.

Level of stress and coping ability can profoundly affect health status. Numerous studies have shown that high stress is associated with a number of illnesses: hypertension, peptic ulcers, diabetes, respiratory infections, and some cancers. However, the data are mixed regarding the effect of stressors on health status of elders, except for widowers. Newly widowed men exhibit an excess illness and death rate following a spousal death (Gerber et al. 1975). Whether this is a psycho-physiological reaction to the stress itself or poor self-care is not known.

Elders experience a number of life changes. However, results of the National Health Interview Survey (National Center for Health Statistics 1986) show that elders report themselves to be under less stress than any other adult age group: 67 percent of those over age sixty-five reported little or no stress in the past two weeks, 50 percent of the forty-five to sixty-four years olds reported little or no stress, and only 40 percent of those age eighteen to forty-four had little or no stress in the past two weeks. Most (65 percent) older people reported that stresses experienced in the past year had little or no effect upon their health. The reason might be that stress is a relatively new term and many older people do not associate mental stress with physiological effects upon health. On the other hand, elders may cope more effectively with stress for a variety of reasons: they anticipate the changes, allow themselves more time to adapt to their stressors, minimize the total number of stressors to those they can control, or have enough experience in coping with stress to have learned effective coping strategies.

At any age, stress demands adaptation and adaptation demands energy. The vast majority of elders are able to cope with life's stresses and need transient psychological assistance at most. When

Chapter 8

Losses

Today I read about a man who slashed his
    wrists because he lost his hat.
He was old, and of course, they say he was crazy.
I think not.
I think he'd just had all the losses he could take.
He said as much.
His last words were, "Oh, God, now I've lost my hat, too."
I know how he felt.
Every time you turn around, time—with a little help from
    your friends—grabs off something else. Something precious.
    At least to you.
Hearing, Sight, Beauty, Job, House. Even the corner
    grocery store turns into a parking lot and is lost.
Finally, you lose the thing you can't do without—hope
    (that it can get better).
Dear God, when he gets to heaven, let that man
    find his hat on the gatepost.

the stress becomes unmanageable, temporary mood disturbance or more serious mental illness may result.

Mental Illness

Older people with mental problems may continue a pattern begun in younger years or may manifest a mental problem for the first time in later life. Mental problems appearing for the first time in an older person are generally due either to a failure to adapt to stresses or to a physiological disorder in brain function that may have taken years to develop. Elders who have sustained multiple losses over a short time period, lack social support, and have adapted poorly to past stresses are particularly vulnerable to the onset of mental disorders in later life. Hospitalization, institutionalization, or the presence of multiple physical illnesses with little chance of recovery can also predispose one to mental problems.

The prevalence of mental illness in elders is difficult to determine because studies use different criteria to define mental illness. Some rely on self-reports of mental illness, others base their results on the number of persons seeking professional assistance. Still others attempt to test for the presence of certain disorders by interviewing elders or administering written psychological surveys. Most studies report an estimated 10 to 20 percent of elders living in the community have some degree of mental impairment. Although elders have fewer mental disorders than other age groups when all categories of mental illness are grouped together, elders as a group have higher rates of cognitive impairment. One study of three communities reported that mild cognitive impairment (mainly attributed to Alzheimer's disease) was present in 14 percent of elder men and women, and severe impairment was noted in 5.6 percent of elder men and 3 percent of the elder women (Myers et al. 1984). Another indicator of mental problems—suicide rate—is highest among the elder population, and widowed males have the highest rates of all. Suicide among elders will be discussed in Chapter 14.

Almost half the nursing home residents in the United States have a significant mental impairment, while another 40 percent have moderate to mild psychiatric difficulty (Blazer 1983). Rovner et al. (1986) randomly interviewed fifty elders in a nursing home and reported that 94 percent of the residents had mental disorders. Dementia was the most common diagnosis.

The types of mental illness to be discussed below are classified according to the *Diagnostic and Statistical Manual of Mental Disorders* (*DSM III*) developed by the American Psychiatric Association in 1980. Mental disorders are divided into two categories: organic and functional. Organic disorders are mental disturbances caused by impaired brain function. Functional disorders are assumed to result from personality and life experience of the individual, not due to brain alterations. However, both organic and functional disorders commonly coexist in elder individuals; symptoms overlap and it is difficult to distinguish one from the other. Those who develop organic impairments may later show functional symptoms. Conversely, those with functional disorders may later have organic disorders.

Functional Disorders

The majority of functional disorders are of long duration, and symptoms only rarely appear for the first time in later life. If a functional disorder is noted for the first time in an older person, it is likely that maladjustments occurred earlier in life but were not noticed until the later years. It is estimated that functional disorders account for almost one-half the admissions of older adults to acute-care psychiatric hospitals (Gurland and Cross 1982).

Functional disorders are difficult to diagnose in elders because they often manifest symptoms that can be easily attributed to physical ailments, adverse drug reactions, and age-associated changes in mental functioning. Whether some functional disorders are the cause or consequence of chronic illness is not known, but they usually occur together. Those functional disorders common in elders will be discussed in this section.

Anxiety

Anxiety may be classified as a symptom or a mental disorder, depending upon the appropriateness of the response, the severity of the symptoms, and the degree to which it affects daily living. Transient anxiety can be a normal state of tension in response to a stressful situation. For anxiety to be considered a disorder, the symptoms must significantly curtail social functioning, intimate relationships, or work. Whereas transient anxiety generally occurs in response to a specific environmental signal, such as an upcoming test, anxiety disorders occur without a specific external trigger. Regardless of the cause, anxiety is characterized by a general fear or agitation, accompanied by such physical signs as dry mouth, restlessness, sweating, upset stomach, heart palpitations, insomnia, diarrhea, hyperventilation, shortness of breath, faintness, obsessive eating, or loss of appetite. Other symptoms of anxiety disorders include a fear of dying, losing control, or going crazy.

Anxiety disorders are of four types: generalized anxiety disorders, panic disorders, phobic disorders, and obsessive-compulsive disorders. Panic and generalized anxiety disorders are the most common forms of anxiety exhibited in elders, while phobic and obsessive-compulsive problems are uncommon. Individuals with panic disorders suffer brief, recurrent attacks of intense anxiety, while those suffering from generalized anxiety disorders have a constant sense of restlessness, heart palpitations, apprehension, and tension unassociated with a dangerous situation. Phobic disorders are characterized by irrational fears that result in avoidance of particular situations or objects. For instance, agoraphobia is an irrational fear of open spaces and claustrophobia is a fear of closed spaces. Finally, those with obsessive-compulsive disorders have recurring unpleasant thoughts that they feel unable to control as well as a need to continually complete senseless behaviors (e.g., washing and rewashing the hands) to reduce anxiety.

Anxiety is very common among American adults. Surveys report that mild anxiety reactions are more prevalent in old age than other age groups (Sallis and Lichstein 1982). It is estimated that about 14 percent of elders in the community experience abnormal anxiety (Lurie et al. 1987).

Diagnosing anxiety in elders is difficult since it commonly occurs with depression and dementia and may be overlooked. Furthermore, symptoms of anxiety mimic symptoms of illness: heart palpitations, shortness of breath, weakness, appetite changes. For this reason, a comprehensive examination is necessary to determine if the anxiety is caused by disease, drug reactions, psychological problems, or transient life events.

Both transient and chronic anxiety should be treated because they increase feelings of helplessness and isolation, raise susceptibility to several illnesses, and decrease ability to withstand stress. Elders already weakened by illness may suffer further physical and mental deterioration because of persistent anxiety. The best treatment is to remove the cause of the anxiety. When this is not possible, mild tranquilizers are commonly prescribed for short-term symptom relief. However, their degree of success in anxiety reduction is questionable (Solomon 1976). These anti-anxiety agents are more potent in elders and commonly cause drowsiness, muscle weakness, dizziness, fatigue, and uncoordination.

Psychotherapy is likely to be effective, both individually and in groups. However, there are no published reports on the value of psychotherapy for anxious elders. Relaxation training, physical exercise, and activity therapy may help to reduce stress levels as they enhance the ability to relax and reduce self-defeating negative thoughts.

Depression

Clinical depression is the most common psychological disorder among older people. However, contrary to earlier belief, the rate of major depression is significantly lower among elders than among younger adult groups. About 4 percent of older people suffer from major depression (Lurie et al. 1987). Further, the reported rate of depression symptoms are three times more common in the under forty-five group than those over sixty-five (Koenig 1986). The lower rate of depression among elders may be due to less stress or more effective coping behavior. In the later years, depressive symptoms are likely to be initiated by adverse social conditions and declining health, as healthy elders who do not encounter adverse social situations are no more depressed than in younger years (Murrell et al. 1983).

Symptoms of depression vary from transient moods of feeling blue to persistent and incapacitating despair and suicidal thoughts. Other symptoms include weight loss, sleeping troubles, loss of energy, feelings of worthlessness, and loss of interest in usual activities. Depression can be a normal response to losses or life changes that cannot be controlled. Despite the intense emotion, few people develop major depression following the loss of a loved one. Depression is considered a clinical problem when there is a prolonged mood disturbance and at least four other symptoms consistently for at least two weeks. Older people who are depressed may withdraw from social participation, refuse to speak, and become unable to care for themselves. In addition, depressed elders commonly manifest cognitive impairment, disorientation, slow speed of movement, angry outbursts, and shortened attention span.

Depression is difficult to diagnose because its symptoms may reflect other problems. It is hard to differentiate clinical depression from depression as a normal reaction to loss. Some physicians do not attempt to determine the underlying cause of depression, preferring to treat its symptoms.

Depression may be a transient reaction to stress or a long term chronic illness.

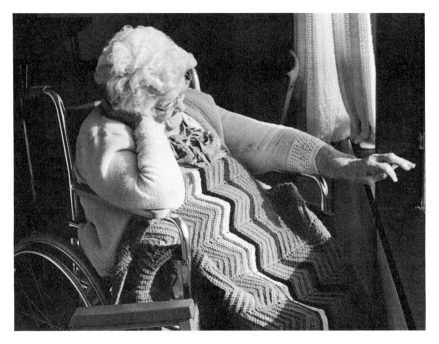

However, depression can be a symptom of disease, especially dementia, cardiovascular disease, cancer, and stroke, so it is important to determine its cause, not only treat the symptom (Jarvik and Noshkes 1985).

A number of treatments may be used for depression but drugs are the most common approach to symptom relief for older people. However, the side effects of disorientation and memory loss may be falsely diagnosed as dementia, prompting treatment with stronger drugs that promote further dependency. It is estimated that 15 percent of the causes of dementia are the result of drug reactions. Often the patient improves when all drugs are removed. Psychotherapy has been shown to be effective in treating depression in elders (Scholomskas et al. 1983). In serious cases, electroconvulsive therapy is utilized.

It is hard to treat depression in later life since there are often real reasons for depression (loss of income, cognitive loss, loss of health, loss of family and friends). In contrast to younger people, depression among elders is more likely a reaction to reality than a distorted view of it. However, proper treatment of depression is crucial because of the high rate of suicide in elders.

Hypochondriasis

Hypochondriasis is an inordinate preoccupation with bodily functions and unrealistic concerns about disease. From 10 to 20 percent of elders residing in the community have some degree of hypochondriasis (Busse and Blazer 1980). People with hypochondriasis often complain of problems with digestion, constipation, shortness of breath, and heart palpitations, and usually believe their multiple symptoms are due to a serious underlying disease. They are not reassured when a physician finds nothing physically wrong. Hypochondriasis almost always accompanies depression, but the hypochondrial patient is generally less socially withdrawn. Hypochondriasis is a response to accumulated stress, mainly due to situations in which the person suffers prolonged criticism, isolation due to economic restrictions, or decline in marital satisfaction due to a partner's disability (Busse 1976). The individual loses interest in others and lapses into self-absorption. Complaints of physical symptoms are used to deal with unacceptable hostile feelings toward significant others. Instead of voicing concern about feelings directly and honestly, the individual focuses on physical disease. Some believe hypochondriasis is used as an escape from feelings of personal failure; taking on the sick role is easier than reinvesting in new goals and interests (Busse and Pfeiffer 1977).

It is generally believed that hypochondriasis becomes more prevalent in later life but no evidence to support that claim has been found (Costa and McCrae 1980). However, this increase may be due to the widely held stereotype that elders are unduly preoccupied with bodily functions and health complaints. Older people do have a higher incidence of health problems with age, so it is reasonable that somatic complaints would increase. In addition, symptoms often associated with hypochondriasis (e.g., heart palpitations, general fatigue, and constipation) are common symptoms of real health problems.

Because of the multiplicity of chronic illnesses and drug reactions in elders, all complaints should be taken seriously before diagnosing hypochondriasis since the complaints often have an organic base. Older persons who are known hypochondriacs may not be properly diagnosed and treated for a real illness because their symptoms are immediately labeled as psychological.

Hypochondriasis may be treated with minor tranquilizers, placebo medications, or harmless home treatments (such as warm baths) to assure the client that the health worker is attempting to relieve the symptoms. Individual, group, or marital psychotherapy may help the hypochondriac to express feelings directly, enhance self-concept, and increase socialization.

Paranoia

Paranoid individuals have delusions that they are being persecuted by others for a perceived wrongdoing. A delusion is a false belief based on mistaken assumptions about external reality that is not changed by obvious evidence to the contrary. The behavior is considered serious if it has continued for at least six months. Paranoia generally develops gradually and intellectual function is not impaired. Mild paranoia is characterized by rigidity in thought, unwarranted suspiciousness, hypersensitivity, exaggerated self-importance, and a tendency to blame others and attribute evil motives to them. Paranoid individuals are seldom seen by mental health workers because they are secretive, or merely viewed as eccentric or senile by those around them. Paranoid psychosis is more serious. These people harbor delusions that may also be accompanied by auditory hallucinations. For instance, a person may believe that someone is trying to poison him or her and may even hear someone in the kitchen doing the deed. When these delusions affect health or social contacts, professional help is warranted.

Among young people, paranoia indicates a severe psychiatric disturbance, but in the old it is considered less serious. Paranoia rarely appears for the first time in elders. When it occurs for the first time in the later years, it is associated with losses and increased vulnerability: institutionalization, hearing or visual impairments, dependence, social isolation, organic brain disorder, stress, or drug reactions. In elders, most reactions are brief with only slight alterations in behavior, mood, and reasoning. It is estimated that 1 to 3 percent of those elders living in the community suffer from paranoia (Post 1980).

Like other functional disorders, paranoia is difficult to diagnose. Although strange behavior occurs, it is not so strange as to attract attention. Before diagnosing paranoia, one should investigate whether the patient's belief is based on fact. Next, the presence of sensory losses, organic problems, and stressful events should be examined. Family therapy is helpful for paranoid disorders; the family can be trained to listen and offer support to counteract the individual's fears, increase the elders' social interaction, and provide a stable environment to reduce paranoid incidents. Drugs, mainly minor tranquilizers, are effective in some cases.

Schizophrenia

There is more confusion about the cause, symptoms, and classification of schizophrenia than any other mental disorder. Schizophrenia is characterized by delusions, persecutory thoughts, hallucinations, and illogical thought sequences. Speech may have reduced intensity, there may be no sign of emotional expression, or inappropriate emotional responses. Confusion regarding personal identity and withdrawal into a fantasy world is common.

Nearly half those in mental institutions are diagnosed as schizophrenic. The majority of institutionalized elder schizophrenics acquired the disorder in late adolescence and have carried the disorder into their later years. A diagnosed schizophrenic is never cured, and interludes of sanity are assumed to be temporary remissions. Symptoms of schizophrenia also occur with alcoholism and depression. In many old persons, schizophrenia may mistakenly be assumed to be organic brain syndrome since the symptoms overlap.

Schizophrenia is difficult to treat because the individual is seldom lucid and capable of responding to psychotherapy. Psychotherapeutic approaches include behavioral interventions to increase positive behaviors and decrease disruptive ones, and the use of small groups to work on social skills and activities of daily living. Most older schizophrenics need a structured environment for survival. Unfortunately many are placed in nursing homes where staff have neither the interest nor training to respond to their needs. Major tranquilizers are the most effective treatment for schizophrenics of all ages to reduce the symptoms of psychotic episodes. Often other drugs must be given simultaneously to counteract side effects of the tranquilizers.

Sleep Disorders

Elders report more sleep complaints than any other age group: difficulty falling asleep, periods of wakefulness in bed, restless sleep, and early morning awakening. Studies have documented that sleep patterns change with age. In the later years, it is more difficult to sustain sleep through the night; night awakenings are more frequent and prolonged. Also, sleep stage periods are shorter. The sleep of older males is more disturbed than their female counterparts (Webb 1982). Despite these complaints, a recent report indicated that, on the average, elders slept slightly more than those age thirty to sixty-four. More than twice as many elders (21 percent) reported that they slept nine or more hours in a twenty-four-hour period as those aged thirty to sixty-four (National Center for Health Statistics 1986).

Sleep disturbances can result from a number of physiological and psychological causes. One of the most common is respiratory disturbances (Bliwise et al. 1983). Unfortunately, the incidence and length of respiratory disturbances are worsened with sleeping pills (Guilleminault 1982). Other reasons for sleep disruption are the need to urinate, bone and joint pain, or drug reactions. Worry, anxiety, stress, grief, or depression can inhibit restful sleep. Worry about the ability to fall asleep further aggravates the problem.

In treating sleep disorders in elders, the presence of illness, alcohol or drug reactions, depression, grief, or organic brain syndrome must be ruled out so that the underlying cause, not the symptoms of insomnia, can be treated. Sleeping patterns can be ascertained by conducting a sleep history that includes self-reported information on symptoms, napping patterns, evidence of recent life changes, diet, exercise, general activity level, and current drug use. If the sleep disorder is severe, observation of sleeping patterns in a sleep laboratory provides further information.

Many sleep disorders can be improved by behavioral modification: going to sleep at the same time each evening, drinking warm milk before bedtime, eliminating caffeine or other stimulants a few hours before bedtime, light exercise during the day, using the bed only for sleeping. Many people nap during the day to compensate for poor night-time sleep, but napping makes it more difficult to fall asleep the following night. If one does not nap, sleep loss improves the deep sleep the next night (Bliwise et al. 1983). If sleep disorders are not improved with behavioral modification, psychotherapy may be utilized. Barbiturates and benzodiazapines (such as Valium) are often prescribed to induce sleep, but there is no evidence that they are effective in long-term use. Further, they suppress deep sleep, affect daytime wakefulness, and, for barbiturates, tolerance builds up after only a few days.

Substance Use Disorders

Elders rarely abuse illegal substances associated with drug abuse in younger groups. They more commonly misuse or become dependent on prescription drugs or alcohol. It is generally agreed that the risk of prescription drug misuse and adverse drug reactions increases proportionally with the frequency and quantity of drug intake. The extent of prescription drug abuse among elders is difficult to determine because it encompasses both drug addiction/dependency and misuse (such as not taking a drug according to label directions).

Elders are less likely to abuse alcohol than younger groups as alcohol consumption decreases with age. In the later years, there is a significant drop in heavy drinkers and a higher percentage of abstainers than in younger adult groups (National Center for Health Statistics 1986). However, as studies are cross-sectional, the lower use of alcohol in old age may reflect generational differences: those who are now old may never have drunk as much as the young. It is predicted that the younger generation as they grow old will have a higher prevalence of alcohol use. Alcohol abuse is more common among elder men than women and those of both sexes who live alone.

Data are extremely variable, but from 2 to 10 percent of elders living in the community abuse alcohol (Shuckit and Pastor 1978). Alcohol abuse is often difficult to confirm in elders. Elder alcoholics are less likely to be detected by an employer or spouse, and since many are retired and live alone, their behavior is not socially disruptive. Further, the definition of a problem drinker varies. Moderate alcohol consumption in a young adult may be manifested as a drinking problem in older persons. For a given amount of alcohol, older people become more readily intoxicated and experience the effects of alcohol longer than young people.

Alcoholism in old age is of two types. Two-thirds of elder alcoholics are *early-onset*—those with a long history of chronic alcoholism. In contrast, *late-onset* alcoholics develop problem drinking habits in their later years, probably in response to the stresses and losses of old age. Insomnia and chronic physical illness accompanied by pain and emotional disorganization may predispose some to abuse alcohol. Major depression may also precede alcoholism, especially among older women. However, the relationship between late-onset alcoholism and such factors are as yet untested. Both types of alcoholism are treated in the same way.

Alcoholism has more subtle manifestations in elders than in younger groups and the problems are often social rather than medical. Younger people who abuse alcohol are likely to have visible signs of alcohol intoxication and withdrawal. However, in older persons, alcohol abuse is more difficult to diagnose and may be missed. The physical signs of alcoholism are more diffuse in elders: depression, dementia-like reactions, poor grooming, incontinence, susceptibility to injury and falls, malnutrition, and general physical deterioration (Wattis 1981). Dementia has been reported to accompany alcoholism in as many as 60 percent of older alcohol abusers admitted to hospitals (Atkinson and Kofoed 1984).

Alcohol abuse is associated with multiple physical and psychological problems. Studies show that excess alcohol consumption shortens life expectancy, contributes to high suicide rates, and antagonizes many chronic illnesses (especially diabetes) and nutritional deficiencies. Additionally, heavy alcohol use can induce dementia, cognitive deficits, depression, and psychosis (Parsons and Leber 1981; Ryan and Butters 1980). When alcohol abuse progresses to the extent that it causes brain damage, it is considered an organic problem. Alcohol affects muscular coordination, reaction time, and equilibrium, increasing susceptibility to accidents. Older alcoholics are also at high risk for adverse reactions when other drugs are mixed with alcohol.

Alcoholism can be treated. In young and middle-aged problem drinkers, hospitalization and detoxification are common methods. However, in older alcoholics, there is usually an absence of physical distress and the need for hospital treatment of alcohol withdrawal is rare. Alcoholics can often be successfully managed by their own physician while living in the community. Therapy directed at social and psychological stresses associated with aging, antidepressant drugs, and medical care for those with problems are the most successful treatment strategies for older adults. Older alcoholics are more likely to complete treatment successfully than younger alcoholics and to maintain sobriety for longer periods (Schuckit 1977). Although older people do participate in Alcoholics Anonymous meetings, intervention and treatment programs with specific focus on elders seem to be the most successful (Zimberg 1983).

Organic Disorders

Significant memory loss and other cognitive impairments are not signs of aging but are symptoms of an underlying physiological problem. It is estimated that about 5 percent of the older population have a moderate to severe organic disorder and 10 percent more have a mild disorder (Gurland and Cross 1982). Organic problems may be caused by a number of factors, such as malnutrition, drug effects, and disease. Organic disorders are difficult to diagnose in elders since symptoms overlap with functional disorders. However, early diagnosis of organic disorders is essential because many are treatable. Diagnostic

procedures should include an assessment of the person's ability to function, selected laboratory tests, and a thorough medical history and physical examination. See Larson et al. (1986a) for information on a proper dementia workup. Even if cognitive impairments are mild, it could be a sign of a more severe disorder. One study found that mild memory impairments were associated with death four years after first being observed (Zarit et al. 1978).

Dementia or Organic Brain Syndrome

Dementia, also called organic brain syndrome, is a progressive brain impairment that interferes with normal intellectual functioning. Classic symptoms include significant losses of at least three of the following: cognition, memory, language, recognition, visual and spatial skills, and personality (Larson et al. 1986b). All behaviors may not be present at all times and they may vary in intensity. Those with mild organic brain syndrome cannot abstract and assimilate new information. In severe cases, the individual loses self-care skills and becomes incontinent (Butler and Lewis 1982).

The incidence of dementia increases with age, afflicting 5 percent of those sixty-five to seventy-five and over 20 percent of those eighty-five and older. Some degree of dementia is present in over half the nursing home residents (Rowe 1985). Although records are not kept on deaths from dementia, it is estimated to be the fourth or fifth leading cause of death since it shortens the life of those with other diseases. It is estimated that by 1990, the cost of maintaining those with organic brain syndrome will be $43 billion a year (Rowe 1985).

In the past, dementia was believed to be an acceleration of the normal aging process caused by hardening of the arteries that supply the brain with oxygen. Researchers now find that dementia can be caused by a number of factors: brain tumors, fever, trauma, environmental toxins, chronic lung disease, alcoholism, drugs, and stroke, to name a few. The majority of dementias are irreversible and result in progressive, permanent mental impairment. Hearing loss, pneumonia, electrolyte imbalances, nutritional deficiencies (especially B12), and certain drugs also have been known to cause temporary dementia. A sudden onset of symptoms often signals a reversible drug reaction or treatable condition, while a progressively worsening deterioration that does not respond to therapy is more likely irreversible. About 10–20 percent of the dementias are totally reversible or can be partially reversed with appropriate drugs or surgical procedures (Smith and Kiloh 1981).

Dementia, or senility, is often used as a catch-all diagnosis for troubled elders and is frequently misdiagnosed. Many elders diagnosed with dementia actually suffer from depression (Garcia 1981). An incorrect diagnosis of dementia can have profound effects on the patient and the family since a diagnosis of senility is often used as a rationale for nursing home placement. Not only is it overdiagnosed, but potentially treatable dementia is often overlooked, perhaps because physicians view its symptoms as an inevitable accompaniment to old age (Sabin et al. 1982). Despite its common usage, the term *senility* should be discouraged.

By far the most common dementia is Alzheimer's disease. Unfortunately, very little is known about its cause, prevention, or treatment. Alzheimer's disease is a devastating syndrome characterized by a gradual, irreversible, and progressive decline in mental functioning that interferes with the activities of daily living. The course of the disease is from about five to ten years.

The presence of Alzheimer's disease can only be diagnosed by eliminating other possibilities through a comprehensive assessment and consultation with the family, if present. The only physiological determinant of the disease is a characteristic tangle of fibers within nerve cells and the presence of senile plaques—abnormal nerve cells wrapped with a waxy waste material—in the part of the brain where higher thought originates. Their effect on brain function is unknown. The extent of these neurological changes can only be determined by autopsy.

Senility

Senility, despite its popularity among lay persons and the medical profession, tells us virtually nothing about the older person's actual condition or prognosis. Confusion, hostility, memory loss, and disorientation are often "explained" by "Well, what can you expect, you are old." Unfortunately, "old" frequently translates into "senile" which in turn often results in no effort at treatment. Senility is too often used as a "wastebasket" term when no identifiable cause can be found for the person's behavior. Its use is to describe age at onset; senility refers to the appearance of a disorder after the age of 65. Realistically, it has no redeeming scientific value as a diagnostic term; it encourages a "give up" approach, making matters much worse for staff, family members and elderly "victims" themselves. Treatment for those who are "senile" often consists of custodial care—in effect, no active treatment.

(From Hayslip, 1983, p. 168)

There are many hypotheses to explain the cause of Alzheimer's disease. Alzheimer's disease may be a variety of diseases, all with the same outcome but differing causes. It is estimated that 10 to 15 percent of the cases have a hereditary base. There seems to be a genetic component since relatives of a person who developed symptoms before age sixty-five are more likely to contract dementia. Further, those with Down's Syndrome (a genetic disorder caused by the presence of an extra chromosome), are at particularly high risk for Alzheimer's disease. Other proposed causes of Alzheimer's disease are: slow-growing virus, biochemical abnormality in

Individuals with Alzheimer's disease need stimulation in a sheltered environment.

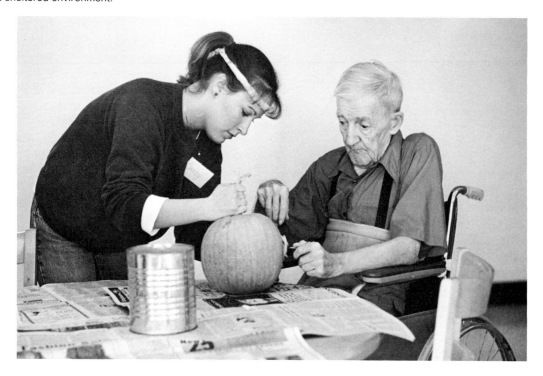

the brain, or accumulation of heavy metals (aluminum and iron) or mineral deficiencies (zinc) in the brain, among others. Even though many of these abnormalities occur, it is difficult to tell which of the above cause Alzheimer's disease and which merely accompany it.

The second most common type of dementia is multi-infarct dementia. Small strokes occur within the brain that cause an insufficiency of blood to some areas and consequent death of the brain tissue. Appearance is sudden, with symptoms of dizziness, headaches, and decreased energy in addition to the classic dementia symptoms. The course of this type of dementia is erratic. Initially, individuals may recover lost function, but as more small strokes occur, the chance of recovery decreases. This type of dementia is associated with high blood pressure. However, overtreatment of hypertension to reduce the incidence of small strokes is risky; if blood pressure is reduced excessively, blood flow to the brain is impaired.

No medication is known to reverse progressive cognitive losses. However, one preliminary study on a drug called THA (tetrahydroaminoacridine) reported significant improvement in memory of sixteen out of seventeen Alzheimer's disease patients. The drug blocks the action of the enzyme that degrades acetylcholine, an important neurotransmitter in the brain (Summers et al. 1986). The researchers caution that the drug is not a cure but has promise in reducing some symptoms for some patients. Until a drug is found to reverse the degeneration caused by the disease, clinicians can only reduce the symptoms. Antidepressant and major tranquilizer drugs are often used to control the most troublesome behavioral disturbances that accompany dementia: sleeplessness, violent behavior, agitation, depression, and paranoia. In the early stages, the patient needs counseling to cope with stress and depression.

　　　　　　　　　　　　　　Chapter 8

Dementia, especially Alzheimer's disease, has a devastating effect on families as they witness a slow, progressive physical and mental decline of a loved one with no hope of treatment or cure. The physical stress resulting from providing around-the-clock personal care, coupled with the psychological stress can be overwhelming. The financial burden of care can leave a family impoverished. Social isolation can be reduced by group activities. Attention to personal hygiene can reduce the risk of other diseases. For more information on the care of those with dementia, see Larson et al. (1986b) and Council of Scientific Affairs, American Medical Association (1986).

Most of those with dementia are cared for at home, mainly by the spouse, but often by a daughter. Caretakers are frequently depressed, isolated from previous friends and outside interests, and are in poor health. The strain on caregivers of demented elders is due to problems of emotional or attentional demands of the patient rather than the number of disabilities of the patient or the level of behavioral disturbances (Gilleard et al. 1982). Despite the stress of caregiving, most caretakers develop a close bond with the patient and continue to care for the patient even to the point of exhaustion or illness.

Those who care for the demented often need outside help to cope with its heavy demands. This assistance may include support to cope with feelings of grief, guilt, and anger; knowledge about the disease, changes to expect, and how to cope; suggestions to restructure the home environment; referrals to community agencies, especially those that provide temporary relief to the caregiver; and finally, support for the family when institutionalization is necessary. Groups composed of families of those with Alzheimer's disease have been organized in many communities for mutual support and education. An excellent source of guidance for families of patients with dementia is *The Thirty Six Hour Day* (Mace and Rabins 1981).

Delirium

Delirium is a temporary malfunction of a significant proportion of brain cells. It is characterized by a well-defined onset of symptoms: confusion, disorientation, memory loss, decreased attention span, insomnia, and excitability. Unlike dementia, delirium begins abruptly and may not progressively worsen. However, if left untreated, it may become irreversible. Delirium can be caused by a number of factors: alcoholism, malnutrition, vitamin deficiencies, viral infections, drug side effects, abrupt drug withdrawal, fever, pneumonia, head trauma, heart attack, diabetes, or dehydration.

Delirium may be difficult to diagnose because it mimics dementia and may occur with it. Because delirium is most often caused by a somatic problem or drug reaction, it is imperative that a thorough medical assessment be undertaken and the underlying problem corrected to restore mental function.

Assessment of Psychological Vulnerability

A thorough assessment of the impaired individual must be conducted to accurately diagnose the cause and extent of mental dysfunction. Assessments should be conducted periodically throughout the treatment process to detect changes. The assessment procedure must be comprehensive. A physical examination and laboratory tests enable illnesses, sensory decrements, and malnutrition to be detected. A drug history can discern medical problems and their impact on cognitive or emotional state. An extensive interview with the impaired individual and a family member helps the clinician to better understand the history, description, and social and psychological context of the problem.

A number of interviewing instruments are available to assist the clinician in assessing mental status and medical and social problems. They utilize client self-report, psychological testing, interviewer observation, and information from significant others to make a diagnosis. The two most popular comprehensive assessment tools used are the Older American's Resources Services (OARS) questionnaire (Pfeiffer 1970) and the Comprehensive Assessment and Referral Evaluation (CARE) (Gurland et al. 1977). The test giver should be aware that there are a number of variables that will affect elders' performance on these tests, including degree of sensory decrements, transient anxiety, motivation, desire to please the test-giver, level of education, and familiarity with testing procedures. A critical part of the assessment is to address the concerns and problems of family members.

Types of Treatment

Treatment of mental disorders may be directed towards a cure, or, if the condition is irreversible, towards improvement of the quality of life to the greatest extent possible. Several types of treatment methods exist: individual and group psychotherapy, drugs, electroconvulsive therapy, or manipulation of the environment. There are no guidelines outlining the best treatment for a particular disorder. Many times, more than one type of treatment is used for a particular mental dysfunction. The capacity of the elder, prognosis of the disorder, preference of the client and family, training of the mental health professional, and financial resources are important considerations.

Because the nature of mental illness in later life is complex, treatment is best accomplished by utilizing the team approach: a general practice physician for organic problems, specialists to reduce vision and hearing deficits, a neurologist, a psychotherapist, and a social worker to link the individual and family to needed community services. In reality, the team approach is not common. Too often an older person with a mental dysfuntion, especially one with limited finances and extensive chronic illness, is prescribed drugs or given only custodial care.

Psychotherapy

There are a number of different types of psychotherapy, but all rely on structured conversation designed to change the client's attitude, feelings, beliefs, defenses, personality, and behavior. Clients may interact one-on-one with a psychotherapist, in a group led by a therapist, or in self-help groups. The techniques used depend upon the physical, emotional, and cognitive state of the impaired individual and the nature of the problem. With older people, as any other age group, the fit between client and therapist is crucial to the success of the therapy.

Evaluative research regarding the effectiveness of particular psychotherapeutic techniques for older people is sparse, but it is generally agreed that they respond as well as other adult age groups. Psychotherapeutic interventions considered here include the traditional techniques, as well as less formal ones without professionals such as self-help groups and peer counselors.

Many experts believe that therapy for older people should focus on problem-solving rather than personality restructuring. For elders, short-term therapy is often the most effective to assist in coping with transient problems. Hayslip and Kooken have developed eight goals of therapy for elders: aid insight into behavior, provide symptom relief, provide relief to relatives, delay deterioration, aid in adaptation to the present situation, improve self-care skills, encourage activity, and facilitate independence. They assert that the most effective treatment a therapist can offer to alleviate a client's stress is to coordinate family, friends, and community resources to assist the client (Hayslip and Kooken 1983).

Most institutionalized elders are either chronic schizophrenics or elders with physical disability, dementia, or both. Therefore, the main goal of psychotherapy in an institutional setting is to provide environmental stimulation to decrease those disabilities above those expected for the illness to facilitate improved morale and/or successful discharge (Kahn 1975).

Psychotherapeutic Techniques

The same types of psychotherapy used with younger clients are helpful for elders. A brief summary of the major types of psychotherapy and their effectiveness with elders follows.

Psychodynamic

The most popular psychodynamic therapy, psychoanalysis, was developed by Sigmund Freud. The therapy is based on the rationale that current mental problems are due to early life experiences and unconscious conflicts. The therapy involves both free association and analysis of the past in order to provide insight into old conflicts. The goal is personality restructuring, which leads to changes in self-concept and enhancement of coping skills. However, the therapy is long-term and may not be useful to elders who have pressing current problems to solve that are caused by forces outside themselves.

Life Review

The tendency for elders to discuss past events is a healthy process thought to be almost universal among elders. Butler (1963) postulated that the reminiscences of elders are not the result of dementia or other mental deficits, but rather the important process of life review. As an elder becomes conscious of the end of life, she or he will mull over past memories, goal fulfillment, and unresolved conflicts, and attempt to integrate and unify life's experiences. Life review therapy relies on this natural tendency to reminisce and encourages the client to systematically review life events with a therapist, either individually or in a group. Through structured or free reminiscing, clients resolve current and past conflicts and increase self-esteem by reviewing life successes (Butler and Lewis 1982).

Behavioral Modification

Behavioral modification therapy is based on the assumption that mental disorders are maladaptive coping strategies that are learned the way all other behavior is learned. Namely, behaviors that are reinforced or rewarded are likely to be repeated. Conversely, behaviors that are ignored or punished are less likely to recur. The behaviorists do not attempt to understand the reasons behind the behavior, but seek to know how the behavior is reinforced. They then attempt to remove that reward and substitute a more healthy behavior. This therapy is effective with elders for a variety of problems including incontinence, attention-getting behaviors, and phobias.

Reality Orientation

This therapy does not have a theoretical base, but is a therapeutic technique based on the assumption that repeated orientation to the immediate environment will reduce disorientation and withdrawal from the environment (Folsom 1967). The technique is commonly practiced in nursing homes with confused elders because it is easy to train staff and implement. At every opportunity the staff offers basic information to the resident regarding present time and place: where they are, what day it is, the weather, the time, activities of the day. It is believed that this practice encourages thinking and prevents further cognitive deterioration. Some studies report it effectively orients elders to the present and improves learning and memory (Schonfield 1980). However, the long-term effectiveness of reality orientation is not known.

Cognitive-Behavioral

The theory behind this therapy is that mental disorders are the result of irrational and self-defeating thinking. Perhaps the most popular is rational-emotive therapy developed by Albert Ellis (Ellis and Harper 1973). The therapist works with the client to uncover distorted thoughts and then confronts the patient with them so the thoughts can be replaced with rational perceptions. One study reported this therapy to significantly decrease anxiety and increase rational thinking in elders (Keller et al. 1975). The therapy is especially effective for those who are depressed, paranoid, or coping with multiple stresses. The patient needs to have adequate cognitive capacity for this therapy to be effective.

Client-Centered

This therapy is based on the theory that when individuals are given unconditional positive support, they can solve their own problems. The therapy was developed by Carl Rogers (1951). The therapist's role is to listen attentively, restate the client's observations, and help the client to bring forth and solve his or her own problems while providing a warm, accepting, supportive, and understanding presence. As in cognitive-behavioral therapy, in order for client-centered therapy to be useful, adequate cognitive function is needed.

Interpersonal

This treatment was developed specifically for depressed clients by Klerman and colleagues (1979). The therapy is based on the premise that depression occurs because of interaction with others, and that understanding and working on interpersonal relations associated with the onset of depression helps one recover from depression and to prevent future episodes. The primary tasks of the therapist are to relieve depressive symptoms and to help the person develop more effective strategies for dealing with the interpersonal problems associated with the onset of depression. The therapy is designed to be short-term and is aimed at symptom reduction and improved interpersonal functioning. Typically the treatment occurs once a week for six weeks with follow-up visits and is often accompanied by drug therapy. Interpersonal therapy has successfully reduced depressive symptoms and enhanced elder's ability to deal with problems associated with depression onset (Scholomskas et al. 1983).

Milieu

This type of therapy is utilized in institutional settings. The rationale is that people change, learn, and mature as a result of relationships and experiences. Hence, all interactions within the institution are important in providing support and help to all its members (Jones 1953). The institutionalized individual is expected to participate, make decisions, assume responsibility and interact with both staff and other patients. The therapy discourages regression and social withdrawal. For example, patients are not allowed to remain in bed or in nightclothes during the day. The climate is geared to help achieve a realistic appraisal of feelings, behavior, and social relationships and to try new skills in a safe environment. This therapy may not be as effective with elders who have inadequate cognitive function and verbal skill since it relies upon multiple interactions. (Gotestam 1980).

Creative Expression

Creative expression uses artistic expression in art, music, or dance to unlock negative feelings and to facilitate social interaction. This therapy is also useful in teaching elders a new skill, and, in the case of dance therapy, encouraging light physical activity. Older people may be more willing to undergo this type of therapy because it is seen more as creative activity than as traditional therapy. Although increased feelings of well-being, self-confidence, and socialization have been reported, there is little documentation regarding its value in reducing or ameliorating mental illness.

Group Therapy

Group therapy integrates a group of clients, generally with similar problems or concerns, in a therapeutic setting under the direction of a skilled leader. Although traditional group therapy is led by a psychotherapist, groups may also be facilitated by trained laypersons, often elders themselves. Group therapy is useful for a wide range of people, from those who are mentally healthy to those who are severely impaired. The focus may be to maintain mental health, to improve adaptation to old age, or to reduce the progression of mental illness in severely impaired elders. Many of the psychotherapeutic approaches listed above may be used in a group setting.

Group therapy has many advantages. It is efficient and less expensive since it reaches a number of people at one time. Further, clients can get support and learn from others with similar problems in varying stages of resolution. The group setting provides a safe place to try out new roles and behaviors. Perhaps the most beneficial aspect of group therapy for elders is that it promotes mutual emotional support and social interaction among its members.

Family and Marital Therapy

Family therapists attribute an individual's mental problems to a breakdown in the family's functioning. They assert that the family, not the individual, should be the treatment focus. As a result, all members of the family are convened, both in groups and individually, to work out the problem.

A number of forces work against this type of therapy for older people including lack of reimbursement, practitioner biases, and resistance of family members to seek treatment. Further, such psychologic problems of elders as dementia or reaction to retirement, although they affect the family, are not directly caused by poor familial relations (Edinburg 1985). Nevertheless, this therapy can assist families in coping with the demands of the impaired family member or to work on relationships that are aggravating the older person's mental condition.

Marital therapy, in which both partners receive counseling, enables them to better cope with life transitions. Elder couples have a number of life stresses that affect the dynamics of a marital partnership including retirement, physical disability, or changes in sexual activity. Marital therapy for elders usually consists of short term crisis intervention that focuses on a particular problem that has arisen. The aim is not to radically change the relationship, but to apply behavior that worked well in the past. Adult children may be brought in as necessary.

Even though it is difficult to attract many elders to marital therapy and lifetime habits may be difficult to change, the need for marital therapy for elder clients is great. Howells (1975) asserts that the ultimate stress in later life is to be left with a "disharmonious spouse." Elders' satisfaction with family life is strongly related to morale and mental health (Mancini 1979).

Self-Help Groups

Self-help groups generally arise spontaneously within a community to answer a specific need and are composed of persons who share mutual concerns. Typically, they are initiated by individuals with the need, although recently agencies and organizations have facilitated their formation. There are over a half-million self-help groups in the United States and the number is increasing. Most groups are formally organized and meet regularly. The meetings usually include group discussions in which members learn from one another as they share the experiences and give advice. The groups may invite professionals as guests when needed. Some groups publish newsletters and many consider public education and advocacy part of their goal.

Self-help groups are available for a wide gamut of needs. Some, such as Alcoholics Anonymous, stop-smoking, and weight-reduction groups, focus on controlling negative behaviors by working on techniques members can use to help themselves. Another type is that in which members in a common stressful predicament support one another (such as families of Alzheimer's patients or widowhood groups). Some groups stress medical care and rehabilitation. Groups composed of those with diabetes, colostomies, or breast surgery, commonly discuss skills to ease the burden of daily living with a disease. Finally, there are self-fulfillment and self-improvement groups designed to maximize personal potential.

Elder Peer Counselors

Elders are likely to avoid the traditional mental health setting and approaches because they are reluctant to accept formal help. One solution is to offer informal, nonthreatening services that establish a personal relationship to prevent or ease a future mental health intervention (Sargent 1980). A relatively new idea in psychotherapy for elders is the use of elder peer counselors who are trained to facilitate groups or work individually with troubled elders. They may visit elders in their own homes or in community or institutional settings. They may provide education, social support, counseling, and referral to appropriate community agencies.

Peer counselors may be as effective as professional mental health workers in many instances. One study compared the effectiveness of professionals with that of trained peer counselors in the delivery of an educational and therapeutic course on depression for elders. Participants had reduced psychological distress after the course, and there was no difference in benefits between those with a trained peer leader and those led by a professional (Thompson et al. 1983). Some experts believe that peer counselors, especially those that reach out into elders' homes and places where great numbers of elders congregate, have greater potential than the traditional approaches in which an elder goes to a mental health facility to be treated by a psychotherapist.

Implementation of elder peer counselors can benefit both the trained elder and the client. Elders may be less threatened by a peer counselor than a professional psychotherapist. This type of therapy reinforces the belief that elders are capable of solving their own problems and the help needed is transient. Additionally, peer counselors are usually responsible and motivated workers, willing to become a friend as well as a helper.

Pet Therapy

Pets are known to give attention, stimulate laughter, encourage regular exercise, and make an owner feel safe and needed. A number of studies report that owning a pet increases many paramenters of physical and mental health. In nursing homes, pet visitation has been reported to expand conversation topics, increase sociability and animation, calm residents, and increase self-esteem (Brickel 1980–81).

For many, pets provide companionship and a reason to stay well.

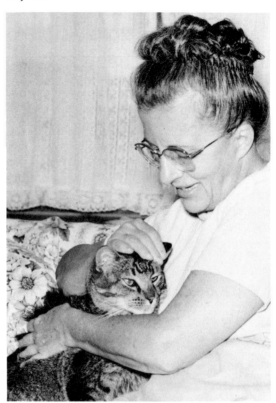

Pet therapy, as opposed to pet ownership or visitation, utilizes pets for more than making people smile. Pet therapy changes a person's behavior by using pets to reinforce positive behaviors. For instance, a person in a nursing home may be rewarded with ten minutes with a pet if he or she refrains from exhibiting a disruptive behavioral problem. In this case, the pet must not live in the home, but is brought by the therapist only during the times when the positive behavior is to be reinforced. After the behavior is established, the patient is gradually weaned from the pet (Andrysco 1985).

Drug Therapy

Psychoactive drugs can be of immense therapeutic value in treating mental disorders. However, they are often overprescribed. Psychoactive drug use accelerates sharply after age twenty-five, hits a peak between age forty-five to fifty-four and begins a gradual descent over the remaining years of life. After age sixty-five, women are prescribed these drugs 60 percent more than men. In 1981, psychoactive drugs were prescribed in 6 percent of office visits to physicians, mainly for mental disorders (National Center for Health Statistics 1983).

Although drugs can be effective in treating mental disorders, they should never represent the sole mode of treatment and should generally be used only after less-invasive methods have been attempted. When drugs are used, therapy should be closely monitored and discontinued when no longer needed. The four drugs most commonly used to treat mental disorders are antipsychotics, antianxiety agents, antidepressants, and sedative/hypnotics. For more information on each of these drug types, see Chapter 7.

Therapeutic use of alcohol can have psychological benefits. A number of studies have documented that modest alcohol use in a controlled setting increases sociability and satisfaction with institutional facilities and food (Kastenbaum and Slater 1964; Sarley 1968). One study in which a geriatric unit served beer in a pub-like setting found that the beer was more effective than strong tranquilizers in improving social interaction and behavior (Chien et al. 1973). It is not certain whether alcohol exerts drug-like effects or whether the major benefit comes from the psychological association of alcohol with sociability and independence.

Electroconvulsive Therapy

Electroconvulsive therapy (ECT), or electroshock therapy, consists of a brief electrical shock applied to the head by an electrode to produce a generalized seizure. The treatment regimen usually consists of six to twelve treatments given two to three times a week while the person is anesthetized. The patient is generally prescribed antidepressant medication to reduce relapse. The treatment may cause short-term confusion and both short- and long-term memory deficits that depend on the number of treatments and placement of the electrodes (National Institute of Mental Health 1985a).

This treatment may sound barbaric, but multiple studies have shown this therapy to be effective in reducing symptoms of severe depression and some types of schizophrenia. The therapy is shown to have faster symptom relief and less danger than some long-term drug therapies. ECT is indicated when severe depression interferes with normal function, especially among the suicidal (Salzman 1982) and those who cannot tolerate the three to four weeks it takes for an antidepressant to exert its influence. ECT is also used for patients who do not respond to other treatments or who suffer severe side effects from drug therapy. This therapy is used in less than 3 percent of all psychiatric admissions (National Institute of Mental Health 1985a).

Environmental Manipulation

Environmental manipulation is the attempt to reduce or remove the external sources that are placing stresses upon the mentally ill. This therapy generally involves an alteration of the physical environment to decrease stress, increase feelings of security, and promote maximum independence and sensory stimulation. For example, moving a bedroom to the first floor, painting a hallway in colors to reduce the confusion of uniformity, arranging furniture for socialization, and installing a handrail for safety may all be considered environmental manipulation. In a broader sense, environmental manipulation is the intervention with a patient's family to assist them in changing their behavior towards a frail elder to reduce disruptive behavior. Moving an impaired elder to a more protective environment may also be considered environmental manipulation.

Private Therapists and Psychiatric Outpatient Clinics

Both private psychotherapists and those working in private clinics rarely see elder clients. It is estimated that older people comprise about 3 percent of the total patient load. One reason for lack of use is that these services are seldom reimbursed by Medicare and Medicaid and paying the hourly costs are prohibitive for many elders. Generally, those elders who do participate are those who can afford it, are in good health, are highly educated and have a positive attitude toward their treatment.

Halfway Houses

Psychiatric halfway houses provide a home environment for the mentally ill who can meet many of their own needs, yet need some support and supervision to be able to live in the community. They have great potential in serving the needs of mentally impaired elders since they prevent or postpone institutionalization for many. However, few provide treatment, staff are poorly trained, there is no reimbursement by Medicare and Medicaid, and there are far fewer houses than are needed. Many homes are located in community neighborhoods and often face problems from neighbors who fear the mentally ill. Currently, board and care homes, and single room occupancy homes house many mentally ill individuals. Treatment, rehabilitation, or supervision is rare in most instances.

Elder Utilization of Mental Health Services

Despite the variety of mental health services, older persons are underserved by all forms of these services (Redick and Taube 1980). In all age groups, only a fraction of those who need mental health services receive them. Elders have an especially low rate of utilization of community psychotherapeutic services; they comprise only about 3 percent of the total patient load (VandenBos et al. 1981). It is estimated that about 80 percent of those residing in the community who might benefit from mental health services are not receiving them (Kramer et al. 1973). Minority group elders are less likely to use formal health services than Caucasians, and Hispanic elders may be the least likely of all (Weeks and Cueller 1981). Many do not use services until their illness has become severe, making it more difficult to treat, and increasing the probability of institutionalization.

Why do older people in the community not seek formal services for mental problems? Experts have attributed low utilization to client factors, professional biases, and barriers created by the mental health system itself.

Client Factors

Bias against the use of mental health services occur among all age groups, but older persons are especially prone to resist psychological help from a stranger. Many believe that those who need a therapist are crazy. Perhaps elders underutilize mental health services because they do not see themselves as having a problem. On the other hand, they may fear that if their mental disorders are fully explored, they may be stigmatized as mentally ill and institutionalized. Many elders value self-reliance, and visits to a therapist may be seen as an inability to solve their own problems. Many older people may attribute poor mental health to physical ailments or the aging process itself, believing that a therapist cannot help. Lack of awareness of available services may also play a role.

Therapist Biases

A therapist may share the cultural ageist view that therapy for older individuals is not worthwhile because they only have a few years left to live. Psychotherapists consistently rate older clients as having less chance of treatment success than younger patients, even though no research has documented this belief. Therapists tend to attribute many symptoms of distress to organic symptoms or old age and may not treat them. Many of the therapists' biases may be due to a lack of knowledge about the characteristics, needs, and concerns of older people and the special considerations in dealing with an older client. Working with elders, particularly the sick or very

Although few elders undergo psychotherapy, it can assist elders to cope with the transitions of later life.

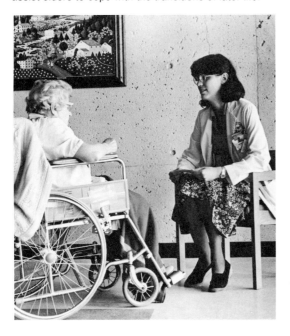

old, may force therapists to confront the difficult, personal questions of their own aging, decline, and eventual death.

Mental Health System Barriers
Financial considerations are perhaps the greatest barrier to availability of mental health services for older people. Psychiatric services are expensive and Medicare and Medicaid provide very little reimbursement for mental health services. Lack of personnel skilled in geriatrics and the shortage of services geared to elders also serve as barriers to care. Many of the services are physically inaccessible to older people because outreach is seldom provided for those who are unable to get to the facility. Physicians seldom refer elders to mental health services. Last, there is little cooperation and coordination among private medical providers, community agencies and institutions. Because of this, the teamwork approach to meeting the multiple needs of mentally ill elders is not an option in most communities.

Summary

Mental health is a difficult term to define for any age group because the differentiation between normal and abnormal behavior is dependent on one's culture, age, and situation. It is thought that mental health in elders can be defined as the ability to successfully adapt to the transitions of old age—including retirement, change in financial status or living arrangement, death of loved ones, and declining health. The ability of an elder to adapt to later life is related to a number of physical, psychological, and situational factors, such as: personality, physical health, financial situation, availability of social support, and coping strategies. Although most elders adjust readily to the stresses and transitions of old age, a few need outside assistance to deal with mental disorders.

In elders, mental disorders may appear for the first time during old age, but most commonly have been continuous throughout life. Mental disorders may be of two types: functional, which are caused by life and personality disturbances, and organic, which result from impaired brain function. Functional disorders include anxiety, depression, hypochondriasis, paranoia, schizophrenia, sleep disorders, and substance abuse. Organic disorders include dementia (both Alzheimer's and multi-infarct) and delirium.

Because a number of conditions may cause symptoms that resemble mental problems, a thorough assessment is necessary to ensure proper treatment. Treatment modalities for elders include both traditional and nontraditional therapies: including psychotherapy, drug therapy, electroconvulsive therapy, and environmental manipulation. There is very little documentation about the effectiveness of mental health therapy with elders; more research is needed in this area.

Mental health services are available for elders in both community and institutional settings. These include public mental health hospitals, wards in general hospitals, nursing homes, community mental health centers, halfway houses, and individual and outpatient psychiatric services. However, these services are underutilized by elders for a number of reasons: client factors, therapist biases, and system barriers.

Activities

1. Develop your own definition of mental health, taking age and cultural background into account. Identify some behaviors that are universally healthy or nonhealthy. Ask several individuals to characterize elders. Do their descriptions define a mentally healthy old age?
2. List the strategies you use to cope with stress, both those that are effective and those that are not. Which strategies work best for you? Share with the class.
3. Conduct a life review interview of an older person. Tape the conversation and write a summary for the class. Be sure to leave a copy with the person interviewed.
4. Question elders about their attitudes toward psychotherapy and compare their views with your classmates. Do their views differ from younger groups? What type of therapy would each undergo and under what circumstances?
5. Seek out the mental health services in your community. Find out the percentage of clients who are over sixty-five. Do they have any specialized services for elders? Do any utilize peer counselors? Do any have preventive programs?
6. Make a list of the self-help groups in your community. If possible, talk with a member to find out the percentage of participants over sixty-five. Attend a group session and report your response to the class.
7. As people live longer, many younger elders spend their retirement years caring for their aging parents or spouse. How will this trend affect your plans for your old age?
8. How many people age sixty-five and older are patients in mental institutions in your state? What is the percentage of elders compared to other age groups? If possible, visit a facility, observe the patients and find out the frequency and types of therapy utilized there.
9. Develop a policy and group of programs to promote mental health and reduce mental deterioration in a nursing home.
10. Interview a nursing home administrator. What is the percentage of mentally ill elders in the facility? How are behavioral problems (e.g., wandering, disruptive behavior) managed? What therapy is available? What is the educational background of the therapist, if present?

Bibliography

Andrysco, R. M. 1985. Pets in the nursing home. *Long-Term Care Currents* 8(1):1–4. Columbus, Ohio: Ross Laboratories.

Atkinson, R. M., and L. L. Kofoed. 1984. Alcohol and drug abuse. In Cassel, C. K., and J. R. Walsh. eds. *Geriatric medicine, vol. II: Fundamentals of geriatric care.* New York: Springer-Verlag, 219–35.

Berkman, L. F., and S. L. Syme. 1979. Social networks, host resistance and mortality: A nine year follow-up study of Alameda county residents. *Am J Epidemiol* 109:186–204.

Birren, J. E., and V. J. Renner. 1979. A brief history of mental health and aging. In *Issues in mental health and aging: Vol. 1 Research.* Washington, D.C.: NIMH.

Birren, J. E., and V. J. Renner. 1980. Concepts and issues of mental health and aging. In J. E. Birren, and R. B. Sloane, eds. *Handbook of mental health and aging.* Englewood Cliffs, N.J.: Prentice-Hall. 3–33.

Blazer, D. B. 1983. The epidemiology of depression in later life. In L. D. Breslaw, and M. R. Haug, eds. *Depression and aging: Causes, cures, care, and consequences.* New York: Springer. 30–50.

Bliwise, D. L., E. Carey, and W. C. Dement. 1983. Nightly variation in sleep-related respiratory disturbance in older adults. *Exp Aging Res* 9:77–81.

Borus, J. F. 1981. Deinstitutionalization of the chronically mentally ill. *N Engl J Med* 305:339–42.

Brickel, C. M. 1980–81. A review of the roles of pet animals in psychotherapy with the elderly. *Intl J Aging and Human Dev* 12:119–29.

Busse, E. W. 1976. Hypochondriasis in the elderly: A reaction to social stress. *J Am Geriatr Soc* 24:145–49.

Busse, E. W., and D. Blazer. 1980. Disorders related to biological functioning. In E. W. Busse and D. Blazer, eds. *Handbook of geriatric psychiatry.* New York: Van Nostrand Reinhold. 390–414.

Busse, E. W., and E. Pfeiffer. 1977. Functional psychiatric disorders in old age. In E. W. Busse and E. Pfeiffer, eds. *Behavior and adaptation in late life.* Boston: Little, Brown.

Butler, R. N. 1963. The life review: An interpretation of reminiscence in the aged. *Psychiatry* 26:65–76.

Butler, R. N., and M. I. Lewis. 1982. *Aging and mental health.* St. Louis, Mo: C. V. Mosby.

Chien, C., B. A. Slotsky, and J. O. Cole. 1973. Psychiatric treatment for nursing home patients: Drug, alcohol or milieu. *Am J Psychiatry* 130:543–48.

Cohen, C. I., J. Teresi, and D. Holmes. 1985. Social networks, stress, and physical health: A longitudinal study of an inner-city elder population. *J Gerontol* 40(4):478–86.

Cohen, E. S. 1979. Nursing homes—the new mental hospitals. *Generations.* Spring. 8–9, 14.

Costa, P. T., and R. R. McCrae. 1980. Somatic complaints in males as a function of age and neuroticism: a longitudinal analysis. *J Behav Med* 3:245–255.

Costa, P. T., R. R. McCrae, and D. Arenberg. 1980. Enduring dispositions in adult males. *J Pers Soc Psychol* 38:793–800.

Council of Scientific Affairs, American Medical Association. 1986. Dementia. *JAMA* 256:2234–2238.

Donahue, W. 1978. What about our responsibility toward the abandoned elderly? *Gerontologist* 18: 102–11.

Edinberg, M A. 1985. *Mental health practice with the elderly.* Englewood Cliffs, N.J.: Prentice-Hall.

Ellis, A., and K. A. Harper. 1973. *A guide to rational living.* Hollywood: Wilshire Books.

Folsom, J. C. 1967. Intensive hospital therapy of geriatric patients. In J. H. Masserman, ed. *Current psychiatric therapies* (Vol. 7). New York: Grune and Stratton. 209–15.

Garcia, C. A. 1981. Overdiagnosis of dementia. *J Am Geriatr Soc* 29(9):407–10.

Gatz, M., M. A. Smyer, and M. P. Lawton. 1980. The mental health system and the older adult. In L. W. Poon, ed. *Aging in the 80s: Psychological issues.* Washington, D.C.: American Psychological Assoc. 5–18.

Gerber, I., R. Rusalem, N. Hannon, et al. 1975. Anticipatory grief and aged widows and widowers. *J Gerontol* 30:225–29.

Gilleard, C. J., W. D. Boyd, and G. Watt. 1982. Problems in caring for the elderly mentally infirm at home. *Arch Gerontol Geriatr* 1:151–58.

Gotestam, K. G. 1980. Behavioral and dynamic psychotherapy with the elderly. In J. E. Birren and R. B. Sloane, eds. *Handbook of mental health and aging.* Englewood Cliffs, N.J.: Prentice-hall. 775–805.

Guilleminault, C. C. 1982. Effect of various pills on sleep and daytime alertness in the elderly. *Gerontologist* 22:187–93.

Gurland, B. J., and P. S. Cross. 1982. Epidemiology of psychopathology in old age. In L. F. Jarvik and G. W. Small, eds. *Psychiatric clinics of North America.* Philadelphia: W. B. Saunders. 11–26.

Gurland, B. J., J. Kurinansky, L. Sharpe, et al. 1977. The comprehensive assessment and referral evaluation (CARE): Rationale, development and reliability. Part II: A factor analysis. *Int J Aging Hum Dev* 8:9–42.

Hayslip, B. 1983. Mental health and aging. In N. S. Ernst and H. R. Glazer-Waldman, eds. *The aged patient.* Chicago: Yearbook Medical Publishers. 158–81.

Hayslip, B., and R. A. Kooken. 1983. Therapeutic interventions—mental health. In M. S. Ernst and H. R. Glasser, eds. *The aged patient.* Chicago: Yearbook Medical Publishers. 282–303.

Howells, J. G. 1975. Family psychopathology. In J. G. Howells, ed. *Modern perspective in the psychiatry of old age.* New York: Brunner-Mazel. 253–68.

Jahoda, M. 1958. *Current concepts of positive mental health.* New York: Basic Books.

Jarvik, L. F., and R. E. Noshkes. 1985. Alterations in mental function with aging and disease. In R. Andres, E. L. Bierman, and W. R. Hazzard, eds. *Principles of geriatric medicine.* San Francisco: McGraw-Hill. 237–47.

Jones, M. 1953. *The therapeutic community.* New York: Basic Books.

Kahn, R. L. 1975. The mental health system and the future aged. *Gerontologist* 15(1, part II):24–31.

Kastenbaum, R., and P. E. Slater. 1964. Effects of wine on the interpersonal behaviors of geriatric patients: An exploratory study. In R. Kastenbaum, ed. *New thoughts on old age.* New York: Springer-Verlag, 191–204.

Keller, J. F., J. W. Croaks, and J. Y. Brooking. 1975. Effects of a program in rational thinking on anxieties in older persons. *J Counseling Psych* 22:54–57.

Klerman, G. L., B. Rounsaville, E. S. Chevron. et al. 1979. *Manual for short-term interpersonal therapy (IPT) of depression.* New Haven-Boston Collaborative Depression Project.

Koenig, H. 1986. Depression and dysphoria among the elderly: dispelling a myth. *J Fam Prac* 23:383–385.

Kramer, M., C. Taub, and R. W. Redick. 1973. Patterns and use of psychiatric facilities by the aged: Past, present and future. In C. Eisendorfer and M. P. Lawton, eds. *Psychology of adult development and aging.* Washington, D.C.: Am. Psychological Assoc.

Larson, E. B., B. V. Reifler, S. M. Sumi, et al. 1986a. Diagnostic tests in the evaluation of dementia: a progressive study of 200 elderly participants. *Arch Intern Med* 146:1917–1922.

Larson, E. B., B. Lo, and M. E. Williams. 1986b. Evaluation and care of elderly patients with dementia. *J Gen Int Med* 1:116–126.

Linn, M. W., L. Gurel, W. O. Williford, et al. 1985. Nursing home care as an alternative to psychiatric hospitalization. *Arch Gen Psychiatry* 42:544–51.

Lurie, E. E., J. H. Swan, and Associates. 1987. *Serving the mentally ill elderly.* Lexington, Ky: Lexington Press.

Mace, N. L., and P. V. Rabins. 1981. *The 36-hour day.* Baltimore: The John Hopkins University Press.

Mancini, J. A 1979. Family relationships and morale among persons 65 years of age and older. *Am J Orthopsychiatry* 49:292–300.

Murrell, S. A., S. Himmelfarb, and K. Wright. 1983. Prevalence of depression and its correlate in older adults. *Am J Epidemiol* 117(2):173–85.

Myers, J. K., M. M. Weissman, G. L. Tischler, et al. 1984. Six-month prevalence of psychiatric disorders in three communities. *Arch Gen Psychiatry* 41:959–67.

National Center for Health Statistics. 1983. Utilization of psychotropic drugs in office-based ambulatory care: National Ambulatory Medical Care Survey, 1980–81. *Advance Data from Vital and Health Statistics* No. 9. June 15. Hyattsville, Md: Public Health Service.

National Center for Health Statistics. 1986. Health promotion and disease prevention: Provisional data from the National Health Interview Study. United States, January-June, 1985. *Advance Data from Vital and Health Statistics* No. 119, May 14, Hyattsville, Md: Public Health Service.

National Institute of Mental Health. 1985a. *Electroconvulsive therapy. Consensus Development Conference Statement.* 15(11). Washington, D.C.: U.S. Govt. Printing Office.

National Institute of Mental Health. 1985b. *Mental Health, United States:* 1985. DHHS Publ. No. (ADM) 85–0000. Rockville, Md.: U.S. Govt. Printing Office.

Neugarten, B. L. 1977. Personality and aging. In J. E. Birren and K. W. Schaie, eds. *Handbook of the psychology of aging.* New York: Van Nostrand Reinhold. 626–49.

Parsons, O. A., and W. R. Leber. 1981. The relationship between cognitive dysfunction and brain damage in alcoholics: causal, interactive or epiphenominal? *Alcoholism: Clin Exp Res* 5:326–43.

Pfeiffer, E. 1970. *Multidimensional functional assessment.: The OARS methodology.* Durham, N.C.: Duke University, Center of the Study of Aging and Human Development.

Post, F. 1980. Paranoid, schizophrenia-like and schizophrenia states in the aged. In J. E. Birren and R. B. Sloane, eds. *Handbook of mental health and aging.* Englewood Cliffs, N.J.: Prentice-Hall. 591–615.

Redick, R. W., and C. A. Taube. 1980. Demography and mental health care of the aged. In J. E. Birren and R. B. Sloane, eds. *Handbook of mental health and aging*. Englewood Cliffs, N.J.: Prentice-Hall. 57–71.

Rogers, C. R. 1951. *Client-centered therapy*. Boston: Houghton Mifflin.

Rovner, B. W., S. Kafonek, L. Filipp. et al. 1986. Prevalence of mental illness in a community nursing home. *Am J Psychiatry* 143(11):1446–49.

Rowe, J. W. 1985. Health care of the elderly. *N Engl J Med* 312(13):827–35.

Ryan, C., and N. Butters. 1980. Further evidence for a continuum of impairment encompassing male alcoholic Korsakoff patients and chronic alcoholic men. *Alcoholism: Clin Exp Res* 4:190–98.

Sabin, T. D., A. J. Vitug, and V. H. Mark. 1982. Are nursing home diagnosis and treatments adequate? *JAMA* 248:321–22.

Sallis, J. F., and K. L. Lichstein. 1982. Analysis and management of geriatric anxiety. *Int J Aging Hum Dev* 15(3):197–211.

Salzman, C. 1982. Electroconvulsive therapy in the elderly patient. In L. F. Jarvik and G. W. Small, eds. *Psychiatr Clin North Am* 5(1):191–97. Philadelphia: W. B. Saunders.

Sargent, S. S. 1980. *Non-traditional therapy and counseling with the aging*. Springer series on adulthood and aging, Volume 7. New York: Springer Publ. Co.

Sarley, V. C. 1968. Use of wine in extended care facilities. In S. P. Lucia, ed. *Wine and health*. Menlo Park, Calif.: Pacific Coast Publ. 28–30.

Scholomskas, A, J., E. S. Chevron, B. A. Prusoff, C. Berry. 1983. Short-term interpersonal therapy (IPT) with the depressed elderly: Case report and discussion. *Am J Psychotherapy* 37(4):552–66.

Schonfield, A. E. 1980. Learning, memory, and aging. In J. E. Birren and R. B. Sloane, eds. *Handbook of mental health and aging*. Englewood Cliffs, N.J.: Prentice-Hall. 214–44.

Schukit, M. A. 1977. Geriatric alcoholism and drug abuse. *Gerontologist* 17:168–74.

Schukit, M. A., and P. A. Pastor. 1978. The elderly as a unique population: Alcoholism. *Alcohol Clin Exp Res* 2:31–38.

Smith, J. S., and I. G. Kiloh. 1981. The investigation of dementia: Results in 200 consecutive admissions. *Lancet* 1:824–27.

Solomon, K. H. 1976. Benzodiazepines and neurotic anxiety: Critique. *NY State J Med* 2156–64.

Summers, W. K., L. V. Majovski, G. M. Marsh, et al. 1986. Oral tetrahydroaminoacridine in long-term treatment of senile dementia, Alzheimer type. *N Engl J Med* 315(20):1241–45.

Thompson, L. W., D. Gallagher, G. Nies, and D. Epstein. 1983. Evaluation of the effectiveness of professionals and nonprofessionals as instructors of "coping with depression" classes for elders. *Gerontologist* 23(4):390–96.

U.S. House of Representatives, Select Commitee on Aging, 1987. *Exploding the myths of caregiving in America*. Washington D.C.: U.S. Govt. Printing Office. Committee Print No. 99–611.

VandenBos, G. R., J. Stapp, and R. R. Kilburg. 1981. Health services providers in psychology: Results of the APA human resources survey. *Am Psychol* 36:1395–1418.

Wattis, J. P. 1981. Alcohol problems in the elderly. *J Am Geriatr Soc* 29:131–34.

Webb, W. B. 1982. Sleep in older persons: Sleep structures of 50- to 60-year-old men and women. *J Gerontol* 37(5):581–86.

Weeks, J. R., and J. B. Cueller. 1981. The role of family members in the helping networks of older people. *Gerontologist* 21:388–94.

Winogrond, I. R. 1982. Health, stress, and coping in the elderly. *Wisc Med J* 81:27–31.

Zarit, S. H., N. E. Miller, and R. L. Kahn. 1978. Brain function, intellectual impairment and education in the aged. *J Amer Geriatr Soc* 26:58–67.

Zarit, S. H. 1980. *Aging and mental disorders*. New York: Free Press.

Zimberg, S. 1983. Alcoholism in the elderly. *Postgrad Med* 74(1):165–73.

9 Nutrition

Dietary habits of youth set the stage for health and disease in old age. The time to nourish your body for late life is now.

Alice Chenault (1984)

Introduction

Nutrition is one of the most significant factors affecting health in the later years. Current and past dietary practices accelerate many age-related decrements. While the same nutrients are essential for all individuals of any age, changes accompanying aging may alter the amount of specific nutrients required by elders. Many chronic diseases of later life are associated with deleterious, long-term eating habits. Many prescription and over-the-counter drugs used to treat chronic diseases and disorders increase elders' nutritional risk. Finally, elders generally reduce the amount of food they eat, further increasing the likelihood of nutrient deficiencies.

This chapter will examine the nutritional needs and nutritional status of elders, factors affecting food intake, and the relationship between nutrition and a number of chronic diseases. Programs to enhance nutritional status among elders will also be discussed.

Essential Nutrients and Energy Requirements

The human body requires more than forty nutrients to carry out its functions, including water, protein, fat, carbohydrates, vitamins, and minerals. The metabolism of protein, carbohydrates, and fat supplies the body with energy for growth and maintenance. Vitamins and minerals are important components of enzymes, used in all body processes. Water is perhaps the most essential element in the body. One can live for over a month without food, but only a few days without water. Even though dietary fiber is not a nutrient because it travels through the digestive system unchanged, it also plays an important role in physical health. Each individual requires a different quantity of various nutrients, depending on activity and stress levels, drug use, age, sex, body size, and health condition.

The Recommended Dietary Allowance (RDA), developed by the Food and Nutrition Board of the National Academy of Sciences, is the recognized standard of nutrition for healthy people of all age groups in the United States. This includes daily recommendations for calories, protein, and seventeen vitamins and minerals. (Table 9.1A). In addition, safe and adequate levels of an additional twelve nutrients are listed in the most recent revision of the RDA (Table 9.1B) (1980). These guidelines do not include all essential nutrients because too little is known about recommended intake levels for many of them.

RDA guidelines for adults are divided into two subsections: twenty-three to fifty and fifty-one and over. Many experts object that the nutritional recommendations for all individuals over age fifty are grouped together, despite the vast differences in activity level and health condition within that group. Further, the RDA values for all nutrients for those over fifty are extrapolated from the allowances of younger groups because there are little available data on the special nutrient needs of elders. Finally, the RDA for three nutrients is reduced for those over age fifty; none

is increased to account for the variety of physiological changes associated with aging. Schneider et al. (1986) discusses the many limitations of the current RDA guidelines for elders.

Elders face reduced energy requirements as they age which decreases their caloric need. For instance, the average man age twenty-three to fifty utilizes 2700 Calories/day; for women, 2000 Calories/day. However, a man age fifty-one to seventy-five needs an estimated 2400 Calories; over age seventy-five, 2050. A woman age fifty-one to seventy-five requires about 1800 Calories, and this value is reduced to 1600 for women over age seventy-five (Food and Nutrition Board 1980).

A number of factors contribute to elders' reduced caloric needs. With age, the proportion of body fat increases and muscle mass decreases. Further, there is a small, progressive reduction in resting metabolic rate after maturity. Finally, as a group, elders are less physically active than other adults, further reducing caloric needs. There may be as much variation as 1000 calories needed within each age group: elders who are very physically active need more calories, whereas those who are bedridden require fewer. Consumption of more calories than the body requires results in storage of that energy as fat deposits to be used in times of increased needs.

Many factors influence elders' nutritional needs. Normal aging, disease states, and drug use are associated with a number of physiological changes that affect food absorption, utilization, excretion, and needs for selected nutrients. Age-related changes in physiology affect nutritional needs. Although there is generally a decrease in caloric need, vitamin and mineral needs do not decrease proportionally. Thus, elders should eat nutrient-rich foods and avoid high-calorie, low-nutrient foods such as processed foods and those high in fat or sugar. Age-associated changes in the gastrointestinal and renal systems may alter absorption and excretion of some nutrients (see

Table 9.1A   Recommended daily dietary allowances, 1980*

Nutrient	Age (yr)	Male	Female
Calories (kcal)	23–50	2700	2000
		(2300–3100)	(1600–2400)
	51–75	2400	1800
		(2000–2800)	(1400–2200)
	76 +	2050	1600
		(1650–2450)	(1200–2000)
Protein (gm)	23–50	56	44
	51 +	56	44
Vitamin A (μg retinol equivalents)	23–50	1000	800
	51 +	1000	800
Vitamin D (μg)	23–50	5.0	5.0
	51 +	5.0	5.0
Vitamin E (mg α-tocopherol	23–50	10	8.0
	51 +	10	8.0
Ascorbic acid (mg)	23–50	60	60
	51 +	60	60
Thiamin (mg)	23–50	1.4	1.0
	51 +	1.2	1.0
Riboflavin (mg)	23–50	1.6	1.2
	51 +	1.4	1.2
Niacin (mg niacin equivalents)	23–50	18	13
	51 +	16	13
Vitamin B_6 (mg)	23–50	2.2	2.0
	51 +	2.2	2.0
Folacin (μg)	23–50	400	400
	51 +	400	400
Vitamin B_{12} (μg)	23–50	3.0	3.0
	51 +	3.0	3.0
Calcium (mg)	23–50	800	800
	51 +	800	800
Phosphorus (mg)	23–50	800	800
	51 +	800	800
Magnesium (mg)	23–50	350	300
	51 +	350	300
Iron (mg)	23–50	10	18
	51 +	10	10
Zinc (mg)	23–50	15	15
	51 +	15	15
Iodine (μg)	23–50	150	150
	51 +	150	150

*Adapted from Food and Nutrition Board, National Academy of Sciences: Recommended Dietary Allowances. Washington, D.C., National Academy of Sciences, 1980.

Nutrient	Age	Male	Female
Vitamin K (μg)	Adult	70–140	70–140
Biotin (μg)	Adult	100–200	100–200
Pantothenic acid (mg)	Adult	4.0–7.0	4.0–7.0
Copper (mg)	Adult	2.0–3.0	2.0–3.0
Manganese (mg)	Adult	2.5–5.0	2.5–5.0
Fluoride (mg)	Adult	1.5–4.0	1.5–4.0
Chromium (mg)	Adult	0.05–0.20	0.05–0.20
Selenium (mg)	Adult	0.05–0.20	0.05–0.20
Molybdenum (mg)	Adult	0.15–0.50	0.15–0.50
Sodium (mg)	Adult	1100–3300	1100–3300
Potassium (mg)	Adult	1875–5625	1875–5626
Chloride (mg)	Adult	1700–5100	1700–5100

Table 9.1B Estimated safe and adequate daily dietary intake*

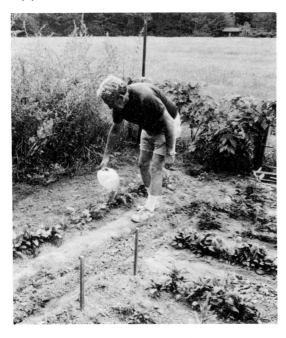

This man will harvest not only fresh vegetables, but the enjoyment of hard work well done.

Chapter 3). Additionally, elders who lack teeth or wear improperly fitted dentures may not eat sufficient fiber because of their inability to chew.

Elders with chronic illnesses and those on medication are also at a nutritional disadvantage since these variables can affect appetite, digestion, absorption, utilization, or excretion of essential nutrients. Some illnesses require special dietary precautions, which may be expensive or difficult to follow. Other illnesses deplete energy, reducing the ability and motivation to shop and prepare meals. The severely ill, bedridden, or institutionalized have special problems because they are dependent upon others for their meals.

Proteins

The body needs many types of protein for maintenance, growth, tissue repair, and energy production. Proteins (e.g., legumes, fish, meat, eggs, and dairy products) consist of various combinations of up to twenty amino acids. The process of

Energy Production from Foods

Energy production is measured in kilocalories (commonly referred to as calories) and represents the amount of energy required to heat one thousand grams (about a quart) of water by one degree Celsius. The burning of carbohydrates and protein yields about four calories per gram, while fat, a more concentrated energy source, yields nine calories per gram. Some high-energy foods contain as much energy as explosives; for instance, a two inch square of fudge (185 calories) contains as much energy as a small stick of dynamite and a double-dip ice cream cone releases energy equivalent to one-half cubic foot of natural gas (334 calories). This huge amount of energy does not explode the body because it is released gradually by the enzyme-coordinated process of metabolism (Chenault, 1984).

digestion splits the proteins we eat into their component amino acids, which the body then uses to build all proteins needed for growth and maintenance of body tissue. Some of these amino acids, called essential, must be ingested because the body cannot make them. Those the body can synthesize are nonessential. The body requires more protein during periods of rapid growth, illness, and recovery from surgery or injury.

Experts disagree about how much protein elders require; some believe they need less than the recommended allowance because of their reduced lean body mass, others assert that more is needed to counteract tissue deterioration. Most surveys reveal that Americans, including elders, consume more protein than their bodies need. However, those with chronic illnesses, the bedridden, and the low-income are at risk for protein deficiency.

Carbohydrates

Carbohydrates provide an immediate source of energy and should comprise at least 60 percent of total caloric intake. Carbohydrates may be simple (sugars) or complex (starches). Foods high in carbohydrates may be eaten in their natural state or refined by a process that removes most vitamins, minerals, and fiber. For example, table sugar is a refined sugar and white bread is made from refined starch. Foods high in unrefined, complex carbohydrates (e.g., bananas, beans, potatoes, and whole grains) are preferable in the diet because they are digested slower and therefore satisfy hunger longer while providing essential vitamins, minerals, and fiber. Carbohydrates provide the major source of calories for elders because they are inexpensive and easy to prepare, store, chew, and digest.

Fats

Despite its negative press, fat is necessary to provide energy, transport fat-soluble vitamins, insulate and cushion the body, and manufacture essential cell components. Fats also provide flavor to food and a feeling of fullness after they are eaten. All animal and plant foods contain fat; foods high in fats include dairy products, vegetable oils, and red meat. The majority of fats produced in the body are triglycerides, which consist of three fatty acids on a carbohydrate backbone. One particular type of fatty acid (Omega three) seems to have a preventive effect on many diseases. Omega three, found in cold water fish (e.g., salmon), is structurally different from the fatty acid commonly found in meat (Omega six). Triglycerides come in two forms, saturated (usually from animals) and unsaturated (plant origin). Saturated fats tend to increase blood cholesterol levels, whereas polyunsaturated fats lower them.

Although cholesterol is a fat, it differs both structurally and functionally from the most common lipids, the triglycerides. Cholesterol is a steroid, similar in structure to testosterone and estrogen. It is an important part of cell membranes and is needed to manufacture bile and many hormones.

but it can also be ingested as it is associated with the saturated animal fats. If too much cholesterol is ingested, the body adjusts by reducing production in the liver and increasing cholesterol excretion. However, in one-third to one-fifth of the population, excess cholesterol accumulates in the arteries, eventually causing atherosclerosis. It is not clear why this occurs, but a genetic defect in cholesterol metabolism, over-consumption of cholesterol, or response to stress may be contributors.

There is little danger of insufficient fat intake; even if one ingests no visible fat, about 10 percent of all calories would still be derived from fat. On the average, Americans consume an average of 40 percent of their calories as fats. Americans

should reduce their fat consumption to 30 percent or less of their total caloric consumption because too much dietary fat is associated with a number of health problems. Excess fat intake is particularly harmful for elders on low-calorie diets since it provides calories in a concentrated form with few vitamins, minerals, fiber, or other nutrients. In addition, some elders have reduced tolerance of fat due to digestive problems and slower metabolism.

Fiber

What grandma called roughage has been renamed fiber and health experts are encouraging many to eat more of it. Fiber is the undigestible parts of plants. It speeds the passage of food through the digestive tract. Five types have been described, each with a unique chemical composition and health benefits: cellulose, hemicellulose, pectin, gums, and lignin (see table 9.2). Individuals should consume between 30–60 grams of fiber a day but the average American eats 10–20 grams of fiber a day. Elders may tend to eat less fiber since foods rich in fiber are often hard to chew.

Table 9.2	The five kinds of fiber and where they are found				
	Cellulose	**Hemicelluloses**	**Gums**	**Pectin**	**Lignin**
Food Sources	Whole-Wheat Flour Bran Cabbage Young Peas Green Beans Wax Beans Broccoli Brussels Sprouts Cucumber Skins Peppers Apples Carrots	Bran Cereals Whole Grains Brussels Sprouts Mustard Greens Beet Root	Oatmeal & Other Rolled-Oat Products Dried Beans	Squash Apples Citrus Fruits Cauliflower Green Beans Cabbage Dried Peas Carrots Strawberries Potatoes	Breakfast Cereals Bran Older Vegetables Strawberries Eggplant Pears Green Beans Radishes
Function	Mechanically smooths function of large bowel: Absorbs water, increasing stool and decreasing transit time. Helps prevent constipation, and may protect against diverticulosis, colon cancer, hemorrhoids and varicose veins.		Influences absorption in stomach and small bowel: Binds with bile acids, thereby decreasing fat absorption and lowering cholesterol levels. Coats gut and delays glucose absorption, smoothing sugar surges for diabetics.		Influences other kinds of fiber: Binds with bile acids to lower cholesterol. Reduces digestibility of other fibers: Helps speed food through gut.

© From Lang, S. 1984 Beyond bran, *American Health*, May, pp. 62–64. Reprinted with permission.

Water

Water is essential for swallowing, digestion, transportation of wastes, and regulation of body temperature. All chemical reactions within the body need water; even small changes in water balance can lead to metabolic problems. In addition, water, especially hard water, provides the body with needed minerals such as zinc, magnesium, calcium, and copper.

The healthy older person requires from 1.5–2 quarts of water each day, some of which is obtained from food. Elders face special problems with water balance because they have a lower body water content, which may be due to decreased fluid intake. Elders are also susceptible to dehydration from diarrhea, diuretic drugs, and a number of diseases. Healthy older people whose bodies need water are not as likely as younger people to complain of dry mouths and tend to drink less than younger people, suggesting that elders cannot rely totally on their thirst mechanism to determine needed water intake (Phillips et al. 1984). Symptoms of mild dehydration include weakness, confusion, dry mouth, and flushed skin. Symptoms of more severe dehydration include sunken eyes, dry, loose skin, and low urinary output.

Vitamins

Vitamins are a diverse group of chemicals needed in small amounts to make the enzymes for many chemical reactions in the body. Vitamins must be included in the diet since they are not synthesized by the body in sufficient amounts. Fat-soluble vitamins (A,E,D, and K) are stored in body fat and the liver. Excessive levels of these vitamins can be toxic. Water-soluble vitamins (vitamin C and the B complex vitamins) do not build up to toxic levels because they are regularly excreted in the urine. However, they need to be ingested more often and are more easily destroyed by cooking than the fat-soluble vitamins.

Little is known about special vitamin requirements for elders. Many nutritionists assert that elders' needs are different than younger adults because of age-associated physiological decrements and the presence of chronic disease. Because elders generally eat fewer calories than other age groups, they must consume foods more concentrated in vitamins to be adequately nourished. The following section will discuss each vitamin, its role in health, signs of deficiency, and common dietary sources. The role of specific vitamins in the prevention and treatment of chronic diseases and disorders of elders will be discussed in a later section. Table 9.1 described the established RDA for each vitamin.

Vitamin A

Vitamin A is available in two forms: pre-formed vitamin A (called retinol) or carotenoids, vitamin A precursors that are converted to vitamin A within the body. Although high doses of vitamin A are toxic, carotenoids are considered safe, even in high quantities. Vitamin A is essential for the rejuvenation of visual pigments. A deficiency in vitamin A can lead to night blindness. Vitamin A is also necessary for skin and mucous membrane function. A deficiency causes reduced mucus production of all membranes and rough and scaly skin. Vitamin A deficiency is also associated with a high incidence of infection and slow healing rates due to decreased immune function. Green and yellow fruits and vegetables are good sources of carotenoids; vitamin A is found in some meats and animal products.

Vitamin A deficiency in elders is likely to be caused by reduced intestinal absorption of the vitamin rather than a low intake. Reduced absorption can be caused by reduced availability of bile to enable fat to be absorbed, liver disease, or use of antibiotics or laxatives.

Vitamin B Complex

The B vitamins differ structurally, but their functions are related. The eight B vitamins used to be identified by numbers, but are now designated by their chemical name, except Vitamin B_{12}.

Thiamine (B_1) enrichment of foods in our country has largely eliminated the dreadful disease beriberi, which leads to paralysis, heart failure, and death. However, between one-third and one-half of all Americans may suffer from mild thiamine deficiencies. Symptoms of a mild deficiency include appetite loss, nausea, constipation, depression, and mental confusion. Alcoholics are often deficient in thiamine, possibly due to inadequate intake, insufficient absorption, and heightened need. Surveys report that low-income Americans commonly receive significantly less thiamine than the RDA. Thiamine-rich foods are whole and enriched grains, dried legumes, and pork products.

The term **niacin** refers to the two forms of vitamin B_3, nicotinic acid and nicotinamide, which work together. The word *niacin* is used because the chemical names may be confused with nicotine, a harmful substance found in cigarettes, which has no relation to the vitamin B_3. Without sufficient niacin, an individual may contract pellagra, characterized by a skin rash, diarrhea, dementia, and death. Pellagra used to be a widespread disease, but now refined carbohydrates are enriched to prevent this deficiency. Mild deficiencies may be manifest as depression and mental confusion. Elders rarely have a niacin deficiency unless they are alcoholics or on heavy aspirin therapy. However, excessive doses of niacin can cause flushed, hot and tingling skin, nausea, headache, cramps, and diarrhea. Niacin is found in meat, poultry, legumes, and peanut butter. If sufficient tryptophan, an essential amino acid, is ingested, the body can manufacture its own niacin.

Pyridoxine (B_6) is essential for antibody production and brain and nerve function. Deficiency of pyridoxine is rare. The need for pyridoxine increases for those who ingest high levels of alcohol or protein, are heavy smokers, or use estrogen supplements. Bananas, vegetables, meat, liver, whole grains, and egg yolks contain high levels of pyridoxine.

Elders, especially the low-income and institutionalized, are commonly deficient in another B vitamin, **folic acid** or **folate.** Heavy alcohol consumption and some drugs (e.g., antibiotics) can decrease folic acid levels. A folacin deficiency is first manifested by anemia-like symptoms that are only reversed with folic acid supplementation. Folic acid is inactivated by sunlight and food storage. The richest sources of folacin are liver, oranges, spinach, wheat germ, and bran.

The primary function of **vitamin B_{12}** is to build nerve tissue and deficiencies cause nerve damage. Even though some people ingest sufficient B_{12}, their bodies cannot absorb it because they lack a particular gastric enzyme called *intrinsic factor*. These people exhibit a B_{12} deficiency called pernicious anemia. This permanent malady mainly affects people over age fifty and is treated with monthly vitamin B_{12} injections. Vitamin B_{12} deficiencies may also occur among strict vegetarians who do not eat meat, eggs, or dairy products. Unlike other water soluble vitamins, B_{12} can be stored in the liver so deficiencies may not show for some time. Liver is an extremely good source of B_{12}, although meat, eggs, and dairy products are also good.

Riboflavin (B_2) is essential for the action of other B vitamins. Marginal riboflavin deficiency is characterized by visual problems, swollen lips, and scaly skin rashes. Strict vegetarians, alcoholics, and those who take estrogen supplements are at higher risk for riboflavin deficiency. Some believe riboflavin to be the most common marginal deficiency among elders and the poor. Liver, dairy products, and whole or enriched grain products are good sources of riboflavin.

A variety of symptoms have been associated with deficiency of another B vitamin, **pantothenic acid** including gastrointestinal difficulties, burning pain in the feet, appetite loss, diarrhea, muscle cramps, skin rashes, and increased susceptibility to infection. Foods high in pantothenic acid include liver, dairy products, avocados, and mushrooms.

Biotin deficiencies may be common because it is lost in processing or refrigeration of food and not added back during enrichment. Symptoms of biotin deficiencies are similar to those of other vitamin B deficiencies: gastrointestinal distress, fatigue, and depression. Deficiencies can be aggravated by persistent diarrhea or long-term therapy with antibiotics or sulfa drugs. Biotin is present in almost all foods. Organ meats, legumes, egg yolks, nuts, and whole grains are particularly rich in this vitamin.

Vitamin C

The primary role of vitamin C (also called ascorbic acid) is to form substances, such as collagen and cartilage. Collagen is an important structural fiber in the walls of cells and cartilage holds bones together. Although its other roles are not well-defined, it also acts as an antioxidant, assists in the manufacture of thyroid hormone, and enhances the absorption of iron and calcium from the small intestine. Major sources of vitamin C are citrus fruits, strawberries, brussels sprouts and broccoli.

Severe vitamin C deficiency causes scurvy. Scurvy is characterized by a loss of appetite, irritability, and depression, followed by sore limbs and hemorrhaging in all parts of the body, including gums, bones, and joints. The disease was first noticed in sailors on long voyages without fresh fruits and vegetables. Although scurvy is now very rare, some experts believe that a mild deficiency can cause increased susceptibility to illness. Use of certain drugs affects the need for vitamin C. Those who take estrogen supplements, high doses of aspirin, smoke cigarettes, or drink alcohol heavily have an increased need for vitamin C.

The amount of vitamin C needed for optimal health is highly debated. Although only minimal levels of vitamin C are needed to prevent scurvy, some experts believe that higher levels of vitamin C in the diet will assist in preventing illness and enhance recovery. Documentation of this claim relies heavily on studies that show vitamin C levels are decreased during infection, surgery, or stress. There is no evidence to substantiate the claim that too much vitamin C can increase the incidence of kidney stones and gout in susceptible individuals. Rather, all excess ingested leaves via the urine. However, large doses may interfere with some diagnostic laboratory tests. For a more complete listing on the studies regarding the role of vitamin C in prevention and treatment, see Pauling (1986).

Vitamin D

Vitamin D (calciferol) is not technically a vitamin, but a hormone because it is manufactured in one part of the body and affects another part. When skin is exposed to sunlight, vitamin D is activated in a complex chain of events that also involves the kidneys and liver. The end product, calciferol, regulates blood calcium levels by allowing calcium from the intestine to be released into the bloodstream to build bones and increase neuron function, among others. Without vitamin D, ingested calcium cannot enter the bloodstream. Instead, the body will maintain blood calcium levels by removing necessary calcium from the bones.

Vitamin D deficiency causes rickets in children and osteomalacia in adults—diseases that severely weaken the bones and increase susceptibility to fractures in adults. Drugs taken for epilepsy, bulk laxatives, antacids containing aluminum, cholesterol-lowering drugs and mineral oil laxatives reduce the effectiveness of vitamin D, increasing the risk of deficiency. In addition to vitamin D production from sunlight, it can be ingested either in the form of oily fish, cod liver oil, eggs, liver, butter, or milk fortified with a form of vitamin D.

Some experts believe the recent concern about skin cancer and cholesterol has led to widespread vitamin D deficiency in elders. A study of healthy retirees from the Southwest revealed that, despite the availability of sunshine, more than 60 percent had reduced blood levels of vitamin D, which worsened in the winter. Not only did elders avoid the sun, but they also consumed fewer fortified dairy products in an effort to lower cholesterol levels and avoid gastrointestinal problems associated with lactose intolerance (reported in *American Health* 1985). Some believe the need

The nutritional requirements of each of these women differ because of health status and activity level.

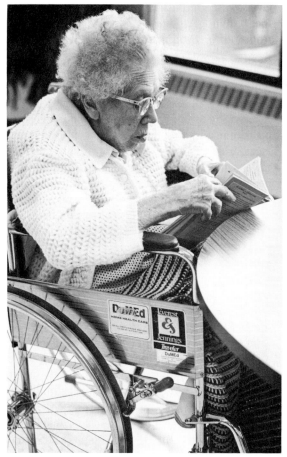
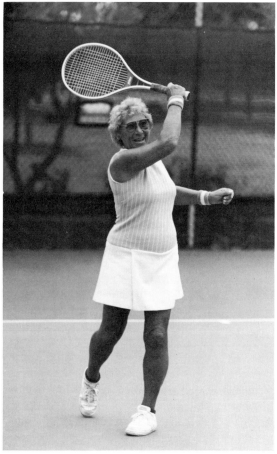

for vitamin D among elders to be significantly more than the current RDA because their bodies are less efficient at converting vitamin D into its active form.

Vitamin E

The only documented role of vitamin E is its antioxidant properties that prevent fat in cell membranes from breaking down. Even if one has sufficient intake of vitamin E, a deficiency may result in those who cannot absorb fat properly. Symptoms are serious and obvious and include anemia and nervous system abnormalities. The majority of vitamin E is obtained from vegetable oils.

Vitamin K

The main function of vitamin K is to promote blood clotting. It can be obtained from vitamin K-rich foods (e.g., leafy green vegetables) or manufactured by special bacteria that live in the colon. Vitamin K deficiency is very rare in adults; however, it can occur in individuals on long-term antibiotic therapy because the antibiotics kill the colon bacteria. Additionally, those who have difficulty absorbing fats or those taking mineral oil are also at higher risk of deficiency. Symptoms of deficiency include anemia, prolonged bleeding, and easy bruising.

Minerals

Minerals are inorganic substances needed in relatively small amounts for proper body function. Macrominerals, such as calcium, magnesium, phosphorus, sodium, potassium, sulfur, and chlorine, are needed in amounts greater than 100 mg/day. Other minerals are needed in trace amounts such as iron, iodine, copper, manganese, zinc, chromium, flourine, and selenium. Further, trace elements, such as tin, vanadium, silicon, arsenic, nickel, and cadmium may be important, but recommended doses have not been established. The quantity of each mineral needed is no measure of its relative importance in the body.

Mineral deficiencies are more common than vitamin deficiencies. Although vitamins are usually present in foods in similar amounts throughout the world, some areas are very poor in specific minerals and trace elements, predisposing residents of these areas to deficiencies. In elders, mineral deficiencies may be related to decreased absorption, marginal diets, drug intake, and the stress of disease. This section will discuss the role of selected minerals, signs of deficiency, and common food sources. The use of specific minerals in the prevention and treatment of chronic diseases and disorders will be covered in a later section. Refer to tables 9.1A and 9.1B for the RDA or estimated safe and adequate dietary intake for a number of minerals.

Calcium

Calcium is the mineral needed in the highest quantities by the body. It is crucial to bone formation, blood clotting, heartbeat regulation, muscle contraction, and neuron function. Blood calcium levels must always remain constant. If levels are low, dietary calcium is absorbed through the small intestine with the help of vitamin D. When dietary intake is insufficient, blood calcium level is maintained by drawing on calcium stores in the bones. Both high calcium intake and physical activity stimulate calcium to deposit in the bones. Conversely, low intake stimulates gradual depletion of calcium from the bones, causing osteoporosis, which may not be obvious for years.

The 1980 RDA suggests a calcium intake of 800 mg/day for all adults, but most experts agree that elders, especially women, need from 1,000–1,500 mg/day to prevent or minimize bone loss (Heaney and Recker 1981). A number of dietary surveys document an insufficient dietary intake of calcium in the American population, especially middle-aged and older women. Not only do older people ingest less calcium, but their activity level is generally lower, aggravating bone loss. Further, they are less able to absorb calcium from the intestine than younger groups. A high-protein diet and some drugs reduce blood calcium levels. Those with low-calorie intake (whether by poverty or dieting) are also at risk of deficiency because dairy products are often reduced or eliminated. The richest sources of calcium are dairy products, green vegetables, and canned bony fish.

Calcium supplementation is now recommended for all women, starting in their 20s or 30s, to reduce the rate of bone demineralization. Calcium carbonate supplements are the most inexpensive, safest, and contain the most available calcium per tablet. Calcium gluconate and lactate are safe, but more tablets are needed to get the same amount of available calcium. Although bone meal, dolomite, and oyster shell have high calcium content, they may be contaminated with lead or other toxins.

Chlorine and Sulfur

Chlorine works with sodium to maintain acid-base and fluid balance of the body and is important in neuron message transmission. Chlorine is part of the hydrochloric acid secreted by the stomach. Almost all chlorine is consumed in the form of sodium chloride (salt). Sulfur is used by the body to produce insulin and other important molecules. Some proteins and vitamins contain sulfur. Although both chlorine and sulfur are important to the body, no dietary deficiency is known.

Chromium

Chromium is needed for the production of glucose tolerance factor. This factor is a chemical that increases the ability of body cells to respond to insulin. Cells stimulated by glucose tolerance factor can take in needed nutrients that flood the bloodstream after a meal. Some experts suggest that long-standing chromium deficiencies common among elders are partially responsible for adult-onset diabetes since body cell sensitivity to insulin decreases with age (Boyle et al. 1977). Food processing drastically decreases the amount of chromium available in foods and it is not replaced by the enrichment process. Chromium-rich foods include brewer's yeast, blackstrap molasses, wheat germ, whole grains, and mushrooms.

Copper

Copper is involved in the transport of oxygen from the lungs to the body tissues. This mineral is also important in the production of the structural fibers collagen and elastin. Symptoms of copper deficiency include anemia, reduced immunity, loss of color in the skin and hair, and damage to the brain and spinal cord. Marginal copper deficiency is thought to increase the risk of heart disease. Foods high in copper include shellfish, nuts, cocoa, dried beans, mushrooms, and whole grains.

Iodine

The main function of iodine is to make the thyroid hormone, thyroxine, which regulates metabolic rate. Iodine deficiencies result in an enlarged thyroid, called a goiter. Goiters are now rare because of the widespread practice of iodizing salt. Iodine is also important in reducing the effects of radiation. Besides iodized salt, other rich sources of iodine are saltwater fish, clams, oysters, and seaweed.

Iron

Iron is the key component of hemoglobin, which transports oxygen from the lungs to peripheral tissues, and myoglobin, which transports oxygen to working muscle. Additionally, iron is part of several enzymes that convert nutrients into energy, is active in production of elastin and collagen, maintains the immune system and is part of several neurotransmitters.

Iron is continuously recycled by the body and is only depleted through blood loss. Iron-deficiency anemia is common among elders and may result from an inadequate intake of iron in the diet, impaired iron absorption, or blood loss due to disease or injury. Inadequate iron causes a shortage of red blood cells, consequently reducing the amount of oxygen available to the tissues. Symptoms of iron deficiency anemia are weakness, headache, and heart palpitations. Those who have a vitamin C deficiency may also be more susceptible to iron deficiencies because ascorbic acid enhances absorption of dietary iron. It is interesting to note that body iron stores increase with age. Liver, dried beans, some meats, prunes, and shellfish are rich in iron.

Magnesium

Magnesium is required for every major biological process, including metabolism of glucose, production of energy, synthesis of DNA and RNA, nerve cell function, and muscle relaxation. Magnesium also lowers blood lipid concentrations, stabilizes heart beat, and decreases blood clotting (Burch and Giles 1977).

Marginal magnesium deficiency is common in the United States due to processing of cereal grains, which removes the magnesium-rich hull and does not replace the mineral in the enrichment process. Magnesium deficiency may be caused by restricted calorie diets, diabetes, alcohol use, heavy exercise, excessive diarrhea and vomiting, and use of diuretics or digitalis. Magnesium deficiency is particularly common among elders. Symptoms of magnesium deficiency are loss of appetite, nausea, diarrhea, tremors, and loss of coordination. Even though a marginal deficiency has no obvious symptoms, it may damage the heart, leading to abnormal cardiac rhythms or heart attack. Magnesium-rich foods include whole grain cereals, molasses, nuts, legumes, and hard water.

Phosphorus

Phosphorus is crucial for every cell reaction that releases or uses energy. This mineral is also an important part of DNA and RNA, cell membranes and bones, and helps balance blood acidity. Vitamin D regulates the levels of phosphorus in the blood by controlling the rate at which it is absorbed and excreted. A phosphorus deficiency is rare because it is abundant in all proteins and is used as an additive in processed foods such as soft drinks. However, an excess can impair calcium absorption.

Potassium

Potassium is involved in nerve conduction, muscle contraction, regulation of heart beat, and body fluid balance. Diarrhea, the use of diuretics, excessive sweating, or fasting can cause potassium deficiencies. Symptoms of deficiency are rapid heartbeat, muscle weakness, nausea, and vomiting. There is growing evidence that low potassium levels may elevate blood pressure. Potatoes, raisins, bananas, avocados, orange juice, sardines, and skim milk are good dietary sources of potassium.

Sodium

Sodium is necessary for nerve transmission and muscle relaxation. It is also important in maintaining water balance and urine production by regulating thirst and water excretion by the kidneys. Sodium deficiencies are rare, although sodium may be lost in excessive quantities due to heavy sweating. In our country, sodium excesses are common because most processed foods are high in sodium due to added salt and preservatives. The association between sodium and hypertension will be discussed in a later section.

Zinc

Zinc is an essential chemical in more than a hundred metabolic enzymes. Zinc deficiency is characterized by decreased sense of smell, delayed wound healing, and increased susceptibility to infection. Although severe zinc deficiency is rare, experts believe marginal zinc deficiencies are common among elders, especially the poor and hospitalized (Garry et al. 1982). Progressive zinc deficiency may play a role in the gradual, age-related decrease in immunity. One study found zinc supplementation increased immune response in elders (Duchateau et al. 1981). The richest dietary sources of zinc include seafood, meats, eggs, and nuts.

Vitamin and Mineral Supplements

There is widespread controversy surrounding the value of vitamin and mineral supplements. Some experts believe that a balanced and varied diet provides all nutrients essential for good health. However, others claim that Americans seldom eat a balanced and varied diet and vitamin or mineral supplements promote better health. While the nutritionists debate, from one-third to one-half of American elders use supplements regularly (Sobal et al. 1986). The public relies on the news media, advice from friends, and advertisements to decide which vitamins and doses to take. Physicians are seldom consulted about vitamin use and prescriptions for vitamins are rare.

It is generally agreed that a well-balanced diet can provide a healthy individual with the recommended daily allowance for each nutrient. Nevertheless a number of nutrition assessments indicate that the general population is not meeting the RDA of many vitamins and minerals by food intake alone. Dieting, processed foods, vitamin-depleting storage and cooking methods, and low income contribute to widespread deficiencies. Further, special groups have an increased need for some vitamins and minerals, such as those recovering from surgery or injury, those taking drugs, those who smoke or drink alcohol, and those with specific chronic diseases. Some researchers feel that the RDA for certain nutrients may protect against deficiency disease but is inadequate for optimal health. Evidence is building that even though an individual does not manifest symptoms of a deficiency disease, marginal deficiencies occur. However, their symptoms may be vague (e.g., fatigue, frequent illness, and slowed wound healing).

Most nutritionists agree that moderate supplementation, combined with a balanced, varied diet, is a convenient way to avoid deficiencies. This method is preferable to large doses of a single vitamin or mineral because people are seldom deficient in only one area. There is little evidence that megadoses (ten or more times the RDA) are beneficial and they may even be dangerous. Vitamin supplements should not replace a balanced diet; it is estimated that there are more than twice as many essential nutrients as those promoted by the Food and Nutrition Board.

Nutritional Status of Elders

Major changes have occurred in the average American diet over the lifetime of the current elder population. From 1910–1976, the consumption of fats increased by almost one-third, complex carbohydrate intake decreased by 20 percent and consumption of processed foods increased 50 percent. Elders are increasingly relying on processed foods, protein, and fats rather than whole grains, fresh fruits, and vegetables (Boykin 1980). Overall, both national and local surveys reveal that a significant proportion of American elders suffer from caloric and other nutrient deficiencies. However, nutrient deficiencies are not likely due to poor dietary practices. More likely the pervasiveness of chronic disease, poverty, and excessive drug consumption are to blame. Those with the greatest nutrient deficiencies are those with low intake of calories, indicating that when food intake falls, it is more difficult to get needed vitamins and minerals.

Surveys that attempt to determine nutritional adequacy of elder populations utilize a number of methods to determine food intake so that the RDA standard may be applied. The most common method used, especially in large studies, is the twenty-four-hour dietary recall whereby individuals are asked to list the type and amount of foods eaten in the last twenty-four hours. A dietary history, in which individuals are requested to answer a variety of questions regarding factors influencing food intake may also

---

Components of a Dietary History

1. **Demographic Characteristics:** ethnicity, sex, age, religion, education.

2. **Living Condition:** family composition, marital status, type of housing, social supports, income, distance to grocery store, available transportation.

3. **Health Conditions:** presence of chronic illness, mobility, quality of teeth, appetite, digestion, elimination, vision, smell, taste.

4. **Health Behaviors:** smoking, drinking, exercising, drug-taking practices, vitamin supplement practices.

5. **Dietary Habits:** special diet information, number of meals/day, who does shopping/cooking, recent changes in dietary habits, food likes and dislikes, allergies, use of certain artificial sweeteners/low-sodium foods.

6. **Regular Diet:** List foods commonly eaten (e.g., fresh vegetables, baked goods, red meat, TV dinners, green and yellow vegetables, ice cream, low-fat dairy products).

---

be useful. A food record may be used to assess an elder's nutritional status. The client is requested to accurately record type and quantity of all foods eaten over a specific time period (three days to a week).

Self-reported information on dietary intake, when combined with a physical assessment, gives even more information regarding nutritional status. Measurements of weight, height, arm circumference, and skinfold thickness, when compared to population norms, can determine malnutrition and obesity. A physical examination can also detect overt signs of nutritional deficiency. Finally, laboratory tests on blood and urine can indicate current levels of essential nurients—such as protein, vitamins, and minerals. However, since norms for elders on these scales are not well-established and their needs are often increased by poor health and drug use, results should be read cautiously.

Three major nationwide dietary surveys have been conducted that have included elders. The most recent, Nationwide Food Consumption Survey (U.S. Department of Agriculture 1980), assessed the food intake of approximately fifteen thousand households, of which five thousand included elders. However, no elders who lived alone were sampled. Elders, especially women, had higher than average rates of calorie deficiency. Other common deficiencies were magnesium and pyridoxine.

The Ten State Nutrition Survey (U.S. Department of Health, Education, and Welfare, 1972) attempted to assess the problem of hunger and malnutrition in our country, intentionally over-representing those at higher risk. Forty thousand individuals underwent medical evaluations, with additional biochemical analysis on a small sub-group supposed to be at high risk for malnutrition. Many outwardly healthy people over fifty were deficient in calories, protein, vitamins A, B, C, iron, and calcium.

The Hanes Health and Nutrition Examination Survey (National Center for Health Statistics 1979) combined biochemical analysis with physical measurements and diet assessment on over twenty thousand people between the ages of one and seventy-four. As a group, elders were reported to be deficient in calories and protein regardless of sex or income. The degree of deficiency was generally greater in those living below the poverty level; 21 percent of elder Caucasians and

Face-to-face interviews serve to gather accurate information regarding daily food intake, but the process is time-consuming.

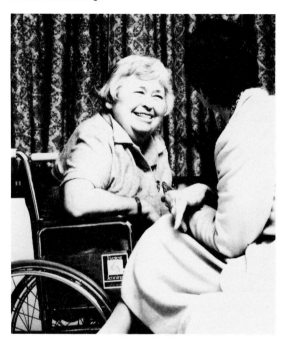

36 percent of black Americans over sixty had a daily calorie intake of under one thousand calories. Elder women were deficient in calcium, iron, and thiamine. Older blacks had a lower vitamin C level than Caucasian elders and over 40 percent of black Americans over age sixty had an indication of anemia.

Population studies of community elders, although important, have a number of limitations that must be addressed. Generally, those most likely to be at high nutritional risk are not included: the institutionalized, bedridden, those who live in isolated areas, and those unable to keep records. Further, the usual dietary assessment tool, the twenty-four hour dietary recall, is not very effective, especially in elders. Foods eaten may be forgotten, estimate of quantities may be inaccurate, and foods eaten over a twenty-four-hour period may not be representative of the usual

Chapter 9

diet. Additionally, the average nutrient intakes for populations tell us little about individual variation within the group. For instance, in one study, elders were reported to consume an adequate amount of dietary protein, but the individual intakes within the population varied from half to double the amount needed (Rozovski 1984). As mentioned earlier, the RDA does not account for increased nutrient requirements among some elders. Further, marginal deficiencies are difficult to assess in population surveys, even though they may affect the state of health. Finally, severe nutritional deficiency is rare in the United States. The major health problems are associated with overnutrition; not only obesity, but over-consumption of some nutrients such as fats (Watkin 1980). The above studies did not address over-consumption of nutrients.

Studies on the nutritional status of institutionalized elders are sparse. One study (Justice et al. 1974) recorded the dietary intake of a group of elders in a nursing home for five consecutive days. They reported that men consumed more calories, carbohydrates, thiamine, and vitamin C than women. Almost all the men and 40 percent of the women were classified as anemic; two-thirds of the women had bone loss suggesting osteoporosis. Because the nutrients provided in the institutional diets of that study equaled or exceeded the RDA, nutrient deficiencies were thought to be caused by a failure of these elders to consume sufficient food offered to them.

Inadequate nutrient intake and the consequent increased death and illness rate are of special concern among hospitalized elders. Studies indicate that 40–60 percent of all patients admitted to hospitals are malnourished. Hospitalization exposes elders to the stresses of disease, surgery, diagnostic and treatment procedures that further deplete their nutritional stores (Lichtenstein 1982). One report indicated that 60 percent of elders hospitalized lost an average of 13.2 pounds during their stay (Butterworth 1974).

Elders in nursing homes and hospitals usually need vitamin or mineral supplements, but these are rarely prescribed. Institution food may be unappetizing and contain low amounts of fiber and fresh fruits and vegetables, further aggravating nutrient deficiencies. Unless the patient's nutritional needs are met, it is unlikely that other therapy will be effective.

Because of the high incidence of nutritional problems of institutionalized elders, individuals should undergo a thorough nutritional assessment upon admittance to a hospital or nursing home. In addition, daily monitoring of weight and dietary intake is necessary.

An individual nutrition assessment utilizes the same tools as population surveys. The difference is that effective individual nutritional assessment utilizes all the methods—twenty-four-hour dietary recall, dietary history, food record, and a physical examination. Additionally, it is important to remember that the RDA, although helpful as a guide for nutrient assessment, is not sufficient to evaluate an elder's nutritional intake. Instead, data from the physical examination combined with knowledge about the individual's food habits, physical activity level, drug intake, and presence of disease should determine optimal nutrient levels (Natow and Heslin 1986).

For institutionalized elders, oral nutrient supplements may be prescribed in addition to regular meals to maintain adequate calorie intake. For elders unable to take in sufficient nutrients by mouth, tube feeding may be necessary. A nasogastric tube, inserted through the nasal passage to the esophagus, allows a continuous drip of nutrients into the stomach. If the gastrointestinal route is not feasible, intravenous tube feeding is necessary. In this case, a nutrient solution is administered into a vein, usually in the arm. Although these methods are acceptable for short-term use (two–three weeks), if long-term feeding is necessary, a tube has to be either inserted directly into the stomach (gastrostomy) or placed into a central vein.

The Functions of Food in American Culture

Attitudes and behaviors surrounding food and eating are learned and shared and are an important part of life. Each culture imparts its own meaning to food and eating. In the United States, food may serve a number of psychological, social, cultural, and even economic functions.

Food may be a manifestation of friendship. Most social events include food and drink, and some—picnics, dinner parties, Thanksgiving, cocktail parties, coffee breaks—center around eating and drinking. Individuals seldom prefer to eat alone. Dinner is the focal point for interaction in many American families.

Food and drink can also serve as status symbols. Filet mignon is more prestigious than macaroni and cheese. For some, the offer of food is a way to show love: a special dessert, a candlelight meal, or an invitation to dinner. Conversely, refusal to eat what another has cooked may be a sign of rejection. Eating can also serve as an outlet for boredom, unhappiness, loneliness, or stress. Nursing home personnel can often detect a resident's stress level by the amount of waste and complaints about the food.

People may use food as a reward for self or others. For instance, the statements, "You mow the lawn and I'll take you for an ice cream," or "I deserve this piece of cake, I worked so hard today."

Food can express individuality and many people are proud of their secret recipes. Some get attention by eating uncommon food combinations while others get attention by not eating at all. Vegetarians may use their food preferences as a political statement or as evidence of their concern for health. Some food habits, such as fasting or avoidance of certain foods, may be a reflection of spiritual beliefs.

Food consumption is an important source of ritual and security. All members of our culture know rules governing American eating: main course comes before dessert, three meals a day, no alcohol before noon, and cereal is a breakfast food. Members of various populations, such as children, vegetarians, teenagers, ethnic groups, or elders, have certain food preferences that establish them as part of a group. Certain foods impart security because of long-standing habit.

Factors Affecting Food Selection

A number of variables profoundly affect food selection and consequent nutritional status. A sample of psychological, physiological, intellectual, socioeconomic, cultural, and environmental factors influencing food selection are illustrated below.

Physiological Factors

Age-associated physiological decrements, chronic illness, and drug side effects can severely affect mobility, energy level, and visual acuity, which decrease interest in eating and ability to shop for and prepare food. Visual decrements can make it difficult for elders to read labels, comparison shop,

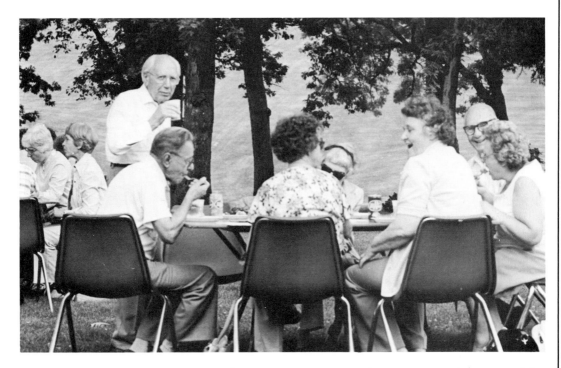

Finally, food serves an economic purpose in America because the provision of foods in supermarkets and restaurants is a profit-making venture. Millions of dollars are spent yearly on advertising that encourages us to buy particular food products even when we are not hungry and the food is not healthful. A disproportionate amount of advertising money is targeted for junk or convenience foods rather than nutritional foods.

and cook. Reduced mobility may force an elder to shop only at nearby stores, which may be expensive or offer little selection. Elders with mobility decrements, especially those using a cane or walker, may have difficulty carrying groceries home from the store. Further, increasing disabilities with advancing age may prohibit elaborate meal preparation and promote high use of pre-packaged food. Age or drug-related decrements in taste or smell acuity, dental problems, poor oral hygeine or appetite can reduce motivation to eat. Dentures or tooth loss can make chewing more difficult. Food intolerances and the necessity of following a prescribed diet can also affect food choices.

Psychological Factors

Emotional state can have profound consequences on motivation to shop for and prepare nutritious meals. Psychological distress can cause either a diminished appetite or overeating. Stress is also known to alter absorption and excretion of nutrients such as calcium, increasing dietary need. Elders who are lonely or grieving may be less likely to cook for themselves and may depend on highly processed snack foods. Those who are depressed or who have low self-esteem may not want to leave the house to shop or may be too lethargic to cook.

Intellectual Factors

Level of education and knowledge about nutrition can affect food choices and methods of meal preparation. Those with a high education level generally have fewer nutrient deficiencies than those with less education. Illiterate elders, those with a minimum of nutrition education, or those who speak English poorly may be unable to read and understand product labels. Elders who are less educated are more subject to food faddism if they select foods that are advertised on television or in magazines. Finally, those with severe intellectual deficits may be incapable of shopping or preparing meals for themselves.

Socio-Economic Factors

Financial status and living arrangement are important variables that influence the quality of food purchased and motivation to eat healthfully. Income is related to diet quality; those who are poor are less likely to have an adequate diet since many high-nutrient foods are expensive. However, a high income does not ensure nutritional adequacy.

Social interaction is positively related to food intake and nutritional status. Those living alone have the poorest diets. Social isolation, especially if involuntary, can also affect the motivation to shop, prepare meals, or eat well. Many elders do not like to prepare and eat a meal alone or go out to eat by themselves. However, the effect of living alone on diet depends on gender. Older men living alone have the poorest diets while those living with a spouse have the best diets. However, living arrangements are not as influential in the diets of older women (Davis et al. 1985). Elder women tend to eat a greater variety of food than men and are more likely to choose fresh fruit, vegetables and milk products, while men eat more meat.

Cultural Attitudes and Behaviors

Differences in eating patterns among age groups are common because each generation grew up in a different cultural milieu. For instance, many elders associate white bread with wealth and beans with poverty. Elders from varied ethnic backgrounds may limit food choices to those traditional foods that are available locally.

Food consumption habits established early in life may be hard to break. However, numerous studies show that elders are not adverse to trying new foods and that eating patterns may change dramatically with age. For instance, many chronic disorders, such as diabetes or cardiovascular disorders, require dietary modifications begun late in life.

Environmental Factors

The availability of community nutrition programs, distance from shopping facilities, transportation availability, and geographical location can also affect food choices and nutritional status. Elders in the inner city may have reduced access to supermarkets and many small grocery stores close to home are expensive. Inner city elders, especially women and those with mobility decrements, may be afraid to shop because of a fear of crime. Climate may affect food choices because winter snows and excessive heat may confine some older people to their homes. Elders in rented rooms or hotels have limited access to cooking or refrigeration facilities.

Effect of Drug Use on Nutritional Status

Many prescription and over-the-counter drugs affect nutritional status. Some drugs may irritate the stomach, cause nausea, vomiting, diarrhea, or alter the absorption or excretion of nutrients. Others alter electrolyte balance, carbohydrate or fat metabolism, or levels of healthful bacteria in the digestive tract. Drugs that alter taste perception can either drive people to overeat in search of satisfaction or to lose their appetite. Appetite may be increased directly by some drugs or indirectly by improving mental status. Current diet, other drugs taken concurrently, and presence of chronic illness must be taken into account when analyzing the effect of drug intake on nutritional status.

Alcohol is the drug that causes the most significant alterations in nutritional status. Heavy alcohol consumption contributes to malnutrition because alcohol diminishes appetite and is often used instead of food. Among heavy drinkers, alcohol can account for up to one-half the caloric intake. Weight loss may occur because of irregular eating or total abstinence from food during or after a drinking episode. This can be devastating for those who are already nutritionally marginal.

Every cell in the body is subject to the effects of alcohol. When alcohol is present, tissues cannot use or store nutrients in their normal manner. Alcohol can damage the gastrointestinal tract leading to impaired absorption and excessive excretion of essential nutrients. Alcohol also damages the liver and pancreas, producing cirrhosis of the liver and pancreatitis. Elders are more susceptible to the toxic effects of alcohol because drug tolerance decreases with age. Age-changes and some chronic illnesses can further prolong the amount of time alcohol circulates in the bloodstream.

Excessive alcohol consumption can lead to deficiencies in proteins, water-soluble vitamins, magnesium, potassium, and zinc. Zinc absorption is decreased and excretion is increased. Magnesium is excreted in abnormal amounts in alcoholics and excessive iron is absorbed, causing liver damage. Heavy drinkers often have inadequate vitamin D production, resulting in calcium deficiency and osteoporosis. Some vitamins and minerals are needed in higher amounts in alcoholics to repair the damage caused by alcohol. Thiamine, and to a lesser degree other B vitamins, are particularly subject to depletion since they are needed to metabolize alcohol.

Relation of Nutrition to Selected Chronic Illnesses

Inadequate nutrition is known to contribute to a number of degenerative diseases and disorders common among older people. In contrast, good eating habits have the potential to prevent and reduce the progression of many of these diseases. The effects of nutrition therapy on the prevention and progression of disease are not fully understood. However, studies report that particular vitamins and minerals have been used successfully to treat some of these diseases. Elders with a particular disease are often found to be deficient in a particular nutrient and when that nutrient is prescribed, the symptoms are reduced. Multiple explanations have been proposed for this phenomenon. Some researchers believe that a nutrient deficiency predisposed the patient to illness in the first place. Others assert that the disease process may have created an increased need for some nutrients. Further, it has been hypothesized that some diseases associated with old age may actually be caused by nutrient deficiencies.

The exact role that proper nutrition or dietary supplementation can play in the prevention and treatment of chronic conditions is not clear.

Nutrient/Drug Interactions

Alcohol: Can lead to deficiencies in all nutrients, especially B vitamins, zinc, iron. Can replace eating.

Antacids: Magnesium salts can cause diarrhea, which can impair intestinal absorption. Reduces acidity of stomach, perhaps altering protein digestion.

Antibiotics: Tetracycline can block absorption of iron, magnesium and calcium salts. Other antibiotics can impair folic acid action in the body.

Anticoagulants: Cause vitamin K deficiency.

Anticonvulsants: Can induce folate and vitamin D deficiency.

Antidepressants: May depress appetite, cause accelerated breakdown of vitamin D. Monoamine oxidase (MAO) inhibitors can cause intolerance to foods containing the chemical tyramine (e.g., aged cheese, red wine, beer, chocolate).

Analgesics: High doses of aspirin may cause gastrointestinal bleeding, which can result in anemia. Can affect status of vitamin C, K, and folic acid. Cause nausea and vomiting.

Barbiturates: Speed breakdown of vitamin D. Excessive sedation may cause missed meals. Impair absorption of folic acid.

Cancer Chemotherapy: Causes nausea and vomiting. Impairs appetite and absorption.

Colchicine: Inhibits secretion of enzymes needed to break down complex sugars.

Corticosteriods: Decrease pancreatic enzymes, decreased digestion. Impair absorption of vitamins C, A, and D, folic acid, pyrioxine, and potassium.

Digitalis: May cause nausea and vomiting.

Diuretics: Cause loss of potassium in the urine. Low levels of potassium in the blood can cause mental confusion. Long-term use may cause magnesium deficiency.

Estrogen: Extended therapy can result in deficiencies of folic acid and vitamin B6.

Laxatives: May cause diarrhea-like effects whereby food passes the intestines too quickly to be totally absorbed. Mineral oil absorbs fat-soluble vitamins, impairing their absorption.

Licorice Candy: Limits potassium absorption.

Some Hypoglycemic Agents: Inhibit absorption of B12.

Narcotics: May cause nausea and vomiting.

Thyroid Preparations: depress appetite.

This section will discuss relevant research on several chronic illnesses that are significantly influenced by nutrition. In some cases, more research needs to be conducted before the results will be accepted by the medical profession.

Arthritis

Nutrition may play a role in both the onset and treatment of osteoarthritis. Those who have osteoarthritis are likely to be obese and weight reduction relieves joint pain and prevents more extensive damage. Drug treatments for osteoarthritis pose nutritional risks. Aspirin, the most common therapy, may cause iron-deficiency anemia or vitamin C deficiency. Steroid therapy may cause bone demineralization and sodium retention, and decrease the absorption of vitamins A, B, and C, and potassium.

Documentation of the effectiveness of vitamin and mineral therapy on osteoarthritis is sparse, but preliminary studies indicate that daily vitamin E supplementation improved some osteoarthritis symptoms (Machtey and Quakmire 1978). Copper may also play a role in relieving symptoms. One study found that those with osteoarthritis who wore copper bracelets had a worsening of symptoms after their removal. A similar phenomenon was not noted for those wearing placebo bracelets. The study also reported evidence that copper can be absorbed through the skin (Walker and Keats 1976). However, these findings are preliminary and not widely accepted by the medical profession. More controlled studies are needed in this area.

Nutrition may play a role in the prevention and treatment of rheumatoid arthritis. Those with rheumatoid arthritis are commonly malnourished and have lower than average levels of zinc (Niedermeier and Griggs 1971). It is thought that zinc may be anti-inflammatory and zinc deficiencies in the joint may cause the rheumatoid condition. Zinc supplements have been shown to significantly reduce joint swelling, morning stiffness, and perceived pain (Simkin 1976). Blood levels of pantothenic acid are also lower in those with rheumatoid arthritis and symptoms have

been reported to improve with supplementation (General Practitioner Research Group 1980). Copper deficiency may also contribute to rheumatoid arthritis symptoms (Sorenson 1978).

Experiments with dietary modification have yielded positive results on arthritis symptoms. One study found that a diet rich in Omega-3, the fatty acid found in cold water fish, reduced arthritis symptoms, and that symptoms worsened drastically when subjects returned to their normal diet (Kremer et al. 1985). It is hypothesized that these acids produce a hormone, prostaglandin, that reduces inflammation. In contrast, the fatty acid found in meat, Omega-6, tends to increase inflammation. Finally, one controlled study found that intolerance to specific foods may aggravate rheumatoid arthritis (Darlington et al. 1986).

Cancer

Epidemiological studies suggest a strong association between diet and some types of cancer—especially of the breast, colon, and stomach. Some experts believe that nutrition may be correlated with more than half the cancers in women and at least one-third in men. Diets low in animal protein and fat and high in fiber are associated with low rates of cancer, especially of the colon. It is hypothesized that diets high in fat or protein increase bile production, which irritates the colon, either causing cancer or making the walls more vulnerable to cancer-causing agents. A number of studies indicate that the higher the rate of colon cancer in a population, the lower their fiber intake and the greater the concentration of bile acids in their feces. In contrast, high-fiber diets reduce bile acid concentration. High animal fat consumption is also correlated with breast cancer (Brammer and DeFelice 1980).

Although the cause of cancer is unknown, some nutrients protect against cancerous growth. Cruciferous vegetables (broccoli, cabbage, and brussels sprouts) may protect against tumor formation by releasing a chemical which helps detoxify carcinogens. Additionally, low vitamin A levels in the blood are correlated with high incidence of many cancers, especially of the liver and intestine (Wald et al. 1980). High blood levels of vitamin A seem to be protective; one study found that smokers with low beta carotene levels were at higher risk of developing lung cancer than those with high levels of this vitamin (Bjelke 1975; Shekelle et al. 1981; Byers et al. 1987).

There is some evidence that vitamin C plays a role in the prevention and treatment of cancer. Vitamin C is believed to increase many immune system defenses by activating white blood cells and may decrease tumor proliferation by strengthening the collagen network between cells. Cameron and Pauling (1978) reported that megadoses of vitamin C increase survival time of cancer patients, but later studies failed to corroborate the results (Moertel et al. 1985). It is well documented that those with cancer have lower vitamin C levels than controls (Cameron et al. 1979).

Calcium and some other minerals may also play a role in cancer prevention and treatment. Colorectal cancer incidence is higher than normal among people drinking water low in calcium; conversely, those with diets high in vitamin D and calcium have lower incidence of this cancer. Calcium may neutralize both fatty and bile acids and control the growth of pre-cancerous cells. A preliminary study of people with early signs of colorectal cancer found that calcium supplementation returned the pre-cancer cells to normal within two to three months (Lipkin and Newmark 1985). Those living in geographical areas with low levels of selenium in the diet seem to be at increased risk for some cancers (Schrauzer et al. 1978) and there is a higher risk of cancer among those with low levels of selenium in their blood (Willett et al. 1983).

Some additives and preservatives are converted to carcinogens during digestion. Sodium nitrate, which is commonly used to preserve meats, is converted into nitrosamine, a cancer-causing agent. Vitamin C can neutralize nitrosamines in the body and is sometimes added to foods containing nitrates to prevent toxin formation. Saccharin, an artificial sweetener, is known to cause cancer in laboratory animals.

Other additives and preservatives might promote cancer, however, insufficient studies have been conducted.

Cancer increases the need for certain nutrients, but the disease and its treatment often diminish ability or desire to eat. Lack of appetite occurs in about 15–25 percent of cancer patients at the time of diagnosis and almost all of those with advanced illness (DeWys 1979). Cachexia, characterized by anorexia (loss of appetite), weight loss, and weakness, is common in advanced cancer victims and is caused by diversion of nutrients to support cancer tissue. Dietary proteins are needed for tissue growth, and if insufficient protein is ingested, the tumor cannibalizes muscle and lung tissue to maintain its rapid growth. It has been suggested that cancer patients need twice as much protein as those without cancer. Although nutritional replenishment is necessary to keep cancer patients from starvation, preliminary studies on laboratory animals suggest that nutrient supplements may actually promote tumor growth. Nevertheless, most agree that cancer patients should consume adequate nutrients to increase tolerance to therapy and prevent starvation.

Nutritional considerations become especially important for those undergoing radiation or chemotherapy treatments. Radiation therapy irritates the small intestine, causing diarrhea and chronic nutrient malabsorption. Those undergoing chemotherapy may experience nausea, vomiting, a full feeling, and changes in smell and taste perception. Altered taste perception cause some to refuse essential foods because they are reported to taste bitter, salty, sour, or spoiled.

Constipation

Epidemiological studies suggest that the lack of fiber in Western diets is the main culprit responsible for constipation and many other gastrointestinal problems. Although constipation may be caused by a number of factors—including inadequate food and fluid intake, lack of exercise, decreased intestinal tone, laxative abuse, medical problems, and some medications—it seems that the presence or absence of fiber in the diet is a major factor. Fiber can soften stools, increase the rate of flow of digested matter through the gastrointestinal tract, and stimulate the colon. When two to three grams of fiber were added to the diets of a group of institutionalized elders, almost none needed laxatives. (Hull et al. 1980).

Diabetes

Obesity is an important contributing factor in adult-onset diabetes. Most adult-onset diabetics in the United States are obese and even those who are only 20 percent overweight are at a significantly higher risk of diabetes than those of normal weight. No specific nutrient is associated with diabetes onset, but those with adult-onset diabetes consume more calories than those who do not have the disease. Conversely, weight loss can correct abnormal glucose tolerance (a prediabetic condition). Dietary modification is essential for those with adult-onset diabetes. Weight loss alone is an effective treatment for 90 percent of all adult-onset diabetics (Flood 1979). A diet high in complex carbohydrates and fiber improved all aspects of diabetic control in both insulin-dependent and nondependent diabetics (Simpson et al. 1981). In addition, preliminary studies indicate that zinc and chromium supplements—minerals associated with insulin action—may also play a role in diabetes management (Kinlaw et al. 1983; Offenbacher and Pisunyer 1980).

Gout

Gout is a genetic disorder in which the body is unable to effectively metabolize a chemical compound called purines, found in meat gravies, broths, organ meats, anchovies, sardines, and mackerel. Because of this malfunction, uric acid crystals are excreted into the bloodstream and precipitate into the joints causing attacks of excruciating pain, swelling, and inflammation. The disorder can be controlled by restricting intake of foods high in purines, especially during an acute attack. A high fat intake should be avoided because it prevents uric acid excretion. In contrast, a high carbohydrate diet and high fluid intake facilitate the elimination of excess uric acid.

Heart Disease

A number of dietary factors have been linked to the development of heart disease: high consumption of animal fat, sugar, and refined carbohydrate, low intake of fiber, and mineral imbalances. However, the data are uneven and sometimes conflicting.

Many believe that an excessive consumption of saturated fats inevitably results in the accumulation of cholesterol in arteries (atherosclerosis), and ultimately to coronary artery disease. However, a low animal fat diet may reduce the risk of heart disease for only one in three to five people—those who are predisposed to accumulate cholesterol in their arteries. The rest of the population do not have this problem.

The literature is replete with contradictory evidence regarding the significance of cholesterol as a risk factor in heart disease. One large longitudinal study demonstrated that for those under 50 years of age, high blood cholesterol was directly related to a higher overall mortality and mortality related to cardiovascular causes. However, for those 60 and above, no such relationship was reported (Anderson et al. 1987). If this is true, efforts to reduce cholesterol in elders with diet or drugs may not significantly alter their mortality rate. In another study, Taylor and colleagues (1987) analyzed the results of several longitudinal studies and reported that even a lifelong program of cholesterol reduction would increase life expectancy as little as three days to three months in those with normal blood pressure who did not smoke. They predicted that for those at high risk (smokers and hypertensives), lowering cholesterol would increase life expectancy from 18 days to one year. They concluded that health education efforts to reduce smoking and hypertension would save more lives among the general public than directives to lower cholesterol intake.

Other nutrients affect cholesterol metabolism. Evidence is mounting that Omega-3 fatty acids, found in cold water fish, lowers blood triglyceride and cholesterol levels and reduces blood clotting. In addition, high sugar consumption by individuals who are genetically more sensitive to sugar produces an increase in blood cholesterol and triglyceride levels in the blood. Stress levels may also influence whether a diet high in sugar and refined carbohydrates leads to high levels of blood triglycerides and heart disease. Conversely, some types of dietary fiber are thought to reduce absorption of dietary cholesterol or modify the cholesterol production in the body.

Low levels of various vitamins and minerals have also been associated with heart disease. For instance, death rates from ischemic heart disease are higher in areas where the water is low in calcium and magnesium. This is reasonable because both minerals are important in maintaining the electrical and physical integrity of heart muscle so that low levels make muscle spasm more likely. Additionally, individuals who die from heart attacks have lower magnesium and potassium levels in the heart than those who died from other causes. This is interesting in light of the fact that those at risk for a heart attack may take diuretics or other drugs that deplete these minerals. Selenium may also protect the heart; strokes and heart attacks are less common in areas with high selenium in the soil. Those with cardiovascular disease have lower than average levels of vitamin C. Animal studies suggest that vitamin C may play a role in reducing high blood cholesterol levels. Additionally, megadoses of niacin are reported to decrease cholesterol and triglycerides and reduce the recurrence rate of heart attacks (Coronary Drug Project Group 1975); but the treatment may cause unpleasant side effects and should not be taken unless under the supervision of a physician. Recent studies conducted with lower niacin levels are promising.

In 1986, the American Heart Association released "Dietary Guidelines for Healthy American Adults," a proposal to reduce the risk of coronary heart disease. They are as follows.

1. Saturated fat intake should be less than 10% of calories.
2. Total fat intake should be less than 30% of calories.
3. Cholesterol intake should be less than 100 mg/1,000 cal, not to exceed 300 mg/day.
4. Protein intake should be approximately 15% of calories.
5. Carbohydrate intake should constitute 50 to 55% or more of calories, with emphasis on increased complex carbohydrates.
6. Sodium intake should be reduced to approximately 1 g/1,000 cal, not to exceed 3g/day.
7. If alcoholic beverages are consumed, the caloric intake from this source should be limited to 15% of total calories but should not exceed 50 ml of ethanol per day.
8. Total calories should be sufficient to maintain the individual's best body weight.
9. A wide variety of foods should be consumed.

Hypertension

The most controversial and publicized factor affecting the development of hypertension is salt intake. Although a number of early, well-publicized studies reported correlations between high salt intake and hypertension, more recent evidence shows that those who are hypertensive do not consume more salt than those with normal blood pressure (Watt et al. 1983). It seems as if high salt intake does not cause hypertension for all individuals, only the 20–30 percent of the population with a sensitivity to salt. For these individuals, salt circulates in the body longer and even a lower intake can boost blood pressure. It is hypothesized that individuals originating from geographical areas distant from the ocean or other sources of salt are more sensitive to salt because they are genetically adapted to retain salt in response to a historical scarcity of salt (Wilson 1986).

Although a sodium-restricted diet is often suggested to treat hypertension, this strategy may only work for those who are sensitive to salt. For most people, severe restriction produces little or no benefit. Some researchers believe there is a salt threshold so that a reduction in salt intake does not reduce blood pressure unless salt is kept to an extremely low level. Therefore, it may be almost impossible to cut sodium consumption to a level that will do any good except in a highly controlled environment such as a hospital. For most of those with normal blood pressure, salt reduction is unnecessary. In fact, diabetics, patients with kidney disease, those with fevers, or those who are at risk for heat stroke may even be harmed by a low-salt diet.

Calcium deficiency is linked to high blood pressure. Those with high blood pressure, especially elders and blacks, have significantly lower calcium intake than those with normal blood pressure. This marginal calcium deficiency is aggravated by the prescribed low-cholesterol diets of most hypertensives that discourage intake of calcium-rich dairy products. Calcium supplements are reported to reduce high blood pressure (McCarron and Morris 1985) and may be more effective than hypertension medication (Johnson et al. 1985).

Preliminary studies on magnesium and potassium show that adequate intake of these minerals may prevent hypertension (Iimura et al. 1981). While diuretics reduce hypertension by expelling salts and decreasing water content of blood, they also cause magnesium deficiencies, which may aggravate hypertension. Diuretics are more effective in treating hypertension when patients receive magnesium supplements (Dyckner and Wesler 1983).

Obesity has also been associated with hypertension. It is thought that obesity aggravates hypertension but may not cause it. Many obese people do not have high blood pressure. On the other hand, a recent study that compared weight loss, drug therapy, and placebo treatment for middle-aged hypertensive men found that weight loss was the most effective treatment at reducing hypertension (McMahon 1986). Weight loss may unload the heart from the double burden of obesity and hypertension.

Some diets seem to offer protection against hypertension. One study found that low-fat and meatless diets significantly lowered blood pressure among hypertensives, but the changes were reversed when subjects reverted to normal diets (Pukka et al. 1983). Additionally, Dodson and Humphreys (1981) reported that a diet high in potassium and fiber and low in fat, sugar, and sodium was so effective in reducing blood pressure that medication was reduced or discontinued in three-fourths of hypertensive patients studied.

Mental Disorders

Malnutrition may cause symptoms of mental illness. One study placed a group of healthy young men on a calorie-deficient diet for six months. The subjects lost weight, and reported feeling insecure, irritable, moody, and depressed. They also had no emotional control, no interest in others, and were unable to make decisions (Keys et al. 1950). Because these traits are often used to characterize elders or to provide reasons for their institutionalization, it is imperative that health workers are aware of the effect of improper nutrition on mental health.

Even marginal nutrient deficiencies can impair mental abilities. One study found that a group of healthy elders with marginal deficiencies in vitamin C and some B-complex vitamins scored poorly on tests of memory and abstract thinking ability (Goodwin et al. 1983). Low levels of B and C vitamins were also reportedly associated with confused states in elders and supplementation reversed the symptoms in most cases (Mitra 1971). Vitamin C and multi-vitamin supplements have been shown to improve the mental status of groups of institutionalized elders (Schokah et al. 1979). In contrast, high levels of zinc and aluminum are found in the brains of those with dementia (Burnet 1981).

Lecithin, a fat found in all plant and animal products, may be useful in the treatment of memory loss that accompanies dementia. Lecithin is a precursor of choline, which stimulates

Nutrition counselors can assist elders in managing many chronic illnesses.

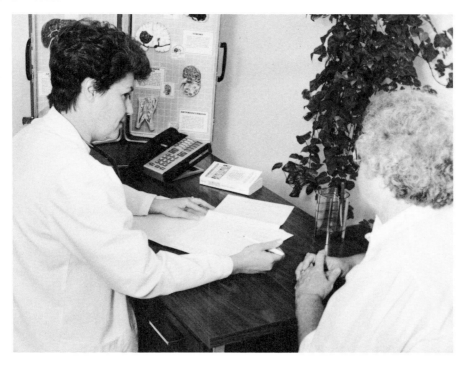

the action of the neurotransmitter acetylcholine, enhancing nerve transmission in the brain. Lecithin and choline supplements have reportedly increased memory in both healthy people and those with Alzheimer's disease (see Reisberg et al. 1984 for a review). Lecithin is also an effective treatment for tardive dyskinesia and it significantly suppressed its symptoms in many cases (Gelenberg et al. 1979). Lecithin-rich foods include egg yolks, liver, soy beans, cauliflower, and cabbage.

Obesity

Obesity, defined as 15 percent or more above desired weight, is known to increase susceptibility to illness and to disability and to decrease life expectancy. It is estimated that from one-fourth to one-half the population in our country is obese. Weight tables compiled by the Metropolitan Life Insurance Company (1983) are the most commonly used standards to determine ideal weights.

The standards are based on weights statistically associated with the lowest mortality rates for various heights and body frames. However, the tables are only accurate for adults under age 60. According to the Food and Nutrition Board (1980), body weight should not increase in old age. However, since elders commonly experience a loss of height with age, their ideal weight can be calculated using table 9.3 if their height when younger is used. Skin-fold measurements, which estimate the amount of fat stored under the skin, are a more accurate means of diagnosing obesity than height-weight tables. An athlete may weigh more than ideal weight because of high muscular content. On the other hand, an older man who fits the ideal weight may be obese because he is carrying a large quantity of fat around his middle. See Frisancho (1981) for the norms on subcutaneous fat and muscle measurements on elders from sixty-five to seventy-four years of age.

Chapter 9

Table 9.3 Metropolitan Life Insurance Company height and weight tables 1983.

Men

Height Feet	Inches	Small Frame	Medium Frame	Large Frame
5	2	128–134	131–141	138–150
5	3	130–136	133–143	140–153
5	4	132–138	135–145	142–156
5	5	134–140	137–148	144–160
5	6	136–142	139–151	146–164
5	7	138–145	142–154	149–168
5	8	140–148	145–157	152–172
5	9	142–151	148–160	155–176
5	10	144–154	151–163	158–180
5	11	146–157	154–166	161–184
6	0	149–160	157–170	164–188
6	1	152–164	160–174	168–192
6	2	155–168	164–178	172–197
6	3	158–172	167–182	176–202
6	4	162–176	171–187	181–207

Weights at ages 25–59 based on lowest mortality. Weight in pounds according to frame (in indoor clothing weighing 5 lb, shoes with 1-in. heels).

Women

Height Feet	Inches	Small Frame	Medium Frame	Large Frame
4	10	102–111	109–121	118–131
4	11	103–113	111–123	120–134
5	0	104–115	113–126	122–137
5	1	106–118	115–129	124–140
5	2	108–121	118–132	128–143
5	3	111–124	121–135	131–147
5	4	114–127	124–138	134–151
5	5	117–130	127–141	137–155
5	6	120–133	130–144	140–159
5	7	123–136	133–147	143–163
5	8	126–139	136–150	146–167
5	9	129–142	139–153	149–170
5	10	132–145	142–156	152–173
5	11	135–148	145–159	155–176
6	0	138–151	148–162	158–179

Weights at ages 25–59 based on lowest mortality. Weight in pounds according to frame (in indoor clothing weighing 3 lb, shoes with 1-in. heels).

Courtesy Metropolitan Life Insurance Company.

Analysis of mortality data for elders indicates that there may be a survival advantage to being slightly overweight when old. Andres (1980) found that mortality was lower among older people who were 10–30 percent above ideal weight than those at or slightly below ideal values. A possible explanation is that the underweight individuals surveyed were very ill, malnourished, smokers, or alcohol abusers. On the other hand, there may be some advantage to having some storage fat.

Although the magnitude of the health risk associated with moderate obesity is much debated, it is clear that those who are severely obese have a higher incidence of chronic disease (especially diabetes, cancer, and hypertension) and higher mortality. Additionally, overweight people are at higher risk for degenerative joint disease and kidney disease. Obese individuals are three to four times more likely to develop gallstones than those of normal weight (Jaspan 1977). Obese people are also more difficult to examine and more prone to surgical complications than those of normal weight.

Obesity is also a hindrance to independence. The obese have decreased mobility because even the mild exertion of everyday activities may leave them short of breath. Accidental injuries are more common among the obese. In addition, obese individuals who are dependent on others to lift or bathe them may receive poorer care because they are so heavy. Obese individuals may also suffer psychologically because of our society's cultural dictum against fat.

Elders are often encouraged to lose weight to reduce the symptoms of many chronic illnesses. Because of the risks of malnutrition and because slightly overweight individuals are not reportedly less healthy, weight loss should not be prescribed for elders unless it is known that the excess weight will reduce the symptoms or progression of chronic illness. Little is known of the effects of dieting in elders, so caloric restriction should be gradual and well-monitored to ensure that the diet supplies all necessary nutrients. A combination of increased physical activity and gradual caloric restriction is the preferred method of weight loss for all age groups, including elders. Strenuous, regular physical activity can assist weight loss efforts by increasing metabolic rate, decreasing appetite, burning calories, and increasing muscle tone.

Assessment and counseling should be provided to ensure the diet includes all essential nutrients and takes food preferences and income into account. It is important that the client be provided with psychological support throughout the weight loss process. Self-help groups such as Weight Watchers or Overeaters Anonymous have had much success in assisting individuals to follow through on a weight loss program. Weight loss programs are the most successful for those with a strong motivation to lose weight such as cardiac patients and newly diagnosed elder diabetics.

Osteoporosis

Calcium intake is perhaps the most important factor implicated to control and prevent osteoporosis. Inadequate calcium intake during middle age results in a slow weakening of bones because needed calcium is extracted from the skeleton to maintain constant blood calcium levels. Age-associated decrease in calcium absorption compounded by the tendency of elders to decrease calcium intake further aggravates bone loss. Although calcium supplementation cannot reverse osteoporosis, it reduces the rate of bone loss. It is believed that long-term calcium supplementation, beginning in the middle years, would reduce the incidence of osteoporosis.

Other vitamin and mineral deficiencies have also been implicated in the development of osteoporosis. High phosphorus intake (soft drinks and meat contain high quantities) can aggravate calcium deficiency by increasing the rate of bone demineralization and increasing calcium excretion. Conversely, a vegetarian diet may decrease bone loss. Long-time vegetarians have denser bones than nonvegetarians and are less susceptible to osteoporosis. Magnesium deficiencies may also contribute to osteoporosis. Vitamin D deficiency reduces calcium absorption and retention and supplements improve calcium absorption. Disease of the liver and kidney, and gastric disorders may interfere with vitamin D absorption and metabolism. The trace element flourine seems to increase formation of new bone as those people in flourine-rich areas have a lower risk of osteoporosis. Evidence suggests flourine may also increase skeletal stability, protecting it against calcium loss.

Parkinson's Disease

Parkinson's disease is caused by a deficiency of the neurotransmitter, dopamine, that reduces the motor function of the brain. To counteract this deficiency, Parkinson's patients are treated with the drug L-dopa, a chemical which is converted to dopamine in the brain. Patients on L-dopa therapy should not take pyridoxine (B_6) supplements because L-dopa is inactivated by the B_6 in the intestines. Additionally, those with Parkinson's disease should not have a high-protein diet since ingested proteins compete for absorption with L-dopa in the intestine. Parkinson's disease is aggravated by obesity, so patients are often prescribed weight loss regimens to improve motor function. Many patients with Parkinson's disease are undernourished because their motor impairments interfere with ability or desire to eat.

Stroke

Recent results of a twelve year longitudinal study of about 850 people between 50 and 79 reported a high correlation between low potassium intake and high incidence of stroke-related deaths. Although high potas-sium intake reduces high blood pres-sure, an important risk factor of stroke, the researchers believe that the decrease of stroke-related deaths from potassium was greater than

its blood pressure lowering effects alone. They assert that one serving of a potassium-rich fruit or vegetable a day is associated with a 40 percent decrease in stroke mortality (Khaw and Barrett-Connor 1987).

Nutrition Counseling and Education

Because nutrition plays such an important role in health maintenance, nutritional counseling is an effective modality to prevent or reduce the progression of disease. The role of the counselor is to work with the client to develop a system of gradual dietary modifications and to support the client through the changes. In order to be effective, nutritional counselors must consider the multiple factors that affect nutritional status— food preferences, economic status, and health condition—when advising clients on dietary practices.

A number of methods can increase the success of dietary modifications. Studies show that nutritional counseling is more effective when continued over a long period of time. In this way the counselor and client are able to regularly review and adapt the diet regimen to the client's changing needs or wants. The usual practice of a physician distributing printed diet information has a very low adherance rate (Zifferblatt and Wilbur 1977). Success is also increased if a spouse or friend is involved in the counseling sessions to assist in motivating the client. For further information on counseling techniques to improve compliance to diet modifications, see Natow and Heslin (1986).

Because elders are at high risk for nutrient deficiencies, and because nutrition influences so many of the diseases common to old age, elders need to be provided with current information regarding proper diet practices. Because proper nutrition can prevent or reduce the impact of many chronic illnesses, many experts believe that proper nutrition education could significantly reduce health care costs. However, helping elders to eat well is often difficult because many elders have reduced incomes. Further, elders may have long-standing food habits or preferences that are difficult to modify. Finally, many may not be motivated to change.

Nutrition education is especially relevant for the elder population because this group knows the least about proper nutrition (National Center of Health Statistics 1975). Unfortunately, people in the United States receive most nutrition information through food industry advertisements designed to sell a particular product. Nutrition education materials and programs are usually no match for these clever, slick, expensive advertisements. Elders can be educated about nutrition by developing activities such as the following:

1. Discussion groups on nutrition-related topics at senior centers, nutrition sites, apartment complexes
2. Cooking classes, potlucks
3. Periodic large-print nutrition newsletter in simple language
4. Nutrition column in local newspaper
5. Public service announcements on radio regarding nutrition education
6. Community garden programs
7. Food cooperatives
8. Programs where elders are trained as peer nutrition outreach counselors
9. Extensive and creative advertising campaigns for nutrition programs
10. Development and distribution of printed information to selected sites

Educational activities for elders must be adapted to geographical location, cultural variation, functional status, education level, and previous experience. Special efforts should be directed toward low-income and minority elders, isolated elders, and rural and inner-city elders.

To be more effective, more state and federal resources need to be allocated to plan and implement effective nutrition education programs. However, it is simplistic to believe that more nutrition education will resolve the problem of malnutrition. Other causes such as depression, isolation, and inability to purchase and prepare food are important barriers to good nutrition.

Additionally, health professionals need training in the role of nutrition in the health in older adults. For instance, nutritionists need specific information on the economic, psychological, and social situation of elders to more effectively counsel them. Physicians and other health professionals must learn the importance of nutrition in the prevention and treatment of chronic diseases as well as important interactions between drugs and diet. Unfortunately, nutrition is seldom thoroughly discussed in medical schools. A recent survey found one-third of all medical schools lacked courses in nutrition. The average time in medical schools spent on nutrition was twenty-one hours in a four year program and 60 percent of students had less than twenty hours total (Longstreet 1985).

In addition to the expansion of nutrition education in medical schools, continuing education programs should be established to update physicians about nutrition therapies and the factors influencing nutrient intake among elders. Results from the National Health Interview Survey indicate that two-thirds of the elders interviewed revealed that diet is rarely discussed in physician visits; fewer than 8 percent reported nutrition was frequently discussed by their physician (National Center of Health Statistics 1985). Finally, long-term studies on elders regarding the relationships between drug use, chronic illness, and nutrition are needed.

Nutrition Programs

A number of federal, state, and local intervention programs have been developed to meet nutritional needs and to promote nutrition education among elders. In addition, private organizations

Government-supported congregate meal sites are located in almost every community and provide elders with nutritious meals and social interaction.

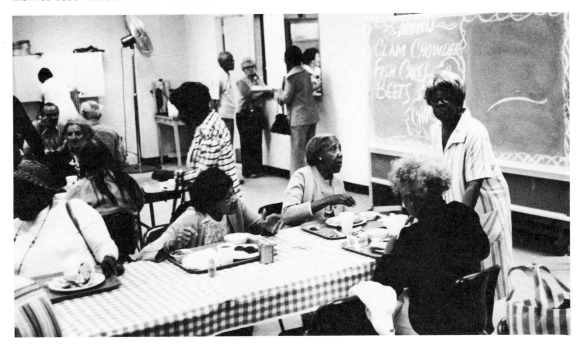

and the food industry have also exerted an effort, especially in the development of health education materials.

The federal Food Stamp Program supplements the food budget of over one and one-half million low-income elders. However, this figure represents less than half those who are eligible to receive the support. It is thought that many elders fail to take advantage of the service because they are unaware of the program, lack transportation to the stamp distribution site, or do not want the stigma of applying for and using the coupons (Hollenbeck and Ohls 1984).

The Older Americans Act allocates federal monies to each state to provide lunch programs and nutrition education to elders. Most communities participate in this program. All sites provide nutritious meals that contain at least one-third the RDA. One report compared the nutritional status of those who attended such a nutrition program with a group who did not. Those

participating in the program had a better quality diet and a higher intake of calories, protein, and calcium, indicating that the program reduced the nutritional vulnerability of the elder participants (Kohrs et al. 1978). However, the quality and number of nutrition education programs offered at the sites are highly variable. Despite their benefit in reducing isolation and improving nutrition, the amount of allocated funds is insufficient in almost every case since there are usually more elders who wish to participate in the program than available funds.

A number of feeding programs are financed locally, either by churches, United Fund, private organizations, local revenue funds, or other means. Free dinners, soup kitchens, and home-delivered meals for the homebound are fairly common. Many restaurants and cooperative grocery stores offer discounts to older people. However, the number and types of programs vary tremendously among communities. Expansion of current programs and the development of new programs are needed to provide quality nutrition to special groups of elders, especially rural, inner-city, ethnic, socially isolated, homebound, and the poor. Adequate financial support and effective publicity are two variables that increase the effectiveness of such programs.

Summary

Nutrition is an important aspect of health in the later years. Normal aging, disease state, drug use, and other variables affect the need for certain nutrients. The recommended daily allowance is the recognized standard of nutritional requirements for healthy people; however, those recommendations may have to be modified in elders to adjust to changing physiology and health status. In general, elders' reduced metabolic rate causes a decreased daily caloric requirement making it harder to ensure adequate levels of essential nutrients. Marginal deficiencies in many nutrients produce symptoms that may be confused with chronic illness or old age.

National studies show that some groups of American elders are deficient in nutrients—especially calories and vitamins. Because of this, there is a need for thorough individual nutrition assessments as part of regular health care. Nutrition has an impact on a number of chronic illnesses common among elders. In some cases, poor food choices encourage the disease process, in others, the disease may cause an increased need for some nutrients. However, some success has been reported in using nutrition supplements to prevent and treat chronic illness. Nutritional counseling and education are effective in increasing elders' knowledge and motivation to eat healthfully.

Activities

1. Record what you ate, when and why you ate each item for at least three days. Compare the nutritional value and caloric intake with the RDA. What type of foods are you eating in excess? Are there some nutrients you are lacking? What psycho-social factors affected your food intake?
2. Eat all meals alone for three to four days. How was your food intake affected? Keep a daily journal to record your feelings.
3. Attend a lunch at a local nutrition site for elders. What is the menu? Describe the associated educational or recreational activities. If you have the opportunity, visit two different sites and compare.
4. Question an elder regarding dietary intake in the last twenty-four hours and analyze nutritional value and caloric intake. What problems do you see with this approach?
5. Design a pamphlet to inform elders about a particular aspect of nutrition.
6. Develop objectives and outline the content of a twenty-minute educational program on some aspect of nutrition for a group of independent elders.
7. What educational programs does your community offer to elders on nutrition? What meal programs are offered?
8. Design a day's menu that includes the RDA for all vitamins and minerals staying within the caloric requirements for an adult age twenty-two to fifty. Now modify it for someone over fifty.
9. Ask five friends or relatives the following questions to determine what information they have about vitamins and minerals: Do you take vitamin or mineral supplements? How often? Which ones? Who told you to take them? What do you believe each does for you? What foods contain high values of these supplements?

Bibliography

American Health. 1985. Vitamin D: Living in the shade. Oct.:35–36.

Anderson, K. M., W. P. Castelli, and D. Levy. 1987. Cholesterol and morality. *JAMA* 257(18):2176–80.

Andres, R. 1980. The effect of obesity in total mortality. *Int J Obesity* 4(4):318–86.

Chapter 9

Bjelke, E. 1975. Dietary vitamin A and human lung cancer. *Int J Cancer* 15:561–5.

Boykin, L. 1980. Problems of the older person in obtaining adequate nutrition. *Aging* 311–312:4–6.

Boyle, E., B. Mondschein, and H. H. Dash. 1977. Chromium depletion in the pathogenesis of diabetes and atherosclerosis. *Southern Med J* 70(12):1449–53.

Brammer, S., and R. L. DeFelice. 1980. Dietary advice in regard to risk for colon and breast cancer. *Prev Med* 9:544–49.

Burch, G. E., and D. Giles. 1977. The importance of magnesium deficiency in cardiovascular disease. *Am Heart J* 94(5):649–57.

Burnet, M. 1981. The possible role of zinc in the pathology of dementia. *Lancet* 1:186–88.

Butterworth, C. 1974. The skeleton in the hospital closet. *Nutr Today* 9:4–8.

Byers, T. E., S. Graham, B. P. Haughey, et al. 1987. Diet and lung cancer risk: findings from the Western New York Diet Study. *Am J Epidem* 125(3):351–363.

Cameron, E., and L. Pauling. 1978. Supplemental ascorbate in the supportive treatment of cancer: Re-evaluation of prolongation of survival time in the terminal human cancer. *Proc Nat Acad Sci USA* 75:4538–42.

Cameron, E., L. Pauling, and B. Leibovitz. 1979. Ascorbic acid and cancer: A review *Cancer Res* 39:663–81.

Chenault, A. 1984. *Nutrition and Health.* New York: Holt, Reinhart and Wilson.

Coronary Drug Project Research Group. 1975. Clofibrate and niacin in coronary heart disease. *JAMA* 231:360–381.

Darlington, L. G., N. W. Ramsey, and J. R. Mansfield. 1986. Placebo-controlled, blind study of dietary manipulation therapy in rheumatoid arthritis. *Lancet,* Feb 1986; 236–238.

Davis, M. A., E. Randall, R. N. Forthofer, et al. 1985. Living arrangements and dietary patterns of older adults in the United States. *J Gerontol* 40(4):434–42.

DeWys, W. D. 1979. Anorexia as a general effect of cancer. *Cancer* 43:2013–19.

Dodson, P., and D. Humphreys. 1981. Hypertension and angina. In Trowell, H. C., and D. Burkitt, eds. *Western diseases: Their emergence and prevention.* London: Edward Arnold.

Duchateau, J., G. Delepresse, R. Vrigens, et al. 1981. Beneficial effects of oral zinc supplementation on the immune responses of old people. *Am J Med* 70:1001–04.

Dyckner, T., and P. O. Wesler. 1983. Effect of magnesium on blood pressure. *Br Med J* 286:1847–9.

Flood, T. M. 1979. Diet and diabetes mellitus. *Hosp Pract* Feb: 61–69.

Food and Nutrition Board, National Academy of Sciences. 1980. *Recommended dietary allowances.* Washington, D.C.: National Academy of Sciences.

Frisancho, A. R. 1981. New norms of upper limb fat and muscle areas for assessment of nutritional status. *Am J Clin Nut* 34:2450–2545.

Garry, P. J., J. S. Goodwin, M. A. Hunt, et al. 1982. Nutritional status in a healthy elder population: Dietary and supplemental intakes. *Am J Clin Nutr* 36:319–31.

Gelenberg, A. J., J. C. Doller-Wojcik, J. H. Growdon. 1979. Choline and lecithin in the treatment of tardive dyskinesia: Preliminary results from a pilot study. *Am J Psychiatry* 136:772–6.

General Practitioner Research Group. 1980. Calcium pantothenate in arthritic conditions. *Practitioner* 224:208–11.

Goodwin, J. S., J. M. Goodwin, and P. J. Garry. 1983. Association between nutrient status and cognitive functioning in a healthy elder population. *JAMA* 249:2917–21.

Heaney, R. P., and R. R. Recker. 1981. *Osteoporosis.* Baltimore: University Park Press.

Hollenbeck, D., and J. C. Ohls. 1984. Participation among the elderly in the food stamp program. *Gerontologist* 24(6):616–21.

Hull, C., R. S. Greco, and D. L. Brooks. 1980. Alleviation of constipation in the elderly by dietary fiber supplements. *J Am Geriatr Soc* 28(9):410–14.

Iimura, O., T. Kijima, K. Kikachi, et al. 1981. Studies on the hypotensive effect of high potassium intake in patients with essential hypertension. *Clin Sci* 61 (Suppl 17):775–805.

Jaspan, J. B. 1977. Obesity and intestinal by-pass. *Comp Ther* 3(10):35.

Johnson, N. E., E. L. Smith, and J. L. Freudenheim. 1985. Effects on blood pressure of calcium supplementation of women. *Am J Clin Nutr* 42:12–17.

Justice, C., J. Howe, and H. Clark. 1974. Dietary intakes and nutritional status of elderly patients. *J Am Diet Assoc* 65:639–46.

Khaw, K. T., and E. Barrett-Connor. 1987. Dietary potassium and stroke-associated mortality. *New Engl J Med* 316(5):235–240.

Keys, A., J. Brozek, A. Henschel, et al. 1950. *The biology of human starvation,* Vol II., Minneapolis: University of Minnesota Press.

Kinlaw, W. B., A. S. Levine, J. E. Morley, et al. 1983. Abnormal zinc metabolism in type II diabetes mellitus. *Am J Med* 25:273–77.

Kohrs, M., P. O'Hanlon, and D. Eklund. 1978. Contribution of the Older American's Nutrition Program to one day's dietary intake. *J Am Diet Assoc* 72:487–92.

Kremer, J. M., J. Bigauoette, A. Michalek. et al. 1985. Effects of manipulation of dietary fatty acids on clinical manifestations of rheumatoid arthritis. *Lancet* 1:184–87.

Lichtenstein, V. 1982. Care of the acutely ill older adult: Part two, nutritional management. *Geriatr Nurs* Nov–Dec:386–91.

Lipkin, M., and H. Newmark. 1985. Effect of added dietary calcium on colonic epithelial cell proliferation in subjects at high risk for familial colonic cancer. *N Engl J Med* 313(22):1381–83.

Longstreet, D. 1985. The sins of omission. *American Health* December.

Machtey, I., and L. Quackmire. 1978. Tocopherol in osteoarthritis: A controlled pilot study. *J Am Geriatr Soc* 26:328–30.

McCarron, D. A., and C. O. Morris. 1985. Blood pressure response to oral calcium in persons with mild to moderate hypertension. *Annals Int Med* 103(6):825–31.

McMahon, S. W., D.E.L. Wilcken, and G. J. MacDonald. 1986. The effect of weight reduction on left ventricular mass: A randomized controlled trial on young, overweight hypertensive patients. *N Engl J Med* 314(6):334–38.

Mitra, M. L. 1971. Confused states in relationship to vitamin deficiencies in the elderly. *J Am Geriatr Soc* 19:536–45.

Moertel, C. G., T. R. Fleming, E. T. Creagan, et al. 1985. High-dose vitamin C versus placebo in the treatment of patients with advanced cancer who had no prior chemotherapy. *N Engl J Med* 312(3):137–41.

National Center for Health Statistics. 1975. Preliminary findings of the first health and nutrition examination survey, U.S., 1971–1972. Anthropometric and clinical findings. DHEW Publ. No. (HRA) 75–1229. Hyattsville, Md: National Center for Health Statistics.

National Center for Health Statistics. 1979. Caloric and selected nutrient values for persons 1–74 years of age, 1971–1974. Series 11, No. 209. Washington, D.C. DHEW Publ. No. PHS 5179–1657. June.

National Center for Health Statistics. 1985. Provisional data from the Health Promotion and Disease Prevention Supplement to the National Health Interview Survey: United States, Jan.–March 1985. *NCHS Advance Data* No. 113, Nov. 15.

Natow, A., and J. Heslin. 1986. *Nutritional care of the older adult.* New York: Macmillan.

Niedermeier, W., and J. H. Griggs. 1971. Trace metal composition of synovial fluid and blood serum of patients with rheumatoid arthritis. *J Chronic Dis* 23:527–36.

Offenbacher, E. G., and F. X. Pisunyer. 1980. Beneficial effects of chromium-rich yeast on glucose tolerance and blood lipids in elderly subjects. *Diabetes* 29:919–25.

Pauling, L. 1986. *How to live longer and feel better.* New York: W. H. Freeman and Co.

Phillips, P. A., B. J. Rolls, J. G. Ledingham, et al. 1984. Reduced thirst after water deprivation in elderly men. *N Engl J Med* 311(12):753–59.

Pukka, P., A. Nissinen, and J. Iacono. 1983. Controlled, randomized trial on the effect of dietary fat on blood pressure. *Lancet* 1:1–5.

Reisberg, B., S. H. Ferris, and S. Gershon. 1984. Dietary treatment of Alzheimer's type senile dementia. In J. M. Ordy, D. Harman, and R. B. Alfin-Slater, eds. *Nutrition in gerontology.* New York: Raven Press. pp. 243–56.

Rozovski, S. J. 1984. Nutrition and aging. *Current Topics Nutr* 13:137–69.

Schneider, E. L., E. M. Vining, E. C. Hadley, et al. 1986. Recommended dietary allowances and the health of the elderly. *N Engl J Med* 314(3):157–60.

Schokah, G. J., A. Newill, D. L. Scott, et al. 1979. Clinical effects of vitamin C in elderly inpatients with low vitamin C levels. *Lancet* 1:408–9.

Schrauzer, G. N., D. A. White, J. E. McGinness, et al. 1978. Arsenic and cancer: Effects of joint administration of arsenite and selenite on the genesis of mammary adenocarcinoma in inbred female C_3H/st mice. *Bioinorganic Chem* 8:245–53.

Shekelle, R. B., M. Lepper, S. Liu, et al. 1981. Dietary vitamin A and the risk of cancer in the Western Electric study. *Lancet* 2:1185–90.

Simkin, P. A. 1976. Oral zinc sulfate in rheumatoid arthritis. *Lancet* 2:539–42.

Simpson, H. C., R. W. Simpson, S. Lousley, et al. 1981. A high carbohydrate leguminous fibre diet improves all aspects of diabetic care. *Lancet* 1:1–5.

Sobal, J., H. L. Muncie, and A. S. Baker. 1986. Use of nutritional supplements in a retirement community. *Gerontologist* 26(2):187–91.

Sorenson, J. R. 1978. Copper complexes—A unique class of anti-arthritic drugs. *Prog in Med and Chem* 15:211–60.

Taylor, W. C., T. M. Pass, D. S. Shephard, and A. L. Komaroff. 1987. Cholesterol reductim and life expectancy: a model incorporating risk factors. *Annal Int Med* 106(4):605–14

U.S. Department of Agriculture. 1980. Food and nutrient intakes of individuals in one day in the United States, Spring, 1972 (Nationwide Food Consumption Survey). Washington, D.C. Preliminary Report No. 2. September.

U.S. Department of Health, Education and Welfare. 1972. Ten-state nutrition survey. DHEW Publ. No. 72–8130–34. Washington, D.C.

Wald, N., M. Idle, J. Boreham, et al. 1980. Low serum vitamin A and subsequent risk of cancer. *Lancet* 1:813–19.

Walker, W. R., and W. M. Keats. 1976. An investigation of the therapuetic value of the copper bracelet—dermal assimilation in arthritic/rheumatoid conditions. *Agents Actions* 6:454–59.

Watkin, D. M. 1980. Better nutrition for those already old: The challenge of the 80s. *Aging* 311–312:21–28.

Watt, G. C., G. J. Foy, and J. T. Hart. 1983. Comparison of blood pressure, sodium intake and other variables in offspring with and without a family history of high blood pressure. *Lancet* 2:1245–50.

Willett, W. C., B. F. Polk, J. S. Morris, et al. 1983. Prediagnostic serum selenium and risk of cancer. *Lancet* Vol II (8342):130–34.

Wilson, T. W. 1986. History of salt supplies in west Africa and blood pressures today. *Lancet* 1:784–86.

Zifferblatt, S. M., and C. S. Wilbur. 1977. Dietary counseling: Some realistic expectations and guidelines. *J Am Diet Assoc* 70:591–95.

10 Physical Activity

If exercise could be packed in a pill, it would be the single most widely prescribed, and beneficial, medicine in the nation.

Robert Butler

Introduction

Before the industrial age, most people were not concerned about getting sufficient physical activity because their daily routine kept their muscles and hearts strong. As the workplace and home becomes more mechanized, fewer people get sufficient physical activity from their occupations and household chores. Most must make an effort to exercise and, for many, it is easier to relax in front of the television than to go out to jog or swim a few laps. This chapter will discuss components of physical fitness, the benefits of keeping active, the pitfalls of inactivity, and the role activity plays in the prevention and treatment of several health problems. Patterns of physical activity in elders, their attitudes toward exercise, and strategies to motivate them to participate in exercise programs will also be addressed.

Components of Physical Fitness

Physical fitness is the ability to work and play without undue fatigue and to have energy reserves to react to a sudden emergency. Fitness has also been defined as the capacity to perform prolonged, heavy work (Astrand and Rodahl 1977). Those who are fit can sustain a higher maximum work load and can expend more energy than those who are not. For elders, fitness may mean the ability to live independently, to do household chores, shop for food, engage in active leisure pursuits, and withstand illness and injury.

Although fitness cannot be achieved by exercise alone, exercise enhances fitness by increasing the capacity of the body to sustain activity. Depending upon the type, exercise can improve endurance by conditioning the heart and lungs, increasing muscular flexibility and strength, improving balance, coordination and agility, restoring normal function to a part of the body damaged by disease or injury, and increasing bone mass.

Cardiovascular endurance is the most important fitness component. An efficient cardiovascular-respiratory system supplies each cell

---

Chopstick-Wielding 'Wrong Old Lady' Nabs Purse-Thief

SAN FRANCISCO (AP)—Pity the poor purse snatcher who made the mistake of picking on 73-year-old Louise Burt.

"I didn't give him a chance. He picked on the wrong old lady," said Burt as she recounted how she chased the would-be thief through San Francisco's Mission District Tuesday.

"Kid, I ran after that son-of-a-b—. I chased him to Hell-and-gone. Then the police caught him."

Burt was en route to a bingo game at a senior citizens' center with a couple of chums when someone grabbed her purse. Dressed in a black pantsuit and pumps with 2 ½-inch heels, her waist-length silver-gold hair anchored with lacquered chopsticks, Burt gave chase.

"That guy took off like a deer and I was right behind him," said the intended victim, whose purse contained her keys, about $10, a transit pass and her police whistle.

"I was so beside myself I wanted to kill him. I pulled out the chopsticks out of my hair to stab him if I could," she said. "My hair fell down and was hanging down to my fanny. I must have looked like a witch but I got superpower from somewhere and kept right after him." Swearing and shouting for help, she chased the thief down one street, through an alley and up another street into a public housing project where police officers Cherelyn Barnett and Melvin Thornton joined the pursuit.

"We were on (foot) patrol when we saw—and heard her—chasing the guy," said Thornton. "Did she run. We finally overtook her and went after him."

Thornton caught the man on a roof-top.

"He took one look at me, dropped the purse and jumped off the roof, two stories down to the ground," said the officer. "It must have been a 20- to 25-foot drop."

Thornton ran downstairs where he found William Jones, 22, cowering beneath a car with two broken ankles.

Table 10.1 Twelve-minute walking/running test. (Distances (miles) covered in twelve minutes)

Fitness Category		Age (years) 13–19	20–29	30–39	40–49	50–59	60+
I. Very Poor	(men)	<1.30*	<1.22	<1.18	<1.14	<1.03	<.87
	(women)	<1.0	< .96	< .94	< .88	< .84	<.78
II. Poor	(men)	1.30–1.37	1.22–1.31	1.18–1.30	1.14–1.24	1.03–1.16	.87–1.02
	(women)	1.00–1.18	.96-1.11	.95–1.05	.88– .98	.84– .93	.78– .86
III. Fair	(men)	1.38–1.56	1.32–1.49	1.31–1.45	1.25–1.39	1.17–1.30	1.03–1.20
	(women)	1.19–1.29	1.12–1.22	1.06–1.18	.99–1.11	.94–1.05	.87– .98
IV. Good	(men)	1.57–1.72	1.50–1.64	1.46–1.56	1.40–1.53	1.31–1.44	1.21–1.32
	(women)	1.30–1.43	1.23–1.34	1.19–1.29	1.12–1.24	1.06–1.18	.99–1.09
V. Excellent	(men	1.73–1.86	1.65–1.76	1.57–1.69	1.54–1.65	1.45–1.58	1.33–1.55
	(women)	1.44–1.51	1.35–1.45	1.30–1.39	1.25–1.34	1.19–1.30	1.10–1.18
VI. Superior	(men)	>1.87	>1.77	>1.70	>1.66	>1.59	>1.56
	(women)	>1.52	>1.46	>1.40	>1.35	>1.31	>1.19

*<Means "less than"; > means "more than."

This simple exercise will help you assess your current level of aerobic fitness. Time yourself for twelve minutes. During that twelve minutes run or walk as far and as fast as you can. You should try and pace yourself so that you are at your maximum effort output at the end of the twelve minutes (i.e., you just can't go any further). Keep track of how far you go and then locate your distance, sex, and age on the chart above. Circle your fitness category.

Source: From *The Aerobics Program for Total Well-Being* by Kenneth H. Cooper, M.D., M.P.H. Copyright © 1982 by Kenneth H. Cooper. Reprinted by permission of Bantam Books.

with sufficient oxygen for growth and maintenance and removes waste efficiently. Certain exercises improve oxygen use and consequent cardiovascular endurance and are called *aerobic* (with oxygen). Aerobic exercises consist of rhythmic or repetitive activity that uses large muscle groups such as the arms or legs. The most common aerobic activities are walking, bicycling, jogging, and swimming.

Aerobic exercise depends on great amounts of inhaled air to supply oxygen to the working muscles. The greater the exercise intensity, the more oxygen an individual requires: highly fit individuals have a higher maximum oxygen consumption than their sedentary counterparts. This means they can utilize more oxygen in an emergency situation so their heart and muscles can work more effectively. Maximal oxygen consumption is the commonly accepted measure of cardiovascular fitness. Although not as precise,

the extent of aerobic fitness can be measured by comparing the maximum distance an individual can cover in twelve minutes (table 10.1).

In contrast, *anaerobic* exercises are those that require so much muscle exertion that oxygen cannot be supplied to muscle tissues fast enough. Thus, the tissues begin to get their energy from a pathway that does not require as much oxygen. Anaerobic exercises include sprinting and weightlifting; these exercises do not increase cardiovascular fitness.

Muscular endurance is the ability of the muscles to work over a period of time—either to keep a muscle contracted or to continually contract and relax the muscle. Muscular endurance is required to hold a heavy object for a long time or to continually repeat a motion, such as hammering, kneading bread, or sawing. Aerobic activities and weight training increase muscular endurance.

Strength is the ability to apply muscular force by muscle contraction. Muscles develop strength when they contract against resistance. Strong muscles are particularly important in the back, shoulders, abdomen, and quadriceps (large thigh muscles) of elders to preserve posture and prevent backache. Kraus (1970) asserts that weakness or stiffness of postural muscles cause most of the disability observed in elder patients. Elders can increase muscle strength with weight training as much as younger individuals (Moritani and deVries 1980). In addition to increasing cardiovascular fitness, bicycling, walking, and jogging also build up abdominal and leg strength. The syndrome of painful knees and tired legs in older people is alleviated considerably by quadriceps strengthening exercises.

Flexibility is the ability to move the joints through a maximum range of motion without undue strain. Flexibility is necessary in all major joints to help avoid muscle pulls and strains. Trunk flexibility prevents low back pain and postural deformities. Inactivity, joint disease, and injuries to the joints and surrounding tissues can also reduce flexibility. Flexibility is especially important for elders because inactivity and illness can cause joints to stiffen, which promotes further immobility, and causes even more stiffness. This may ultimately result in a severe loss of mobility and independence in elders. Flexibility can be enhanced by exercising each joint separately with slow, regular, repeated stretching exercises.

Problems with balance are a major reason for falls and other accidents among elders. Balance can be improved with use. Dancing, some types of calisthenics, yoga, and standing or hopping on one foot are ways to improve balance. For exercises to improve balance among elders, see Overstall (1980).

Coordination is the ability to synchronize different actions of the body with each other and with the eyes. Agility is the ability to coordinate such movements and change directions quickly and safely. Raquet sports, swimming, and dancing may provide the highest degree of training for coordination and agility.

Vigorous physical activity can be enjoyed at any age.

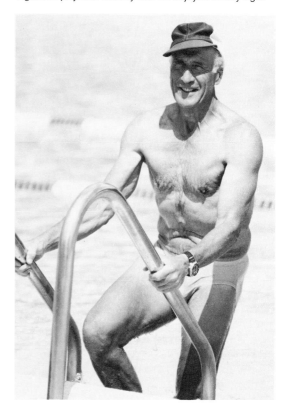

Whether young or old, the goal of developing a personal fitness plan is to seek a balance among different fitness components. Exercise activities which provide a balance of fitness components are swimming, ballet, rhythmic dancing, tennis, and cycling. Even those with physical limitations can find some form of activity that is enjoyable and beneficial (Pardini 1984).

Benefits of Physical Activity

A life of physical activity has been correlated with increased health and life expectancy in the later years. A study of Harvard alumni found that those who regularly engaged in walking, stair climbing, and sports play had a lower mortality rate, especially from cardiovascular or respiratory conditions, than their more sedentary counterparts. By age eighty, the amount of additional

Table 10.3 Modifiable aspects of aging

Aging Marker	Personal Decision(s) Required
Cardiac reserve	Exercise, nonsmoking
Dental decay	Brushing and flossing, diet
Glucose tolerance	Weight control, diet, exercise
Intelligence tests	Training, practice
Memory	Training, practice
Osteoporosis	Weight-bearing exercise, diet
Physical endurance	Exercise, weight control
Physical strength	Exercise
Pulmonary reserve	Exercise, nonsmoking
Reaction time	Training, practice
Serum cholesterol	Diet, weight control, exercise
Social ability	Practice
Skin aging	Sun avoidance
Systolic blood pressure	Salt limitation, weight control, exercise

Source: Fries, J. E., and L. M. Crapo, *Vitality and Aging.*
Copyright © 1981 W. H. Freeman and Company. Reprinted with permission.

life attributable to adequate exercise was up to two years (Paffenbarger et al. 1986). Exercise, even begun late in life, is also known to reduce the effects of aging on the body. Fries and Crapo (1981) list fourteen modifiable aspects of aging and note that eight can be modified by exercise (table 10.3).

This section discusses some of the benefits associated with high physical activity: changes in fat and energy metabolism, changes in fat metabolism, increased cardiovascular endurance, increased bone mass and joint mobility, and psychological and intellectual benefits. However, many reported studies have a number of limitations. Most studies are conducted on young and middle-aged men and may not be applicable to women and older people. Further, many studies of physical activity have methodological problems that affect the interpretation of the results. For instance, health condition of the subjects is generally not considered. Even studies with elders have some drawbacks. Older people who volunteer to participate in exercise research are more likely to be health conscious. The question must be addressed: are those who choose high levels of physical activity healthier to begin with, or does exercise enhance health? Exercise often leads to greater health consciousness that can result in a reduction in cigarette smoking or a dietary change that may make as significant a contribution to physical fitness measures as exercise itself.

Increased Metabolic Rate

Exercise causes an increase in metabolic rate, the speed at which the body burns calories, consequently reducing the level of body fat. DeVries and Gray (1963) reported a 7.5 to 28 percent increase in metabolic rate (from the normal on a nonexercise day) four hours after a vigorous workout. The higher metabolic rate persisted for at least six hours after exercise. If daily exercise continued, the researchers estimated the increased metabolic rate would result in a weight loss of four or five pounds a year. This calorie loss was in addition to the caloric expenditure of the exercise itself. In contrast, dieting without exercise has been reported to reduce metabolic rate, thus burning fewer calories (Schultz et al. 1980).

High levels of physical activity are also correlated with a reduced percentage of body fat. The body fat of the average older person is generally about 30 percent while that of a professional may be only 14 percent (Kavenaugh and Shephard 1977).

Changes in Fat Metabolism

Exercise may reduce the incidence of cardiovascular disease by slowing the progression of atherosclerosis. As discussed earlier, atherosclerosis is caused by deposits of cholesterol on the inner wall of the artery that restrict blood flow. Both triglycerides and cholesterol in the bloodstream are correlated with atherosclerosis and both are affected by exercise. Blood cholesterol levels do not decrease with exercise unless one also loses weight. However, the levels of some cholesterol carriers, specifically HDL (high-density lipoprotein), do increase. High levels of HDL are associated with a lower risk of heart disease. Aerobic exercise increases levels of HDL in the blood, at least in men (Roundy et al. 1978). Further, people with high cardiovascular endurance and high occupational activity have significantly higher HDL levels than their more sedentary counterparts (Wood et al. 1983).

High blood triglycerides increase the risk of cardiovascular disease. In addition to increasing the level of HDL, endurance training may also decrease the level of free triglycerides in the blood (Holloszy et al. 1964). However, the effects last only two days, indicating that one must exercise every other day to maintain a low triglyceride level. Interestingly, when initial triglyceride levels are relatively low, no further lowering effect is achieved (Wood et al. 1983). Further, endurance-trained athletes usually have low blood levels of triglycerides compared with others their age. For instance, older runners may have one-half the triglycerides in their blood as sedentary men (Martin et al. 1977).

The greater the intensity, frequency, and duration of exercise, the more likely blood levels of triglycerides and low-density lipoproteins will decrease. High levels of low-density lipoproteins (LDL) are believed to increase cardiovascular risk. However, the minimum amount of exercise necessary to alter blood lipid levels is unknown. One researcher estimates that one thousand calories of aerobic exercise expenditure a week is sufficient to alter blood lipid levels (Haskell 1984). This accounts for approximately twelve miles of walking or eight miles of running a week.

Increased Cardiovascular Endurance

Between age twenty and fifty, the average American loses 1 percent a year in work capacity of the heart. Some of the decline in cardiovascular fitness may be attributed to aging, but a significant portion is believed to be due to weight gain and atrophy due to inactivity (Bortz 1982). Vigorous aerobic exercise improves a number of the variables affecting cardiovascular system function. Aerobic exercise strengthens the heart, increases the volume of blood the heart can expel with each beat, and increases the efficiency of the system, allowing one to perform the same amount of physical activity with less strain. In adulthood, the decline in cardiovascular measures can be slowed, or even reversed, with regular, vigorous physical activity. A commitment to an active lifestyle retards the decline in aerobic capacity by one-half in elders who exercise (Kasch and Kulberg 1981). The improvements are even greater in elders who were formerly sedentary (Shephard 1977).

A number of reports indicate that an aerobic exercise program can significantly improve elders' cardiovascular endurance. DeVries (1970) exercised 112 men between the ages of fifty-two and eighty-eight for one hour, three times a week for six weeks and reported a significant improvement in oxygen transport and work capacity and reductions in blood pressure and body fat. A subsequent study with older women reported similar improvements (Adams and deVries 1973). Other studies on elders, using a control group, have reported similar gains.

How does exercise increase cardiovascular endurance? In animals, physical activity conditions the heart muscle, increases the size of coronary vessels, and develops collateral circulation (greater capillary development) around blocked coronary vessels (Eckstein 1957). However, this effect has not been demonstrated in humans (Nolewajka et al. 1979). In humans, exercise increases the pumping efficiency of the heart by reducing resting heart rate, increasing maximum oxygen uptake, increasing the amount of blood the heart can pump out per beat, and physical work capacity (Wilmore 1977). Exercise also strengthens the skeletal muscles, enhancing blood return to the heart. Further, exercise may reduce the risk of blood clotting associated with the development of atherosclerosis (Williams et al.

The nature and extent of the benefits of exercise are determined by its type, duration, intensity, and frequency. However, when exercise is decreased or discontinued, gains are rapidly lost, especially among elders. One study indicated that when an exercise program was discontinued, all gains in cardiovascular fitness were lost in ten weeks (Fringer and Stull 1974).

Increase in Bone Mass and Joint Mobility

A decrease in bone mass is correlated with age and inactivity. Donaldson et al. (1970) reported that a sample of young men immobilized for thirty to thirty-six weeks lost up to 39 percent of their bone mineral. Loss of bone mass, whether by age, inactivity, or both affects elders by increasing minor aches and pains and the incidence of debilitating fractures. Elders with brittle bones may become overly cautious about physical activity, inadvertently promoting further decline. When older bones are injured, they take longer to heal. The immobility necessary for healing further exacerbates bone loss.

Exercise increases bone mineral content and consequent bone strength. By submitting weight bearing bones to the pull of muscle contraction and force of gravity, metabolic changes occur that enhance bone remineralization. Those with a high level of physical activity have greater bone mineral content than sedentary individuals. A group of long-distance runners age fifty to seventy-two were compared with a matched group of inactive people. Both male and female runners had 40 percent more bone mineral than the control (Lane et al. 1986). An earlier study analyzing the leg bones in athletes reported that the greater the load placed on the legs, the more bone density increased (Nilsson and Westlin 1971). A number of studies have demonstrated an increase in bone mass in elders after a program of physical exercise (Aloia et al. 1978; Smith et al. 1981).

Lack of exercise contributes to decreased flexibility in many joints. A number of studies have reported that exercise increased joint mobility. Frekany and Leslie (1975) reported that fifteen elder females exercising one half hour twice a week for seven months significantly increased hamstring (the muscle behind the upper thigh) and lower back flexibility. Munns (1981) directed a group of elders in a twelve-week exercise and dance program for one hour three times a week. She reported a significant improvement in range of joint motion in neck, wrist, shoulder, hip and back, knee and ankle as compared with a control group. Bassett et al. (1982) reported that a ten-week nonstrenuous, progressive exercise program for elder men and women provided significant increases in shoulder, hip, and knee joint flexibility. For flexibility exercises, refer to deVries and Hales (1982) and Lonnerblad (1984).

Psychological Effects

We often read reports of the natural highs of vigorous exercise or that exercise promotes mental well-being. However, most studies investigating these phenomena have serious methodological problems; most used no control group, no randomization, no long-term follow-up, and poor measurement devices. Hughes (1984) reviewed over 1100 studies in this area and found only twelve that had at least ten subjects, a control group, and an exercise regime that lasted at least three times a week for three weeks or more. More

Most people assert that exercise makes them feel good.

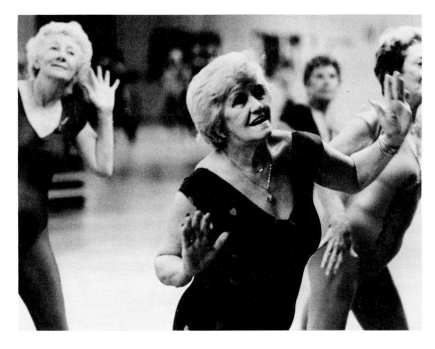

methodologically sound studies are needed in this vital area to corroborate the subjective feeling that exercise is a contributor to psychological health at all ages. One recent work (Perri and Templer 1984–85) reported a significant increase in measures of self-confidence and mastery over the environment in a group of elders. The elders had increased self-image compared to a control group after a fourteen-week program of aerobic and flexibility exercise.

Despite the paucity of experimental evidence, it seems reasonable that if exercise improves physical health, it should do the same for mental health, since mind and body are inextricably linked. In addition, most people agree exercise reduces stress and increases feelings of well-being. Although not documented, exercise may cause biochemical changes that produce a positive psychological effect. For instance, Howley (1976) suggested that strenuous aerobic exercise increases the production of norepinepherine in the

central nervous system. As some types of depression are associated with low levels of norepinepherine, exercise might offer relief. Exercise has also been reported to increase the level of endorphins (natural painkillers) in the body (Gambert et al. 1981). Although it is doubtful whether they produce a high in itself, it is likely they have a pain-relieving effect. In addition, the positive psychological effects associated with exercise—distraction from problems, social reinforcement, feeling of mastery—may also serve to make one feel better after exercise (Hughes 1984).

Increased Intellectual Function

Few studies have analyzed the effects of exercise on cognition in geriatric populations. Powell (1974) compared the effect of exercise on memory and intellectual ability of thirty elder nursing home patients. He divided them into a mild exercise group, attention-control group (interaction but no exercise), and a noncontact control group.

After twelve weeks, the exercise group improved scores on two of three memory tests; no change was reported in the other two groups. Elsayed et al. (1980) reported that highly fit older individuals scored higher on intelligence tests than less fit subjects. Dustman et al. (1984) reported that elders participating in a four-month exercise program had significantly greater improvement on a number of cognitive scores including response time, visual organization, memory, and mental flexibility. They also reported that those participating in aerobic activities—such as fast walking and jogging—improved significantly more than those who did only strength and flexibility exercises. In another study, response times of older men who had participated in physical activities were significantly faster than those of age-matched sedentary men (Sherwood and Selder 1979).

Exercise may help cognitive function by increasing the amount of circulating nutrients to the brain; habitual exercisers generally have high levels of glucose and oxygen in their blood. However, improved cognition in elders undergoing exercise programs may be partially caused by psychological factors. Selection for and participation in exercise programs may make individuals feel better about themselves, resulting in improved intellectual performance and function. Whether mental deterioration is preventable or reversible through exercise is not known.

Physical Activity to Reduce Chronic Illness

In addition to the benefits of physical activity outlined above, exercise is being increasingly advocated to prevent and treat several chronic diseases (Kottke et al. 1984). Life-long patterns of activity as well as exercise programs begun later in life significantly affect the degree and progression of many chronic conditions among elders.

No matter what the specific disease, an individual suffering from a chronic disease is likely to enter into a cycle of reduced physical activity, which results in deconditioning and a number of symptoms associated with decreased fitness. This decrease in fitness leads to increased fatigue and further decreases in physical activity. In addition, characteristics of the disease itself tend to speed the debilitative cycle. Intervening with exercise therapy may delay onset or progression of disease, reduce debilitating symptoms, and maximize independence. However, motivating the chronically ill to initiate and maintain a systematic exercise program is very difficult (Carmody et al. 1980). They may believe their situation to be hopeless, or the exercise itself may cause discomfort, such as fatigue, pain, and breathlessness.

Heart Disease

Heart disease is the primary cause of death and disability in the United States. Although no one knows exactly what causes heart disease, physical inactivity has been implicated in its development. Vigorous physical activity not only decreases the risk of heart disease, but also indirectly reduces a number of other risk factors, such as obesity, hypertension, and blood lipid concentrations.

A number of studies suggest that those who are physically active have less coronary heart disease than their sedentary counterparts. A well-known study by Paffenbarger and Hale (1975) followed San Francisco longshoremen for twenty-two years and compared the heart attack rate of those with high- and low-activity jobs. The workers were matched on personal characteristics and recognized cornonary risk factors. The researchers reported that men who had high activity jobs were at significantly lower risk of fatal heart attack than those whose jobs required little physical activity. The activity variable overrode other cardiac risks such as heavy smoking, hypertension, obesity, and high levels of cholesterol in the blood. Paffenbarger estimates that if all longshoremen worked in high-activity jobs, death rates might have been cut in half. However, whether those who were originally more fit gravitated toward the more active work and vice versa cannot be determined. In another longitudinal study, Harvard alumni with low and high leisure activity patterns reported results similar to the longshoreman study (Paffenbarger et al. 1978). For a review of studies on the relationship of physical activity and cardiac disease, see Paffenbarger and Hyde (1984).

Does a cardiac patient's participation in an exercise program reduce the likelihood of a recurrent heart attack? Blackburn (1983) reviewed the literature and reported that studies to date have not yet answered this question. Small sample size, difficulty in obtaining equivalent control subjects, high dropout rate, and short follow-up time make it difficult to find a significant effect in postcoronary exercise groups. However, Shephard (1983) combined the results of three studies on post-coronary exercise programs and reported that those heart patients who regularly participated in exercise programs lived one-fourth to one-third longer than those who did not.

Evidence indicates that those with angina pain can be helped by regular exercise. Exercise enables angina victims to do more work before feeling chest pain by reducing heart rate and subsequent oxygen requirement. One study indicated that a prescribed aerobic exercise program was as effective as taking nitroglycerine constantly to reduce anginal pain in postcoronary patients (Clausen and Trap-Jensen 1976).

Older cardiac patients can benefit from cardiac rehabilitation exercise programs and should not be excluded on the basis of age. Williams et al. (1985) exercised a group of male elder cardiac patients who had recently suffered a heart attack or coronary bypass operation. He reported that elder patients improved physical capacity and response to exertion as much as younger patients. These elders lost weight, decreased resting heart rate, decreased percentage of body fat, and could tolerate a greater maximum exertion. Further, exercise decreased their breathlessness symptoms, improving their quality of life. For specific exercise-training protocol to rehabilitate patients with coronary heart disease, see Pollock et al. (1984, pp. 298–373) and Williams et al. (1984).

Hypertension

Many studies document a correlation between regular exercise and a low incidence of hypertension. Paffenbarger and colleagues (1983) studied the prevalence of hypertension in two groups of Harvard alumni: those who reported high leisure exercise and their more sedentary cohorts. They reported that two to four hours a week of vigorous activity among overweight individuals reduced the probability of becoming hypertensive by 20 to 50 percent. The more hours of activity, the lower the risk.

Studies also report that a systematic, aerobic exercise program can decrease blood pressure in hypertensive subjects. Most research found that exercising three times a week or more will significantly lower resting blood pressures in hypertensives if trained to at least 70 percent of maximum heart rate. Significant lowering of blood pressure is more likely in those with initial elevated blood pressure (Wilmore et al. 1970). In general, the older the hypertensive subject and the longer the training program, the more extensive the benefits. Hypertensive individuals experience a reduced morbidity and mortality when their resting blood pressures are reduced, even if values are still above normal. Despite this information, inclusion of exercise training in the management of hypertension is not well-accepted by medical authorities and specific guidelines on implementing a therapeutic exercise program are sparse (Tipton 1984).

Diabetes

Regular exercise plays a significant role in diabetes prevention and treatment. It is documented to increase glucose tolerance and insulin sensitivity (Rauramaa 1984; Thomas et al. 1981). Because exercising muscles need less insulin than those at rest in order to take glucose into the cells, diabetics who exercise daily generally need less insulin (Berger et al. 1975). However, the usefulness of an exercise regimen is dependent upon the type of diabetes.

In patients with Type I diabetes (no insulin production/dependent on insulin injections), it is difficult to take advantage of the benefits of exercise because so many variables influence blood glucose levels (food intake, time of day, duration, intensity of exercise, state of training, type and dose of insulin injected). Type I diabetics need to carefully plan to exercise every day for a certain period of time at a certain intensity so that insulin dosage can be adjusted for such activity. Although Type I diabetics are encouraged to exercise for recreation whenever they want, they need to learn to adjust their insulin intake to reduce the risk of metabolic complications (Kemmer and Berger 1984). Thus far, no research has documented a long-term positive effect of exercise to control Type I diabetes.

In contrast, the most common type of diabetes among elders, Type II or adult-onset diabetes, responds well to an exercise prescription. The main method of diabetic control is an exercise and diet regimen. Saltin et al. (1979) conducted one-hour aerobic exercise sessions twice a week for three months on middle-aged male diabetics and reported the subjects had increased insulin sensitivity and normalized glucose tolerance as well as improvement of cardiovascular health. Since these diabetics are often obese and are at risk of cardiovascular disease, exercise prevents or retards complications of cardiovascular disease in diabetes.

For more detailed information on the physiological effects of exercise upon the diabetic, refer to Jette (1984). Hanson and Kochan (1983) suggest exercise regimens for those with diabetes.

Obesity

Obesity is implicated directly or indirectly in a number of chronic health problems including premature death, adult-onset diabetes, hypertension, vascular disease, and respiratory problems (Buskirk 1974). Physical activity can promote weight loss and positively affect the other variables associated with obesity. Mayer (1968) asserts that physical inactivity is the single most important factor responsible for the increasing number of overweight people in Western society. Although obese individuals are not always less active than those of average weight, inactivity is associated with obesity in all age groups (Stern 1984).

Weight is a function of energy output and input. Those who increase food intake and maintain identical activity levels will gain weight. Conversely, those who maintain the same caloric intake and increase activity will lose weight. Exercise is a major factor in regulating body fat content. One pound of body fat is lost for every 3,500 Kcal of energy expended. The American College of Sports Medicine (1980) describes the amount of exercise necessary to decrease body weight or body fat. Exercise must be performed at least three days a week for at least twenty minutes a session with intensity enough to burn three hundred calories a session. If fewer calories are expended, the number of sessions must be increased. Daily exercise increases weight loss.

Numerous studies report that exercise decreases total body fat and increases lean body mass (see Stern 1984 for a review). Those on calorie-restriction diets without exercise often lose muscle tissue as well as fat. However, when exercise is combined with dieting, lean body mass is preserved and even increased, but body fat is decreased (Zuti and Golding 1976). Further, those who exercise frequently are most likely to retain weight loss (Gormally et al. 1980). Because of the high dropout rate in exercise intervention programs for weight control, Bjorntorp (1978) suggests exercise be performed in a group under close supervision and frequent feedback of results of body measurement and blood lipid changes be given to participants.

Respiratory Diseases

Exercise cannot repair damaged lung tissue or replace lost respiratory tissues (Petty and Cherniak 1981), but it can improve other factors associated with efficient respiratory function. Exercise can increase oxygen consumption and utilization, improve ventilation, reduce resting heart rate, and increase the tolerance for work (Moser et al. 1980). Because individuals with pulmonary disease often lose additional lung capacity because of lack of physical activity, exercise is highly recommended to counteract that effect. However, exercise can cause shortness of breath and fatigue in individuals who have pulmonary disease, so a closely supervised program is recommended.

Osteoporosis

A major contributor to the rate and degree of bone loss in osteoporosis is physical inactivity. A number of studies show a high correlation between level of physical activity and bone mass in older women (Black-Sandler et al. 1982; Oyster et al. 1984). Even when an exercise regimen is begun later in life, it can slow the rate of bone demineralization. Smith et al. (1981) studied the effects of exercise on elder female nursing home residents. One group of women participated in a light to moderate exercise program for thirty minutes a day, three days a week. Another group did not exercise. At the end of three years, the bone mineral content of the untreated group declined 3.29 percent. However, in the group that exercised, bone loss was reversed and subjects realized a bone mineral gain of approximately 2 percent.

Lower Back Pain

Physical inactivity is an important contributor to chronic back pain. A back with poor muscle tone is especially susceptible to fatigue, strain, injury, and tension. Although a number of health professionals prescribe exercises for back pain, generally the type, gradation, and duration of these exercises is poorly monitored and exercises are either haphazardly done or overdone. Although manipulative treatment may temporarily allay back pain, an exercise program designed to strengthen the abdomen and back muscles is necessary for lasting improvement. Kraus and colleagues (1977) developed an exercise program to treat back pain related to muscle weakness and

reported an 80 percent success rate in reducing back pain. Woolbright (1983) details exercise protocols for those with chronic low back pain.

Depression and Anxiety

Exercise regimens are increasingly used to alleviate anxiety and depressive disorders despite the lack of documented evidence that exercise offers such relief. The most commonly cited evidence that exercise reduces depression is that of Greist et al. (1979) who compared running with psychotherapy as a treatment for mild to moderate depression. Depressed persons were assigned to running therapy, long-term psychotherapy, or time-limited psychotherapy, and depression was assessed at the beginning and end of the treatment period. Because those in running therapy had reductions in depression as great as that evidenced by those in the two psychotherapy groups, the authors concluded that running was effective in reducing depression. However, because of the absence of a placebo or no-treatment condition, it is impossible to determine if subjects would have improved regardless of any therapeutic intervention.

A recent controlled study of depressed undergraduate women by McCann and Holmes (1984) found a relationship between strenuous aerobic exercise and decreases in depression. Forty-seven mild to moderately depressed women were randomly assigned to an aerobic exercise treatment, a placebo treatment (relaxation training), or a no-treatment condition. The subjects in the aerobic exercise condition had significantly lower depression scores than those in the placebo or no-treatment condition and their improvement was achieved within the first five weeks of treatment.

Limited research on elders has shown that exercise can have a tranquilizing effect. DeVries and Adams (1972) compared the effects of single doses of exercise and a tranquilizer on reducing muscle tension in ten elderly anxious subjects. They reported that the only treatment that significantly lowered electrical activity in muscles was mild exercise. They concluded a fifteen

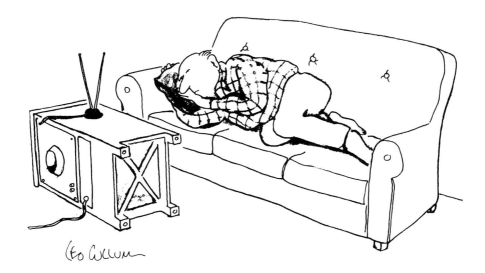

minute walk at a moderate rate (one hundred heart beats/minute) was sufficient to bring about the desired muscle relaxant effect, which persisted for an hour. They assert that it is better to prescribe exercise than tranquilizers because exercise does not impair motor coordination, reaction time, and driving performance like some tranquilizers do. See Hayden & Allen (1984) for a review of relevant literature on the relationship between aerobic exercise, anxiety, and depression.

Colon Cancer

Garabrant et al. (1984) studied the records of almost three thousand colon cancer cases (ages twenty to sixty-four) in Los Angeles between 1972 and 1981 and concluded that physical inactivity may play a major role in the development of colon cancer. Men with sedentary jobs had a colon cancer risk at least 1.6 times that of men whose jobs required a high level of activity. Risk increased as activity level decreased in every socioeconomic and racial group. Studies in this area are still in the early stages.

Hazards of Inactivity

The most common aging complaints are difficulty experienced with minor exertion, diminished muscle strength, a general stiffening of the joints, and loss of bone. While many consider these to be consequences of aging, an unknown proportion of these decrements are due to a sedentary lifestyle. Although some decline in body function with age is inevitable, inactivity makes matters worse. Many gerontologists are convinced that inactivity plays a greater role in the development of such decrements than old age. Kraus and Raub (1961) coined the term "hypokinetic disease" to describe physical and mental dysfunctions caused by insufficient physical activity. Bortz (1982) believes many so-called age changes can be improved by a regular vigorous exercise program.

A number of studies have documented the physiological decrements associated with lack of activity. Anyone who has had a limb immobilized by a cast or has been confined to bed has experienced the detrimental effects of immobility firsthand. The adjacent box outlines the major physiological decrements caused by immobility (adapted from Olson 1967). Note that many of these changes are believed to be associated with the aging process.

Effects of Immobility Upon the Body

Cardiovascular System

Orthostatic hypotension (dizziness upon rising

Heart works 30 percent harder when body is in flat position than sitting position

Heart rate progressively increases with prolonged rest

Blood changes, including clots, anemia, increased triglycerides and low density lipoproteins (LDL)

Respiratory System

Decreased maximum oxygen consumption

Decreased chest expansion, reducing breathing

Decreased mucus movement, predisposing to infections

Oxygen/carbon dioxide imbalance leading to reduced gas exchange

Gastrointestinal System

Lack of appetite

Slowed bowel function, leading to constipation

Musculoskeletal System

Increased susceptibility to fractures due to decreased bone buildup and accelerated bone breakdown

Decreased strength and reduced range of joint motion due to muscle shortening and atrophy

Muscle wastage decreases blood flow to tissues resulting in pressure sores

Urinary System

Reduced function of urinary excretion leading to incontinence

Increased calcium breakdown may create kidney stones

Metabolism

Reduced metabolic rate

Altered drug metabolism

Tissue atrophy and protein deficiency

Alterations in exchange of nutrients and wastes

Increased loss of fluids and sodium

Decreased glucose tolerance

Psychosocial Factors

Decreased learning capacity and problem-solving ability

Decreased motivation

Exaggerated or inappropriate emotional reactions

Sensory deprivation

Depression and diminished feelings of personal worth

Because the effects of immobility are so extensive and debilitating, elders, even those with physical disabilities, should exercise to minimize the physiological and psychological consequences. Even slight limitations in movement will become greater if the elder does not exercise, because inactivity promotes further decline. Elders should be encouraged to begin exercise programs compatible with their ability and interest. One good rule for those who work with older people to follow is that suggested by Asher (1947), a physician:

Teach us that we may dread
Unnecessary time in bed
Get people up and we may save
Our patient from an early grave.

Exercise Promotion

Although it is important to maintain a high level of physical activity throughout life, many benefits can be realized even when an exercise program is started late in life. Despite the data supporting the benefits of regular physical activity in the prevention and management of chronic illnesses, seldom do people begin an exercise program on their own. To promote exercise among elders, physicians must discuss the benefits and risks of exercise and prescribe specific exercise regimens to their patients. Further, techniques to motivate elders to exercise must be developed. Accessible, low-cost education and fitness programs geared toward this group are needed to motivate elders to become more physically active. This section will discuss the role of the physician in exercise promotion. Factors affecting the motivation to start and continue an exercise program will also be addressed.

The Physician's Role

Exercise is invaluable in the prevention and treatment of many of the chronic conditions common to elders and in postponing deterioration. Physicians are in a prime position to educate elders on the benefits of exercise, to prescribe and monitor an individualized exercise regimen, and to motivate the elder to begin exercising. Despite the clear benefits of long-term, regular exercise in prevention and rehabilitation, physicians seldom prescribe exercise for their patients and are more likely to rely on drug or surgical treatments (Thomas et al. 1981). Physicians may actually discourage exercise by advising their elder patients to 'take it easy' or avoid stairs or overexertion. When exercise is prescribed, instructions are seldom specific in terms of duration, frequency, and intensity and monitoring is rare.

Why aren't physicians more aggressive in prescribing exercise, especially for elders? The predominant reason seems to be ignorance of the beneficial effects of physical activity to prevent and treat chronic conditions. Physicians may erroneously believe the risks of sudden death or musculoskeletal injuries that accompany exercise are too great for elders. Or, they may be unaware of the techniques used to assess fitness level, prescribe an exercise regimen, or motivate patients. Unfortunately, information on exercise, especially exercise and aging, is seldom a significant part of the medical school curriculum and continuing medical education courses (Thomas et al. 1981). Further, some physicians may not value physical exercise as evidenced by their own low level of fitness. Additionally, an exercise prescription, like other preventive therapies, consumes more physician time than a drug prescription.

The blame should not be placed solely on the physician because the problem may also be attributed to the patient's attitude. Most would rather take a pill to reduce their disease symptoms than perform daily, perhaps initially painful, exercises, especially when the benefits may not be immediate. Many patients may be dissatisfied when exercise is prescribed. Some believe that doctors are trained and paid to provide modern drugs, not exercise that the patients must do themselves. An exercise prescription forces patients to take control of their own symptoms, instead of relying passively on a cure by drug or surgical intervention.

Physicians are being encouraged to prescribe exercise for their patients by several professional organizations. The American Heart Association developed two booklets for physicians, one for prescribing exercise for healthy individuals (1972b) and another for prescribing for those with or at risk for heart disease (1972a). The American College of Sports Medicine also issued *Guidelines for Graded Exercise Testing and Exercise Prescription* (1980) for physicians. The American Medical Association's Council on Scientific Affairs (1981) makes the following recommendations to physicians:

1. Stress the importance of exercise for older persons, explaining in detail its physiological and psychological benefits.
2. Obtain a complete and reliable medical history and perform a physical examination, employing exercise testing for quantification of cardiovascular and physical fitness as appropriate, before the specific exercise prescription.
3. Maintain an active interest in patients' exercise practices by appropriate follow-up.
4. Encourage all patients to establish an exercise program as a lifetime commitment in preparation for their later years.

With the current public interest in exercise, physicians and other health professionals will play a key role in evaluating physical fitness and prescribing exercise programs for all age groups. Professionals will be more likely to extend their influence if they exercise regularly and are physically fit themselves.

Medical Assessment

A medical assessment is an important tool for the physician to encourage physical activity among elders. An assessment allows the professional to prescribe an individualized exercise program consistent with the patient's current health status and fitness level. An assessment may also detect diseases or disorders that may inhibit exercise or require special precautions. A medical assessment includes a medical history, physical examination, laboratory work, and exercise testing. A medical history requests information concerning present and past levels of physical activity, physical symptoms suggesting conditions that would limit exercise ability, and current medications that affect duration and type of exercise prescribed. In a physical examination, resting heart rate, blood pressure, body weight, and signs of cardiovascular disease can be observed. Laboratory studies might include blood count, urine analysis, fasting blood sugar, blood lipids, and perhaps a resting electrocardiogram. Exercise tests, such as performance on a treadmill or bicycle, may be used as part of a medical assessment to determine a person's capacity for strenuous exercise.

There are conflicting views on who should have a medical assessment before starting an exercise program. The American Medical Association and the American Heart Association recommend those over thirty-five see a physician first. However, these standards may have inadvertently contributed to the view that exercise is dangerous, preventing many healthy people from starting a fitness program. The consensus seems to be moving toward the recommendations in the pamphlet *Exercise and your Heart* (Levy 1981), which suggests persons can begin a gradual, sensible exercise program on their own without seeing a doctor if they have (1) no history of heart trouble, heart murmur, heart attack, hypertension, arthritis, or diabetes; (2) no family history of premature coronary artery disease; and (3) no exercise-related breathlessness, faintness, dizziness, pain or pressure in the chest, neck, shoulder, or arm.

The Exercise Prescription

An exercise prescription is an exercise program tailored to an individual's physical condition by a physician or skilled professional. The exercise prescription may be utilized for prevention, treatment, or rehabilitation. Specific exercises may be suggested to improve muscular strength

A Typical Exercise Prescription

Name: Josephine Doe

Age: 76

Expected outcome: Increased cardio-respiratory functioning and increased bone mass

Type of exercise: Walking

Intensity: Target heart rate between 110 and 130

Frequency: Four times per week

Duration: Twenty minutes of target heart rate, plus five minutes each of warm-up and cool down

Possible complications: Chest, arm, neck, or jaw pain, significant increase in shortness of breath

Motivation: Suggest walking with grandchildren, friend, dog, or to a specific destination

and endurance, increase joint flexibility, reduce bone loss, or improve cardiovascular endurance. For instance, one might prescribe weight lifting to increase muscular strength and endurance, jogging to enhance cardiorespiratory endurance and bone mass, and range of motion exercises to improve joint flexibility. Exercise may also be prescribed as part of a weight reduction plan.

The exercise prescription should include the type of exercise, its intensity, frequency, and duration, as well as the expected outcome (see box above). The prescription should be realistic, since too much exercise may cause discomfort, fatigue, and feelings of failure and too little may not produce a gain in fitness. Further, the prescription should be developed mutually by the client and the health professional. The client needs to be held accountable for meeting his/her goals and the professional should give frequent feedback about progress, and reinforce success (Serfass and Gerberich 1984). See Pollock (1984) for sample exercise prescriptions to improve cardiovascular fitness, muscle strength, and coordination.

Exercise intensity can be monitored by measuring heart rate during exercise. To increase fitness, exercise must be performed at a target heart rate of 70 to 85 percent of maximum heart rate for at least twenty minutes three to four times a week. Elders who have been sedentary may begin a lower intensity program, such as walking at 60 percent of maximum heart rate, and later progress to the 70 to 85 percent range. In any case, in addition to the twenty minutes or more of aerobic activity at the target heart rate, warming up and cooling down periods are necessary for all age groups.

Estimation of target heart rate requires measurement of resting heart rate (taken while lying in bed) and maximum heart rate. Although exact determination of maximum heart rate requires an exercise stress test, one's age subtracted from 220 is a good estimate. To calculate target heart rate, insert maximum heart rate, resting heart rate, and percentage of maximum heart rate desired in the following formula (Karvonen et al. 1957):

| Target Heart Rate | = | percent of max. heart rate desired | × | (maximum heart rate | − | resting heart rate | + | resting heart rate |

For instance, a sixty-eight year old man (maximum heart rate is $220 - 68 = 152$) with a resting heart rate of seventy-two desires to work out at 75 percent of his maximum capacity. He should maintain a target heart rate of 132 beats/minute for twenty minutes.

$$132 = .75 \,(152 - 72) + 72$$

Pulse measurements are the best way to measure heart rate. The middle and ring fingers should be placed lightly over the artery located to the side of the throat and heart beats should be counted for a minute. Heart rate can be monitored quickly when exercising by counting beats for six seconds and multiplying by ten to get an approximation of the number of beats per minute.

Intensity, duration, and frequency of exercise should increase with time so the demands on the body keep ahead of the improvement made. Such overloading can develop muscle strength and improve cardiovascular endurance. However, deVries (1983) underscores the importance of gradual progression in exercising previously sedentary elders. Several in his exercise training program actually decreased in functional capacity after six weeks of exercise because the exercise prescription was too rigorous.

Risks and Complications of Exercise

Like a drug prescription, an exercise prescription has risks and complications that depend on one's health and fitness level. A few health conditions prohibit vigorous exercise: some types of angina, irregular heartbeat, congestive heart failure, or severe cases of hypertension, anemia, or obesity. A number of others require medical supervision before and during a rigorous exercise program. These include acute or chronic infections, poorly controlled diabetes, pulmonary disease, severe mental illness, angina, or recent heart attack. See American College of Sports Medicine (1980) for a complete list. Milhorn (1984) recommends those on particular therapeutic drugs, such as beta blockers or digitalis, be closely observed during an exercise program. The above list underscores the need for an individualized, supervised exercise prescription to optimize the benefit and minimize the risks of exercise for those with health problems.

The most common risks of exercise for all age groups are musculoskeletal problems due to too much stress: muscle soreness, shin splints, tension strains, stress fractures, bone bruises, joint pain, and low back pain (Pollock 1978). In elders, previous injuries of the musculoskeletal system, previous inactivity, osteoporosis, illness, degenerative changes, nutritional deficiencies, hormone imbalances, or diabetes may affect the response to exercise. However, the benefits of a regular exercise program heavily outweigh the risks, and carefully prescribed, moderate, regular exercise is beneficial for almost everyone.

As part of the exercise prescription, the professional must discuss symptoms that may occur during an exercise workout that may be hazardous: chest, arm, neck, or jaw pain, significant increase in shortness of breath, lightheadedness or fainting, irregular heart beat, nausea or vomiting during or after exercise, prolonged fatigue after exercise, weakness or uncoordinated movements, or unexplained weight or exercise tolerance changes. These warning signs could indicate an underlying disease or a need to alter the exercise prescription. If any of the above symptoms occur, the elder should be directed to stop exercising and contact a physician.

The fear that exercise will induce a heart attack inhibits many elders from exercising. There is no evidence to suggest that even strenuous exercise harms the normal heart (Eichner 1983). Heart attack victims are slightly more likely to have a heart attack during exercise than those who have not (Kala et al. 1978). However, habitual, vigorous exercise is associated with a decreased risk of heart attack when not exercising (Siscovick et al. 1984). Thus, the small risk while exercising should not preclude exercising for almost everyone (Thompson et al. 1982). For a review of literature on the risk of exercise, see Eichner (1983).

Motivation to Exercise

The number of young adults who exercise regularly has increased dramatically within the last few decades and the proliferation of articles and books on the subject reflect a new exercise-consciousness. Unfortunately, most elders have not been affected by this exercise trend. The National Health Interview Survey found only about 30 percent of those age forty-five and older reported that they exercised regularly, as compared with 42 percent of those age thirty to forty-four (Thornberry et al. 1986).

Why do so many elders shun exercise? Part of the answer lies in their attitude toward exercise and fitness. In general, they believe their need for exercise diminishes as they grow older. Elders also tend to vastly exaggerate the risks involved in vigorous exercise after middle age. Further, they overrate the health benefits of light, sporadic exercise and underrate their own athletic capabilities (Conrad 1976). These attitudes may reflect the common belief that one should slow down in old age. In addition, older people do not have the same opportunities for exercise as younger people and many are hampered by illness or fear of accidents.

Many elders may not know the benefits and importance of exercise because schools had no physical fitness programs when they were growing up. Many maintained physical fitness during their youth through daily activities so exercise for the sake of exercise was uncommon. Further, much of the information about the benefits of exercise has only been recently understood. It will be interesting to see whether the exercise patterns of the next generation of elders will differ.

Although most people might agree that exercise is "good for you," few actually are motivated to engage in a regular exercise program. Because exercise should be a life-long habit to gain maximum benefit, the health professional needs to learn to motivate people of all ages to include regular exercise as part of their daily routine.

Those most likely to begin and maintain an exercise program are internally motivated: they gain enough pleasure and reinforcement from the physical activity itself. Others may need external reinforcement, such as noticeable weight loss, attention from staff, or socialization from peers to maintain their physical conditioning program. Sidney and Shephard (1977a) reported that those elders who thought they were in poor health (whether or not their belief was based on fact) were unlikely to participate in an exercise program.

Serfass and Gerberich (1984) assert that the lack of knowledge of the effects of exercise, and how much and what type of exercises are needed to increase fitness, contribute to a low level of motivation to exercise. The National Health Interview Survey revealed that elders are significantly less knowledgeable about the cardiovascular benefits of exercise than those in other age groups. Over 80 percent did not know how often to exercise to strengthen the heart and lungs or the minimum duration and intensity needed to benefit the heart and lungs (Thornberry et al. 1986).

Many elders mistakenly believe they are getting all the exercise they need. In one survey, approximately half the elders polled reported they were very physically active (National Council on Aging 1975). In another survey, 71 percent reported they got enough exercise through regular activities (Clark 1974). It is likely that many elders have an inaccurate perception of physical activity; they consider a walk to the mailbox or light housework to be sufficient. Sidney and Shephard (1977a) support this hypothesis by noting their elder subjects rated themselves more active than others their age, but, upon monitoring, their perceptions were not supported. Sidney and Shephard reported that elders, even those in good physical shape, overestimated their amount of physical exertion more than younger individuals (1977b).

Chapter 10

One of the greatest challenges for the health professional is to motivate people to begin and continue an exercise regimen. Many individuals who begin a fitness program exercise sporadically and often tire of the activity within a few months. Less than half those who begin an exercise regimen are still participating after three or six months (Dishman 1982). In programs for those who have had a heart attack, exercisers are likely to drop out even more quickly, possibly because the initial fear of another heart attack that originally motivated them to start an exercise program has subsided. Like others who stop exercising, common reasons post-coronary patients give for terminating an exercise program include: difficulty in arriving to class on time, inconvenient location, parking problems, insufficient staff attention, and belief that exercise had little value (Andrew et al. 1981).

Persistence in a physical conditioning program often depends on whether the program and its results meet initial expectations. Danielson and Wanzel (1977) found that participants who failed to reach their own goals dropped out twice as fast as those who did attain them. Pollock (1978) reported that those who trained at high intensity levels were more than twice as likely to discontinue exercise as those who trained at more moderate levels. These studies underscore the need for health professionals to assist the client in setting realistic goals in order to continue the exercise program.

Social support also increases adherance to an exercise regimen. Individuals who exercise in a group are less likely to drop out than those who exercise alone. Massie and Shephard (1971) reported that only 41 percent of their adult sample who participated in an individualized exercise regimen adhered to the program as compared to 82 percent who entered into a group exercise program. Heizelmann and Bagley (1970) reported that 90 percent of their clients preferred group to individual exercise. Spouses are also an important variable in exercise persistence. Reported attrition rates were three times higher for those

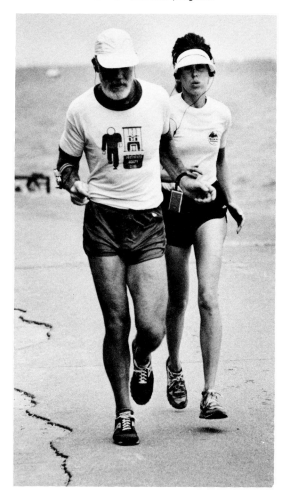

For young and old alike, socialization increases the incentive to maintain an exercise program.

whose spouses were indifferent or negative about the client's exercise program (Andrew et al. 1981).

Sidney and Shephard (1977a) reported their subjects said a lack of facilities and programs were reasons they did not exercise. Communities seldom have adequate facilities or programs attuned to the needs or preferences of elders. Our cultural attitude that elders should take it easy may discourage exercise programs for elders in a community. To encourage elders to participate, the facility must be physically accessible—within walking distance or serviced by public transportation—because transportation problems prohibit many individuals from participating in programs (Trela and Simmons 1974).

Support from the health professional also motivates a client to continue an exercise regimen. Clients respond well to individual attention from the staff and adhere to an exercise program more readily when the professional and client mutually agree on an exercise contract including objectives of the exercise program, specific instructions, time frame, and goal setting (Epstein et al. 1980). Mobily (1982) suggests a number of strategies for professionals to increase elder participation in exercise:

1. Reassure and educate elders that exercise can be done safely, taking medical history into account.
2. Make exercise prescription benefits obvious. Continue with routine evaluations to sustain the elder's interest in and motivation to exercise with emphasis on the elder's physical gains and attitude about exercise.
3. Alter elders' perception about the exercise prescription and help them maintain an accurate appraisal of the benefits and risks of exercise and set realistic expectations.
4. Create opportunities, including times and places, to exercise.

Summary

Regular physical activity can slow many physiological changes associated with age as well as prevent or control deterioration caused by chronic illness. A number of positive health benefits result from regular physical activity: reduction of body fat, increased cardiovascular efficiency, decreased fat in the bloodstream, and increased bone mass and joint mobility. Psychological and intellectual benefits have also been noted. Physical activity plays a significant role in the prevention and treatment of a number of chronic illnesses (including obesity, heart disease, hypertension, pulmonary disease, osteoporosis, lower back pain, and depression). The negative effects of physical inactivity are significant and affect many body systems. The physician has a significant role in directing people to exercise. However, the individual's motivation to begin and continue in an exercise program is the final indicator of success.

Activities

1. If you plan to work with elders, you will be a better role model if you are physically fit and have a positive attitude about exercise. To better understand your own fitness level, monitor the amount and type of exercise you engage in for two consecutive days using the following chart:

A. Type of exercise: Intensity:

   Duration: Frequency:

  Is this usual?

B. Do you feel you get enough exercise per day?

If not, why don't you exercise more?

What activities could you add to your schedule?

What other activities might you omit to make room to exercise?

Which exercise activities may carry on through old age?

C. Assess your physical fitness level by measuring how far you can walk or jog in twelve minutes: Use Table 10.1 to see how fit you are. Did your expectations coincide with your actual performance?

2. Interview five elders regarding their exercise beliefs and practices. Ask them to compare the amount and type of physical activity they currently undergo with what they did ten, twenty, and thirty years ago. Has their activity level changed? What are their reasons for changing their activity level?

3. Visit four places where you can observe individuals of all ages participating in physical activities (e.g., tennis court, swimming pool, health club, bowling alley, jogging or bike trails, aerobics class). What proportion of elders are present? What factors might prohibit their participation? How might participation be encouraged in those locations?

4. Visit a local nursing home. What physical activity programs does it offer? Who attends? How might attendance be increased?

5. Visit a local convalescent hospital. Find out how much time is spent per day per resident in physical activity. You may wish to compare the activity programs in several convalescent hospitals.

6. Using references given in this chapter, design an exercise program for a group of elders in a community setting that improves endurance, strength, flexibility, balance, coordination, and agility. Do you have variety in the program? How much can be done in a social setting? How would you motivate elders to continue the program? How does it differ from an exercise program you would be willing to participate in?

7. Design a thirty-second television or radio spot to encourage exercise in elders. What approach do you take? Who might sponsor such an advertisement?

8. Discuss exercise concepts with people of different ages: a child, a teenager, a young adult, and an older adult. Compare their perceptions of how much exercise is enough, what exercises are effective and how much they do.

9. Create a fifteen-minute educational module to educate elders in a community setting about the value of exercise for older people. Develop objectives, outline, and methodology.

10. Find out if a local hospital offers a post-coronary exercise/rehabilitation program. Interview staff to determine the clientele, kinds of exercises, drop-out rate, and ways professionals motivate clients to stay in the program.

11. Talk to a nurse or a physician in a local hospital or nursing home and find out the protocol for treatment and rehabilitation of bedridden patients. Using Olson's guidelines discussed in this chapter, outline a plan to improve their care, keeping in mind the resources available at the site.

12. You have just been hired by a local fitness center to develop a fitness program for older adults. What type of program will you design? How will you motivate elders to join and continue with the program? What types of advertisements will you use? What are some strategies you could use to motivate a chronically ill, post-coronary, bedridden, or sedentary elder to exercise?

13. What exercise programs does your community have for older adults?

Bibliography

Adams, G. M., and H. A. deVries. 1973. Physiological effects of an exercise training regimen upon females aged 52–79. *J Gerontol* 28: 50–55.

Aloia, J. F., S. H. Cohen, J. A. Ostuni, et al. 1978. Prevention of involutional bone loss by exercise. *Ann Int Med* 89: 356–58.

American College of Sports Medicine. 1980. *Guidelines for graded exercise testing and exercise prescription.* Philadelphia: Lea and Febiger.

American Heart Association. 1972a. *Exercise testing and training of individuals with heart disease or at high risk for its development: A handbook for physicians.* Dallas, Texas.

American Heart Association. 1972b. *Exercise testing and training of apparently healthy individuals: A handbook for physicians.* New York.

American Medical Association, Council on Scientific Affairs. 1981. Indications and contraindications for exercise testing. *JAMA* 246: 1015–18.

Andrew, G. W., N. B. Oldridge, and J. O. Parker. 1981. Reasons for drop-out from exercise programs in post-coronary patients. *Med Sci Sports Exerc* 13: 164–68.

Asher, R. A. 1947. The dangers of going to bed. *Br Med J* 2:967–68.

Astrand, P. O., and K. Rodahl. 1977. *Textbook of work physiology: Physiological bases of exercise.* New York: McGraw-Hill.

Bassett, C., E. McClamrock, and M. Scheizer. 1982. A 10-week exercise program for senior citizens. *Geriatr Nurs* 3: 103–5.

Berger, M., S. Haag, and N. B. Ruderman. 1975. Glucose metabolism in perfused skeletal muscle: Interaction of insulin and exercise on glucose uptake. *Biochem J* 146: 231–38.

Bjorntorp. P. 1978. Physical training in the treatment of obesity. *Int J of Obesity* 2: 149–51.

Blackburn, H. 1983. Physical activity and coronary heart disease: A brief update and population view (Parts I and II). *Cardiac Rehab* 3:101–11, 171–74.

Black-Sandler, R., R. LaPorte, D. Sashin, et al. 1982. Determinants of bone mass in menopause. *Prev Med* 11:269–80.

Bortz, W. M. 1982. Disuse and aging. *JAMA* 248: 1203–07.

Buskirk, E. R. 1974. Obesity: A brief overview with emphasis on exercise. *Fed Proc* 33: 1948–51.

Carmody, T., J. Senner, M. Malinow, and G. Matarazzo. 1980. Physical exercise rehabilitation: Long-term drop-out rate in cardiac patients. *J Behav Med* 3: 163–68.

Clark, H. H. 1974. National adult fitness survey. *Physical Fitness Research Digest* April. Washington, D.C.: President's Council on Physical Fitness and Sports.

Clausen, J. P., and J. Trap-Jensen. 1976. Heart rate and arterial blood pressure during exercise in patients with angina pectoris: Effects of training and nitroglycerin. *Circulation* 53: 436–42.

Conrad, C. 1976. When you're young at heart. *Aging.* Admin. on Aging, U.S. Dept. of HEW.

Cooper, K. H. 1982. *The aerobics program for total well-being.* New York: Bantam Books.

Danielson, R. R., and R. S. Wanzel. 1977. Exercise objectives of fitness program drop-outs. D. M. Landers and R. W. Christina, eds. In *Psychology of motor behavior and sports.* Champaign, Ill.: Human Kinetics Publ.

deVries, H. A. 1970. Physiological effects of an exercise training regimen upon men age 52–88 *J Gerontol* 25: 325–36.

deVries, H. A. 1983. Physiology of exercise and aging. D. Woodruff and J. E. Birren, eds. In *Aging.* New York: Van Nostrand. 285–304.

deVries, H. A., and G. M. Adams. 1972. Electromyographic comparison of single doses of exercise and meprobomate as to effects on muscle relaxation. *Am J Phys Med* 51: 130–41.

deVries, H. A., and D. E. Gray. 1963. Aftereffects of exercise upon resting metabolic rate. *Res Quarterly* 34: 314–21.

deVries, H. A. with D. Hales. 1982. *Fitness after 50.* New York: Charles Scribner's Sons.

Dishman, R. K. 1982. Compliance/adherance in health-related exercise. *Health Psychol* 1:237–67.

Donaldson, C., S. B. Hulley, J. M. Vogel, et al. 1970. Effect of prolonged bedrest on bone mineral. *Metabolism* 19 (12): 1071–84.

Dustman, R. E., R. O. Ruhling, E. M. Russell, at al. 1984. Aerobic exercise training and improved neurophysiological function of older individuals. *Neurobiol Aging* 5: 35–42.

Eckstein, R. W. 1957. Effects of exercise and coronary artery narrowing on collateral circulation. *Circ Res* 5: 230–35.

Eichner, E. R. 1983. Exercise and heart disease: Epidemiology of the "exercise hypothesis." *Amer J Med* 75: 1008–23.

Elsayed, M., A. H. Ismail, and R. J. Young. 1980. Intellectual differences of adult men related to age and physical fitness before and after an exercise program. *J Gerontol* 35: 383–87.

Epstein, H. E., R. R. Wing, J. K. Thompson, and W. Griffen. 1980. Attendance and fitness in aerobic exercise: The effects of contracts and lottery procedures. *Behav Modif* 4: 465–79.

Frekany, G. A., and D. K. Leslie. 1975. Effects of exercise program on selected flexibility measurements of senior citizens. *Gerontologist* 15: 182–83.

Fries, J. E., and L. M. Crapo. 1981. *Vitality and aging*. San Francisco: W. H. Freeman and Co.

Fringer, M. N., and A. G. Stull. 1974. Changes in cardiorespiratory parameters during periods of training and detraining in young female athletes. *Med Sci Sports Exerc* 6: 20–25.

Gambert, S. R., T. L. Garthwaite, T. L. Pontzer, et al. 1981. Running elevates plasma B-endorphin immuno-reactivity and ACTH on untrained human subjects. *Proc Soc Exp Biol Med* 168: 1–4.

Garabrant, D. H., J. M. Peters, T. M. Mack, and L. Bernstein. 1984. Job activity and colon cancer risk. *Am J Epidemiol* 119 (6): 1005–14.

Gormally, J., D. Rardin, and S. Black. 1980. Correlates of successful response to a behavioral weight control clinic. *J Counsel Psychol* 27: 179–91.

Greist, J., M. Kleen, R. Eischens, et al. 1979. Running as a treatment for depression. *Comp Psychiatry* 20: 41–54.

Hanson, P., and R. Kochan. 1983. Exercise and diabetes. *Primary Care* 10(4): 653–62.

Haskell, W. L. 1984. Exercise-induced changes in plasma lipids and lipoproteins. *Prev Med* 13: 23–36.

Hayden, R. M., and G. J. Allen. 1984. Relationship between aerobic exercise, anxiety, and depression. *J Sports Med* 24 (1): 69–74.

Heizelmann, F., and R. W. Bagley. 1970. Responses to physical activity and their effects on health behavior. *Public Health Rep* 85: 905–11.

Holloszy, J. O., J. S. Skinner, G. Toro, and T. K. Curetin. 1964. Effects of a six month program for endurance exercise on serum levels lipids of middle-aged men. *Am J Cardiol* 14: 753–60.

Howley, E. T. 1976. The effects of different intensities of exercise on the excretion of epinephrine and norepinephrine. *Med Sci Sports Exerc* 8: 219–22.

Hughes, J. R. 1984. Psychological effects of habitual aerobic exercise: A critical review. *Prev Med* 13: 66–68.

Jette, D. V. 1984. Physiological effects of exercise in the diabetic. *Phys Ther* 64 (3): 339–42.

Kala, R., M. Romo, P. Stiltanen, and P. Halonen. 1978. Physical activity and sudden cardiac death. *Adv Cardiol* 25: 27–34.

Karvonen, M. S., E. Kentala, and O. Mustala. 1957. The effects of training heart rate: A longitudinal study. *Ann Med Exp Biol Fenn* 35: 307–15.

Kasch, F. W., and J. Kulberg. 1981. Physiological variables during 15 years of endurance exercise. *Scand J Sports Sci* 3 (2): 59–62.

Kavenaugh, T., and R. J. Shephard. 1977. The effects of continued training and the aging process. *Ann NY Acad Sci* 301: 656–70.

Kemmer, F. W., and M. Berger. 1984. Exercise in therapy and the life of diabetic patients. *Clin Sci* 67: 279–83.

Kottke, T. E., C. J. Caspersen, and C. S. Hill. 1984. Exercise in the management and rehabilitation of selected chronic diseases. *Prev Med* 13: 47–65.

Kraus, H. 1970. *Clinical treatment of back and neck pain*. New York: McGraw-Hill.

Kraus, H., A. Melleby, and S. R. Gaston. 1977. Back pain correction and prevention: National voluntary organizational approach. *NY State J Med* 7: 1335–38.

Kraus, H., and W. Raab. 1961. *Hypokinetic disease*. Springfield, Ill.: Charles C. Thomas Publisher.

Lane, N. E., D. A. Block, H. H. Jones, et al. 1986. Long distance running, bone density and osteoarthritis. *JAMA* 255(9): 1147–51.

Levy, R. I. 1981. *Exercise and your heart*. (NIH publ. 81–1677). Washington: U.S. Dept. of HHS.

Lonnerblad, L. 1984. Exercises to promote independent living in older patients. *Geriatrics* 39 (2): 93–101.

Martin, R. P., W. L. Haskell, and P. D. Wood. 1977. Blood chemistry and lipid profiles of elite distance runners. *Ann NY Acad Sci* 301: 346–60.

Massie, J. F., and R. J. Shephard. 1971. Physiological and psychological effects of training: A comparison of individual and gymnasium programs with a characterization of the exercise "drop out." *Med Sci Sports Exerc* 3: 110–17.

Mayer, J. 1968. *Overweight: Causes, cost and control*. Englewood Cliffs, N.J.: Prentice-Hall Inc.

McCann, L., and D. S. Holmes. 1984. Influence of aerobic exercise on depression. *J Pers Soc Psychol* 46 (5): 1142–47.

Milhorn, H. T. 1984. Prescribing a cardiovascular fitness program. *Comp Ther* 10 (2): 46–53.

Mobily, K. E. 1982. Motivational aspects of exercise for the elderly: Barriers and solutions. *Phys Occ Ther Geriatr* 1 (4): 43–53.

Moritani, T., and H. A. deVries. 1980. Potential for gross muscle hypertrophy in older men. *J Gerontol* 35(5): 672–82.

Moser, K., G. Bokensky, R. Savage, et al. 1980. Results of a comprehensive rehabilitation program: Physiological and functional effects on patients with chronic obstructive pulmonary disease. *Arch Intern Med* 140: 1596–1601.

Munns, K. 1981. Effects of exercise on the range of joint motion in elderly subjects. L. Smith and R. C. Serfass, eds. In *Exercise and aging.* Hillside, N.J.: Enslow Publishers. 167–78.

National Council on Aging. 1975. *The myth and reality of aging in America.* Washington, D.C.

Nilsson, B., and N. Westlin. 1971. Bone density in athletes. *Clin Orthoped* 77: 179–82.

Nolewajka, A. J., W. J. Kostuk, P. A. Rechnitzer, et al. 1979. Exercise and human collaterization: An angina graphic with scientigraphic assessment. *Circulation* 60: 114–21.

Olson, E. V. 1967. The hazards of immobility. *Am J Nurs* 67(2): 779–97.

Overstall, P. W. 1980. Prevention of falls in the elderly. *J Am Geriatr Soc* 18 (11): 481–84.

Oyster, N., M. Morton, and S. Linnell. 1984. Physical activity and osteoporosis in post-menopausal women. *Med Sci Sports Exerc* 16 (1): 44–50.

Paffenbarger, R. S., and W. E. Hale. 1975. Work activity and coronary heart mortality. *N Engl J Med* 292 (11): 545–50.

Paffenbarger, R. S., and R. T. Hyde. 1984. Exercise in the prevention of coronary heart disease. *Prev Med* 13: 3–22.

Paffenbarger, R. S., R. T. Hyde, A. L. Wing, and C. Hseih. 1986. Physical activity, all-cause mortality and longevity of college alumni. *N Engl J Med* 314(10): 605–612.

Paffenbarger, R. S., A. L. Wing, and R. T. Hyde. 1978. Physical activity as an index of heart attack risk in college alumni. *Am J Epidemiol* 108: 161–75.

Paffenbarger, R. S., A. L. Wing, R. T. Hyde, and D. L. Jung. 1983. Physical activity and incidence of hypertension in college alumni. *Am J of Epidemiol* 117 (3): 245–57.

Pardini, A. 1984. Exercise, vitality and aging. *Aging* Apr–May, No. 344, 20–29.

Perri, S., and D. I. Templer, 1984–1985. The effects of an aerobic exercise program on psychological variables in older adults. *Int J Aging and Hum Dev* 20(3): 167–72.

Petty, T. L., and R. M. Cherniak. 1981. Comprehensive care of COPD. *Clin Notes Resp Care* 20 (3): 3–12.

Pollock, M. L. 1978. How much exercise is enough? *Phys Sport Med* 6 (6): 50–64.

Pollock, M. L., J. H. Wilmore, and S. M. Fox. 1984. *Exercise in health and disease.* Philadelphia: W. B. Saunders Co.

Powell, E. 1974. Physiological effects of exercise therapy on institutionalized geriatric mental patients. *J Gerontol* 29: 157–61.

Rauramaa, R. 1984. Relationship of physical activity, glucose tolerance, and weight management. *Prev Med* 13: 37–46.

Roundy, E. S., G. A. Fisher, and S. Anderson. 1978. Effect of exercise on serum lipids and lipoproteins. *Med Sci Sports Exerc* 10:55.

Saltin, B. Lindgarde, F. M. Housten, et al. 1979. Physical training and glucose tolerance in middle-aged men with chemical disabilities. *Diabetes* 288 (suppl. 1): 30–32.

Schultz, C., E. Bernaur, P. A. Mole, et al. 1980. Effects of severe caloric restriction and moderate exercise in basal metabolic rate and hormonal status in adult humans. *Fed of Am Soc Exp Biol* 39: 783.

Serfass, R. C., and S. G. Gerberich. 1984. Exercise for optimal health: Strategies and motivational considerations. *Prev Med* 13: 79–99.

Shephard, R. J. 1983. The value of exercise in ischemic heart disease: A cumulative analysis. *J Cardiac Rehab* 3:294–98.

Chapter 10

Shephard, R. J. 1977. *Endurance and fitness.* Toronto: University of Toronto Press.

Sherwood, D. E., and D. J. Selder. 1979. Cardiorespiratory health, reaction time, and aging. *Med Sci Sports Exerc* 11: 186–89.

Sidney, K. H., and R. J. Shephard. 1977a. Activity patterns of elderly men and women. *J Gerontol* 32: 25–32.

Sidney, K. H., and R. J. Shephard. 1977b. Perception of exertion in the elderly: Effects of aging, mode of exercise and physical training. *Percept Mot Skills* 44: 999–1010.

Siscovick, R., N. S. Weiss, R. H. Fletcher, and T. Lasky, 1984. The incidence of primary cardiac arrest during vigorous exercise. *N Engl J Med* 311 (14): 874–77.

Smith, E. L., W. Redden, and P. E. Smith. 1981. Physical activity and calcium modalities for bone mineral increase in aged women. *Med Sci Sports Exerc* 13: 60–64.

Stern, J. S. 1984. Is obesity a disease of inactivity? *Eating and its disorders* 62: 131–39.

Thomas, G. S., P. R. Lee, P. Franks, and R. S. Paffenbarger. 1981. *Exercise and health, the evidence and the implications.* Cambridge, Mass.: Oelgeschlager, Gunn & Hain, Inc.

Thompson, P. D., E. J. Funk, R. A. Carleton, and W. Q. Sturner. 1982. Incidence of death during jogging in Rhode Island from 1975 to 1980. *JAMA* 247: 2535–38.

Thornberry, O. T., R. W. Wilson, and P. M Golden. 1986. Health promotion data for the 1990 objectives: Estimates from the Health Interview Survey of Health Promotion and Disease Prevention. United States 1985. *NCHS Advance Data for Vital and Health Statistics.* No. 126, Sept. 19, 1986.

Tipton, C. M. 1984. Exercise, training, and hypertension. *Exerc Sport Sci Rev* 12: 245–306.

Trela, J. E., and L. W. Simmons. 1971. Health and other factors affecting membership and attrition in a senior center. *J Gerontol* 26: 46–51.

Williams, M. A., D. J. Esterbrooks, and M. H. Sketch. 1984. Guidelines for exercise therapy of the elderly after myocardial infarction. *Eur Heart J* 5: 121–23.

Williams, M. A., C. M. Maresh, D. J. Esterbrooks, et al. 1985. Early exercise training in patients older than age 65 years compared with that in younger patients after acute myocardial infarction or coronary artery bypass grafting. *Am J Cardiol* 55: 263–66.

Williams, R. S., E. E. Logue, J. L. Lewis, et al. 1980. Physical conditioning augments the fibronolytic response to venus occlusion in healthy adults. *N Engl J Med* 302 (18) 987–91.

Wilmore, J. H. 1977. Acute and chronic physiological responses to exercise. E. A. Amsterdam, J. H. Wilmore, and A. N. De Maria, eds. In *Exercise in cardiovascular health and disease.* New York: York Medical Books. 26–63.

Wilmore, J. H., J. Royce, R. N. Girandola, et al. 1970. Physiological alteration resulting from a 10 week program of jogging. *Med Sci Sports Exerc* 2: 7–14.

Wood, P. D., W. L. Haskell, S. N. Blair, et al. 1983. Increased exercise level and plasma lipoprotein concentrations: A one-year randomized, controlled study on sedentary middle-aged men. *Metabolism* 32: 31–39.

Woolbright, J. L. 1983. Exercise protocol for patients with chronic back pain. *J Am Osteopath Assoc* 82 (12): 919–32.

Zuti, W. B., and L. A. Golding. 1976. Comparing diet and exercise as weight reduction tools. *Physi Sport Med* 4: 49–53.

11

Sexuality

I think sex should be confined to one's lifetime.
Woody Allen

Introduction

Sexuality includes a broad range of erotic feelings and behaviors expressed in various ways throughout life. Expressions of sexuality encompass a wide range of activities including sexual fantasy, a child nursing at the breast, affectionate hugs among friends, flirtatious glances, and genital intercourse among lovers. Attitudes and behaviors regarding sexuality are an integral part of personality. Early sexual attitudes and experiences have a significant impact on our expression of sexuality at all levels. The views of families, peers, and culture also tremendously influence sexuality by defining which behavior is acceptable and which is not.

While most people have little trouble understanding that young adults have sexual needs, their idealized view of the older adult does not include sex. However, elders do have sexual desires and the capacity to enjoy sexual intercourse. This chapter discusses the misconceptions of elder sexuality and explores the gamut of sexual behavior in later years, including variations in sexual behavior among sub-groups. Sexual dysfunction, its causes, diagnosis, and treatment will also be addressed. Accurate information about sexuality in later life will enable professionals to better relate to elders and provide an accepting atmosphere to meet their range of sexual needs. Such knowledge also facilitates a realistic perspective of sexuality in our own later years.

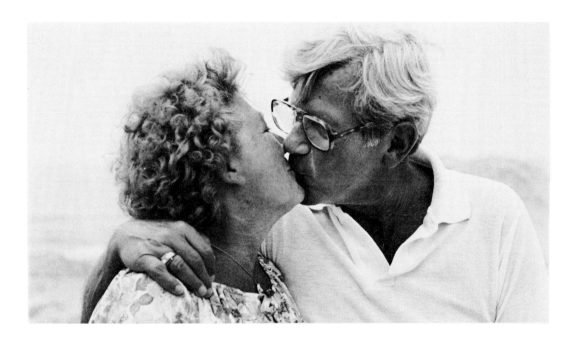

Stereotypes of Elder Sexuality

The topic of elder sexuality is wrought with misinformation and bias, which, in turn, affect our attitudes towards older people, and ultimately our sexual feelings and behavior in later life. These myths also add to our fear of losing sexual function with age. A discussion of some of the more common misconceptions about aging and sexuality follows.

"Sexuality is reserved for the young"

Americans generally associate sexuality with the physical characteristics of youth: beautiful young women with firm and shapely bodies, and muscular, slim-hipped men are the archetype of sexual attractiveness. To a much larger extent than we may realize, images on television, motion pictures, and magazines both shape and reflect our impressions of what is beautiful or sexy. Because older persons (and most of the younger population) do not conform to the popular conception of sex appeal, nobody wants to grow old. The cosmetic industry takes advantage of this fear of growing old by turning our fear into their profit.

A preponderance of products—face creams, age spot removers, hair dyes to cover the grey—reinforce our fear of aging and consequent loss of sexual attractiveness.

The belief that only the young are sexually appealing damages young and old alike. The prejudices of the young against growing old will continue as the young age, eventually making them the victims of their own negative attitudes. Older women seem to be especially affected by society's narrow image of female sexuality. Revised definitions of sex appeal that can withstand the physical changes of age (e.g., grace, competence, sexual energy, playfulness) are necessary to ease the fear of the inevitable changes in appearance that accompany aging.

"Elders' sexual needs are amusing or insignificant"

Elder lovers expressing affection in public are often described as "cute" and commented on as if they were children—amusing, but not to be taken seriously. Physicians may also consider elder sexuality inconsequential. Few take a sexual history or discuss sexual concerns with older patients. They may respond to a patient's concerns in this area with comments such as, "It's not that important at your age," or "That's natural. You're just growing old." As sexual dysfunction may be a symptom or consequence of disease or a side-effect of many common medications, the discussion of sexual issues is critical to accurate diagnosis and treatment.

On a research level, early studies of sexuality did not give elder sexuality adequate attention. Kinsey and colleagues, one of the first human sexuality researchers, devoted only three pages of 1700 to describe the sexuality of those over sixty (1948, 1953). Later, Masters and Johnson's classic work (1966) studied the physiology of the human sexual response, but only thirty-one of a total of 694 subjects were over sixty. These scholars admitted that more studies needed to be conducted on elders. Nevertheless, little subsequent research has expanded or replicated their preliminary impressions.

"Older people don't enjoy sex. If they do, it's abnormal"

Many younger people find it difficult to accept emotionally that older people engage in sexual intercourse. Perhaps this occurs because they unconsciously envision the old as an extension of their parents. In 1977, a large group of college students were requested to estimate the frequency of sexual intercourse of their parents. Even though 90 percent of those students believed their parents to be happily married, when the students' estimates of frequency of sexual intercourse of their parents were compared to Kinsey's data, the students consistently underrated their parents' sexual activity (Pocs et al. 1977). If students underestimate sexual frequency of their parents, it is likely that inconsistencies between the expected and actual frequency of sexual interaction of their grandparents is even greater.

Young people may underestimate the frequency that older people have intercourse because they find sexual intercourse among older people to be immoral, disgraceful, or distasteful. Adult children often have difficulty seeing their parents as adults with sexual feelings. This belief is especially common among adult children with a sexually active parent who is widowed. (For example, see the play, "It's Time We Sat Down and Talked about Sex—Again" page 308.

Data from Starr and Weiner (1981) contradict the attitude that older people do not think about or enjoy sex. When over eight hundred elders between sixty and ninety-one were asked, "Do you like sex?", 96 percent of the women and 99 percent of the men answered affirmatively. Eighty-four percent of both men and women believed touching and cuddling to be very important in their lives. Seventy-five percent of men and 55 percent of women responded that they got excited looking at sexy pictures, books, and movies. On the average, both men and women in the sample said they would like intercourse twice weekly.

"Sexual ability is lost with age"

The misconception that elders have a diminished ability to have sexual relations is often promoted on television and in the print media. For instance, a joke book, *Sex over Sixty,* had nothing but hundreds of empty pages, implying that older people don't have sex—or any sex worth writing about. Verses in birthday cards also perpetuate the view that sex and age are mutually exclusive. The following are only a few of the many light-hearted, but insidious, verses describing sexual inactivity in the later years.

At our age, sex is like birthdays, it happens once a year.

Don't worry about another birthday: you're not old until your whoop-de-doo turns to whoop-de-don't.

Don't worry about being a year older. You still know where it's at—the hard part is remembering what it's for.

On your birthday, remember: you're never too old to do it. 'Course you may be too old to survive the experience.

A common belief about aging and sexual activity is that older men can't have intercourse even if they want to because impotence is a natural part of growing older. Many believe the decline in ability to have an erection starts in the forties, worsens in the fifties, and by sixty, men are "over the hill." In fact, impotence is not a result of the aging process, but is due to factors that can happen at any age. Studies consistently show sexual activity is possible into the eighties and nineties.

Many individuals mistakenly believe that women do not enjoy intercourse after menopause. Data from the Starr-Weiner study (1981) disprove the misconception: about 40 percent of females over sixty reported sex to be better than when they were younger. Almost half said it was the same and less than one-tenth said it worsened. Women retain the capacity to become sexually excited and orgasmic throughout life.

The belief that sexual ability is lost with age is harmful because it may act as a self-fulfilling prophecy. If sexual activity is expected to decline, it probably will.

Sexual Activity in Later Life

Although sexual behavior encompasses more than intercourse and masturbation, these behaviors capture researchers' attention because they are isolated, easily measured events. However, numerical data on frequency of sexual intercourse and masturbation present a limited view of sexuality. Other sexual behaviors such as cuddling and kissing are important, but seldom measured. As one grows older, these other sexual activities may occur more frequently, even though intercourse frequency may decrease. Thus, if other activities were measured, elders may have as much or more sexual activity than younger adults.

Intercourse

Kinsey and colleagues (1948, 1953) were the first to systematically explore the frequency of intercourse in the adult years. They reported that, although sexual intercourse persisted in later life,

both men and women exhibited a general decline in that activity with age. The sexual frequency of males age sixty–sixty-nine was 1.3 times a week; ages seventy and over, once a week. Twenty percent of his male sample were sexually inactive at age sixty. By age seventy, 30 percent were inactive, and by eighty, 75 percent were sexually inactive (1948). Men were reportedly more sexually active than women, likely because women's sexual activity was dependent on the presence and interest of a male partner.

More recently, Starr and Weiner's sample of more than eight hundred elders reported an average frequency of intercourse of 1.4 times per week for those who reported sexual activity (1981). Approximately 7 percent of their male sample were sexually inactive; almost 30 percent of their female sample were inactive. When the data were separated by age, a drastic difference occurred in the number of women who were sexually inactive. Of those women between the ages of sixty–sixty-nine, 22 percent were inactive, in the age group seventy–seventy-nine, 38 percent were inactive, and in those age eighty–ninety-one, 57 percent did not engage in sexual intercourse. As in earlier studies, these data reflect the lack of a male partner for most elder females. Among elder males, 7.2 percent of males in their sixties were inactive, compared to 15 percent in their eighties.

However, the decline in sexual activity may not be as great as was once assumed. Some researchers assert that elders may have intercourse less often than younger groups, but this does not reflect a change with age but rather that those who are now old engaged in intercourse less frequently when young than today's younger adults. George and Weiler (1981) reanalyzed the data from the Duke Longitudinal Study and reported that levels of sexual activity tend to remain stable over middle and later life. Martin (1981) reviewed the data from the subjects in the Baltimore Longitudinal Study and reported similar findings. His sample of 750 older respondents did not appreciably differ from a comparable group fourteen years younger with respect to a number of sexual activity variables. He demonstrated that many older men are as sexually vigorous as much younger men and that male sexual vigor is sustained by factors that are not necessarily related to age.

Reports on the frequency of sexual intercourse in elders raise serious questions as to whether samples are representative of the elder population. Some samples obtain elders from outpatient clinics while others use middle-class white community volunteers. Samples may include a greater proportion of elders who have diseases, ones who volunteer for studies, or those who have an interest in disclosing information about their sex life. Further, it is questionable whether younger or older subjects may lie about their frequency of intercourse. Cross-sectional studies do not take cohort differences into account. Does intercourse frequency decrease with age or did today's elders have less intercourse when younger? More longitudinal studies are needed to determine whether or not frequency of intercourse changes with age. Further, studies should control for marital status when analyzing the relationship between age and sexual activity. Unless marital status is controlled, studies may attribute lower levels of sexual activity to age when in fact reduced levels of activity are due to a lack of a partner.

The frequency of sexual intercourse has a strong cultural component. For instance Marshall's study (1971) of the sexual activity of Mangaian men in Polynesia reported a decrease in frequency of sexual intercourse with age. In Polynesian men, the average number of orgasms decreased from three per night in eighteen year old males to once a night in males in their late forties. However, even with the drop in frequency, the average frequency of sexual intercourse among elder men was still significantly higher than their North American counterparts. In another culture, Merriam (1971) questioned eleven men from Bala whose ages ranged from twenty-two to sixty-six. He reported the lowest frequency of intercourse in the sample to be 1.2 times per day. The average frequency reported

by the oldest subject was 1.5 times per day. Winn and Newton (1982) reported coital frequency of the sexual activity of the Mayurbhanj Santal of India to be once a day for males at sixty, often maintaining that frequency at age seventy. The average sexual frequency of young males was two to four times a day.

These data support the findings that those who engage in high activity in early life maintain high levels in their later years. Further, it suggests that cultural constraints may have more effect on frequency of intercourse than physiological changes due to age. However, as in all studies using self-reports, the subjects may have exaggerated their actual frequencies.

Factors Influencing Intercourse Frequency

The most obvious factor influencing the frequency of intercourse in the later years is the availability of a partner, especially for women. Kinsey (1953) interviewed fifty-six women over age sixty and reported that 80 percent of those who were married reported intercourse at least once in two weeks, but only 20 percent of those who were unmarried reported coitus, all reporting a frequency of less than once weekly. Christenson and Gagnon (1965) studied a group of 241 women age fifty and older and reported that although age had an effect on sexual frequency, marital status was an even better predictor of frequency of coitus. Sexual frequency decreased with advancing age among those who were married (80 percent had intercourse at least once a week at age fifty; at age sixty-five, 50 percent engaged in intercourse at least once a week). Less than 40 percent of unmarried women at age fifty had intercourse at least once a week and all unmarried women over age sixty-five in their study reported no intercourse. These researchers reported that the husband's age was a significant factor in determining the frequency of coitus in married women. Women whose husbands were younger than they reported higher rates of intercourse than those with older husbands. Later reports by Pfeiffer et al. (1968) reiterated the point that cessation of sexual activity for both sexes is dependent on the interest and ability of the male partner.

Even if a partner is available, other factors influence intercourse frequency. Masters and Johnson (1966) attribute decreased frequency in all age groups to six variables: boredom with partner, preoccupation with career or economic pursuits, mental or physical fatigue, overindulgence in food or drink, physical and mental infirmities of individual or partner, and fear of impotence. Butler and Lewis (1976) suggest that marital tension in the later years reduces sexual desire and frequency. A number of studies indicate that past sexual experience, interest, and enjoyment is highly correlated with present sexual interest and activity in older men (Masters and Johnson 1966; Pfeiffer et al. 1972; Martin 1981) For older women, past sexual enjoyment (Pfeiffer et al. 1972) and a secure and warm relationship with a socially appropriate male (Masters and Johnson 1966) were significantly correlated with current sexual activity.

Martin (1981) asserts that much of the variation in sexual frequency among men can be explained by the variation in intensity of their sexual desire. He found no correlation between frequency of sexual expression and marital adjustment, sexual attractiveness of wives, or negative sexual attitudes. Subjects who had infrequent intercourse did not feel performance anxiety, sexual deprivation, or low self-esteem. He reports that the decline of their sexual functioning was due to a corresponding decline in motivation. Thus, those men who did not engage in sexual intercourse were inactive by choice, not because of inability.

Elders who are not motivated to engage in sexual activity may encounter pressure from those who believe intercourse to be one of life's necessities. A number of gerontologists espouse the value of genital sex and describe the negative effects of sexual deprivation (Genevay 1978; Masters and Johnson 1966; Kaplan 1979). When intercourse is seen as therapy or important preventive medicine, it may generate a subtle pressure for elders to keep up sexual performance as

> Aging makes sex less imperative. You can take it or leave it, and that uncovers something that is precious. I can report that women look better to me now than they did when I was young because when I was young, sex was demanding. It was ego; I could be attracted to a woman that I despised, and then not feel good about myself. Now it seems possible to admire only women whom I like, which feels good. It feels cleaner and purer.

Abraham Maslow (1972)

a kind of health insurance (Thomas 1982). It can be very threatening if a partner stops sexual activity or has lessened sexual desire. It is especially harmful to tell older women that intercourse is needed to maintain genital health, especially since most do not have partners. There is no doubt that sexual intercourse is pleasurable. However, other activities promote intimacy and sexual feelings. Thomas (1982) asserts that gerontologists must not project the sexual agendas of the younger years onto older people, but rather should consult with elders about what sexuality means to them.

Masturbation

The frequency of masturbation has not been widely investigated in older people despite the benefits that may be associated with this form of sexual expression. Because it is such a sensitive topic, it is difficult to obtain accurate information about elders' masturbatory practices. Although the vast majority of men and women have masturbated sometime in their life, there are severe prejudices against it. Masturbation, or auto-erotocism, has been considered a sin throughout Christian history and many religious groups still believe it to be immoral. Only during the last few years has auto-erotocism been acknowledged as a normal and beneficial activity for all age groups.

The frequency of masturbation among elders depends upon marital status: those with partners masturbate less frequently than those without. Christenson and Gagnon (1965) interviewed 241 women over fifty and reported that masturbation decreased with age, but twice as many single women masturbated than married women. Starr and Weiner (1981) reported in their sample of over eight hundred elders that 43 percent of the men and 47 percent of the women masturbated. Of those men and women who masturbated, over half reported that they engaged in the activity once a month or more. For men, masturbation occurred in 40 percent of the married group, 44 percent of those widowed, 57 percent of those divorced, and 69 percent of those who were never married. For women, masturbation was practiced in 39 percent of those who were married, 47 percent of those widowed, 66 percent of those divorced, and 81 percent of those who were never married. It is evident by the data that lack of a partner influences masturbatory frequency. Further, Catania and White (1982) reported that older people who feel more in control of their lives masturbate more frequently.

Masturbation is beneficial, both physiologically and psychologically. It maintains the elasticity and lubrication of the vagina for women and preserves erectile ability for men. During orgasm, the adrenal glands release cortisol, a natural painkiller. Orgasms are also known to reduce stress and induce sleep. Masturbation allows individuals to control their own sexuality. Catania and White (1982) hypothesize that masturbation maintains sexual identity. For those elderly persons who have lost a sexual partner through death or infirmity, masturbation offers a form of sexual release that can prevent depression, frustration, and hostility (Masters and Johnson 1966: Barbach 1975). Masturbation also stimulates sexual appetite and is a way to enjoy sexuality without relying on a partner. Despite its benefits, few health professionals are willing to broach the topic

with elders. Discussion of the option of masturbation for those without a functioning partner would assist elders to be more comfortable with this aspect of their sexual expression.

Sexuality in Special Elder Populations

Although frequency statistics are helpful in gaining a general picture of elder sexuality, many ignore the sexual needs of special elder populations. This section will examine the sexual practices of older unmarried women, elder homosexuals, institutionalized elders, and the chronically ill.

Older Unmarried Women

Women without spouses comprise a large proportion of the elder population and include the never-married, divorced, and widowed. Older women are less likely to have a male partner than women of other age groups. The fact that women live longer than men accounts for a great deal of this imbalance. Women outnumber men at all ages over sixty-five and the gap widens with advancing age. In 1985, there were eighty-two men between age sixty-five–sixty-nine for every one hundred women in that age group. There were only forty men for every one hundred women at age eighty-five and older. Women tend to marry men older than they, making the probability of widowhood even greater. In 1985, older men were twice as likely to be married as older women. There were five times as many older widows as widowers. Black women are even more likely to be widowed; in 1982 almost eight of ten American black women seventy-five and over were widowed (U.S. Bureau of the Census 1982). The average age of widowhood in our country is fifty-nine. Because of this sex differential, older men are seven times more likely to remarry than older women, usually to younger women (U.S. Senate, Special Committee on Aging 1984).

Societal attitudes are also responsible for the lack of male partners for older women. Older men are more likely to seek relationships with younger women than women their age or older. This has been attributed largely to our cultural attitude that a man's value is determined more by career success than a youthful appearance, but a woman's value is determined more by how young she looks than what she does (Sontag 1972). Although there are many advantages of older women-younger men relationships, the trend in that direction is not significant and is unlikely to affect those already in their later years.

Not all older women are seeking a husband. Many older widows are not willing to forgo their independence to nurse an older man or to deal with problems of adult stepchildren (Solnick and Corby 1983).

As heterosexual relationships may not be a viable alternative for many older women, they may explore other avenues of sexual satisfaction to increase control of their sexuality. The alternatives include a range of physical and emotional expressions, such as expanding affectional relationships with men and women, exploring sexual fantasy, erotic books and movies, and masturbation. When 518 elder women were asked how older women can deal with their sexual feelings if they do not have partners, 43 percent suggested diversionary activities, such as hobbies, exercise, community affairs, or keeping busy in general. Eleven percent suggested masturbation and about 20 percent suggested finding a partner. Kassel (1966) suggests that polygamy be encouraged in later years. Maggie Kuhn, the founder of the Gray Panthers, suggests that older women experiment with bisexuality and homosexuality to meet their needs for sexual expression since few men are available to older women (1977). However, it is unlikely that the last two options will receive serious consideration among most older women.

Elder Homosexuality

Kimmel (1978) estimates that 10 percent of the older population are homosexuals. However, the vast majority of elder homosexuals have not come out of the closet to identify themselves with the gay rights movement. Thus, many have no support for their orientation and must deal with aging and the added stigma of societal prejudices and fear of being found out.

Most older lesbian couples have been partners for many years.

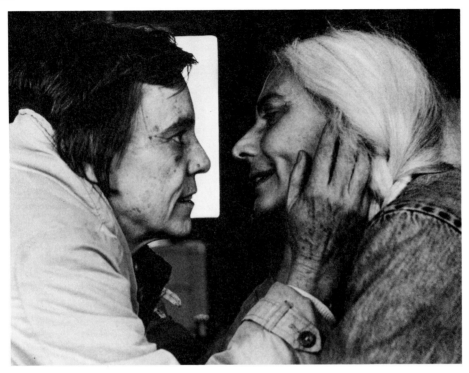

Prejudices and stereotypes about older gays (term usually used for male homosexuals) and lesbians (female homosexuals) abound in our culture. Until 1973, the American Psychiatric Association considered homosexuality to be a mental disorder. It wasn't until 1975 that its members declared that homosexuality implied no impairment in judgement, stability, reliability, or general social or vocational capabilities. Despite this long-overdue declaration, myths about lesbians and gays persist. The image of older lesbians is that they are a lonely, pathetic, and troubled group that somehow missed having a relationship with "a good man," "the right man," or just "any man" (Almvig 1982). For gay males, the stereotype persists that they are unhappy and have no close relationships. Although research on elder homosexuals is sparse, evidence is accumulating to dispute those stereotypes.

An extensive study by Almvig (1982) explored the lives of seventy-four lesbians over fifty. The subjects were members of lesbian organizations and were generally white middle-class. Almost half had been married and one-third had children. The sample represented a picture of healthy adjustment: over half reported themselves to be in excellent mental health (only 2 percent felt unstable or unhappy). Lesbians in this sample were likely to practice serial monogamy—a series of long-term, monogamous relationships with other women throughout their lives. About three-fourths of the sample had five or fewer serious lovers in their lifetime. Almost half were currently in relationships that had lasted from six months to over thirty years; most had been in the same relationship for five years or more, and half had relationships that had lasted at least fifteen years. About one-third reported they had no sex partners within the past year. However, a number of lesbians in the study were not monogamous.

It is generally reported that women's goals in intimate relationships are similar whether their partners are males or females. They look for personality, hygiene, intelligence, and manners. One researcher asserted that lesbian relationships resemble close friendships with the added component of romantic and erotic attraction (Peplau 1981).

Research on elder gays is also sparse. The largest elder study (Berger 1982), questioned 112 highly educated homosexual men between the ages of forty and seventy-nine. The men reported levels of life satisfaction as high or higher than those of older men and women in the general population. Three-fourths of the men were at least somewhat satisfied with their sex lives. Older gay men seemed less anxious about their sexual orientation when compared with younger gays. Most men in the study (86.6 percent) rated themselves as exclusively homosexual. This figure differs from younger samples. Whether older men become more exclusive with age or whether younger men feel freer to express both homosexual and heterosexual tendencies is not known. Almost three-fourths of the men in Berger's study never married. Those who did marry unrealistically expected that marriage would change their sexual orientation. Contrary to popular belief, the older homosexual man is not isolated. Over 60 percent lived with others. Most lived only with their lovers although combinations of lover, roommates, and family were reported.

With regard to sexual attitudes and behavior, the vast majority of elder gay men continued interest and participation in sexual activity at a high level. Over 60 percent engaged in same-sex relations about once a week or more. Only 6.3 percent reported no sexual activity within the past six months. The group was very diverse: many engaged in sexual activity several times a week and many others did so only a few times a year

or less. The number of same-sex partners reported within the past six months varied considerably. Although the majority (60 percent) limited their activity to one partner, almost one-fourth reported three or more partners within the six-month period. Most were not currently in an exclusive relationship, but had been in the past. It is generally agreed that older gays maintain their frequency of sexual activity through their later years, but with fewer partners than when young (Berger 1982).

Most health and social service personnel lack consideration and sensitivity regarding the special needs of elder gays and lesbians. Staff of hospitals and nursing homes need to be sensitized that a same-sex lover may not be a legal partner, but is important to the resident's well-being. Providing space for conjugal visits in group homes for gay/lesbian couples is important. Losing a same-sex partner after many years has as much impact on an individual as losing a spouse. However, widowhood groups seldom, if ever, include grieving gay or lesbian partners. Programs to help the bereaved deal with legal problems that are unique to lesbians and gay men are seldom addressed.

Many elder gay and lesbian couples do not use traditional services offered to elders for fear of disclosure of their sexual orientation. To counteract this tendency, a number of services for gay and lesbian elders have been initiated in big cities; for instance, services to homebound elderly gays, hospice programs, housing programs, and an information and referral service. Although some agencies have initiated services specifically for elder homosexuals, some existing agencies (e.g., YMCA and Senior Multipurpose Centers) are expanding their services to meet the needs of elder homosexuals (Raphael and Robinson 1981). Lesbians and gays who are active in professional organizations (psychologists, social workers, nurses) are working to enlighten their peers on the needs of lesbian and gay people. The National Association for Lesbian and Gay Gerontologists (3312

Descanso Drive, Los Angeles, Ca. 90026) was formed to provide information and support for persons concerned with lesbian and gay aging issues.

Institutionalized Elders

The sexual needs of institutionalized elders are seldom addressed. Reports on sexual behavior in nursing homes suggest that many residents have unmet sexual needs. A study of 250 elders in fifteen nursing homes across the country (White 1982) reported 91 percent of the respondents had neither masturbated nor had sexual intercourse in the month prior to the interview. However, one-sixth of the inactive group reported that they would be interested, but lacked the opportunity (e.g., had no willing or desirable partner, lacked privacy). The study also indicated that elders' sexual attitudes, sexual knowledge, and history of frequent sexual activity was a strong predictor of sexual activity while in the nursing home.

It is unrealistic to expect that all, or even most, institutionalized elders have the interest or capacity for genital sexuality. The majority of the residents have a number of serious disabling illnesses that impact upon their sexuality. Brain damage and medications interfere with sexual desire and potency. Most are more concerned with the day-to-day living, eating, and body care than thoughts of sexual activity. Nevertheless, a number of institutionalized elders might participate in a broader range of sexual activity given a supportive environment.

Research indicates that most institutionalized elders believe themselves to have aged beyond an active sex life for themselves but see it as acceptable for others in the facility. In one study, the residents ranked "remaining physically attractive" as the most important and acceptable way for themselves to express sexuality. However, the majority report they do not feel sexually attractive (Kaas 1978). White (1982) reported the institutionalized females in his study unanimously reported they felt unattractive to the opposite sex. These findings are likely a reflection of the connection our culture envisions between youthful beauty and sexuality for women. These studies point to the importance of assisting elders to be clean and well-dressed, with attention to hair, face, nails, and skin in order to maintain feelings of masculinity and femininity. Such care may be especially important to older women in order for them to maintain or increase feelings of sexual attractiveness and sexual identity.

The nursing home setting, directly or indirectly, deprives elders of their sexual rights. Lack of privacy is commonly reported to influence sexual activity within nursing homes (White 1982; Kaas 1978). Few places offer privacy for married couples, and even fewer attend to the needs of the unmarried. Privacy is created in some homes by setting aside a room in the facility for couples. Privacy can also be increased by allowing the doors of residents' rooms to be closed and by lifting restrictions on personal visits. Segregation of men and women residents by wings or floors reduces the amount and kinds of sexual expression of the residents. One study reported that when the isolation of men and women was ended in one nursing home, residents became better socially adjusted, improved grooming, reduced profanity, and increased sexual relations and contacts between the sexes (Silverstone and Wynter 1975).

Staff attitude toward elder sexuality may reduce many forms of sexual expression in a facility. Even though staff may voice their acceptance of elder sexual expression, their actions are often not as supportive (Wasow and Loeb 1979; Kaas 1978). Staff may help meet elders' sexual needs in a number of ways: holding or touching elders, providing opportunities for both sexes to mingle, discussing with families the sexual needs of their older relatives, and allowing privacy for sexual intercourse or masturbation (Steffl 1984). In-service education for staff has been successful in changing their attitudes toward sexuality and aging (White and Catania 1982).

The Chronically Ill

Sexuality may be compromised by physical decrements accompanying chronic disease or by psychological reactions associated with being ill.

Some symptoms associated with chronic illness can cause discomfort during intercourse. Skeletal pain, angina pain, or breathing difficulty during intercourse tend to make the individual hesitant about the sexual act. Those who are in constant pain may not be interested in intercourse. Chronic illness also has a significant emotional component. The illness may cause an individual to feel tired, depressed, and disinterested in sexual activity. Further, chronic illness may alter personal appearance, which may affect body image and self esteem. However, intercourse can provide intimacy and relaxation, reduce isolation and depression, and take attention off physical incapacities. The degree to which chronic illness affects sexual capacity and interest is highly dependent upon the extent of disability, coping skills, sexual attitude, and motivation for sexual activity.

Couples vary in their support for one another during periods of illness and disability. The degree of acceptance of altered sexual activity is related to the strength and previous communication patterns of the marriage. The well partner may lose sexual interest because of fear of causing more pain, lack of interest by the ill partner, or fear of contracting the disease. Chronic illness also promotes dependence. If the ill person was traditionally the initiator of sexual activity, subsequent sexual activity may be affected.

Human service professionals need to be cognizant of the effects of various diseases upon sexuality. It is important that such information be shared with the patient and partner. Unfortunately, seldom is such education and counseling offered.

Changes in Sexual Response with Age

Although documentation is sparse on the effects of age on the genital system, the physiological changes with age are minimal and do not affect sexual capacity in either aging females or males (see Chapter 4). However, preliminary studies by Masters and Johnson (1966) suggested small changes in sexual response in the later years.

Masters and Johnson pioneered the work on human physiological sexual response. They brought subjects of various ages into the laboratory and quantitatively measured sexual response. Their research showed four distinct phases of sexual response in both males and females: (1) *excitement,* the development and increase of sexual tension in response to stimulation, (2) *plateau,* sexual tension is intensified and subsequently reaches the extreme level, (3) *orgasm,* those few seconds of sexual release with primary focus on the pelvic area, and (4) *resolution,* the move from the height of orgasmic stimulation to the unstimulated state. As part of their study, Masters and Johnson studied twenty males and eleven females over age sixty and made preliminary observations regarding the difference in sexual response between their young and old samples.

Among the twenty older males studied, sexual excitement developed more slowly, the intensity of penile sensation was lessened and increased time and more direct stimulation were needed to achieve an erection. The plateau period was longer in older men, allowing them to maintain an erection longer before the need to ejaculate. Often a full erection was not achieved until ejaculation was imminent. Ejaculatory force was reduced and orgasm intensity and length was shorter in older men. During orgasm, elder men also had fewer pelvic muscle contractions, diminished sexual flush, and less nipple and testes engorgement with arousal than younger subjects. After ejaculation, the erection subsided more rapidly and a longer time was needed to achieve another erection. Older men also frequently went from the plateau phase to the resolution phase without ejaculation.

In their sample of eleven women over sixty, Masters and Johnson reported that vaginal lubrication in response to stimulation was delayed and less profuse. The vagina did not expand as much in response to stimuli in older women. Further, there was a smaller increase in breast size during stimulation among older women. However, nipple erection and clitoral responses to stimulation were no different than in younger women. Both the orgasmic and resolution phases were shorter in older women. However, the capacity to achieve orgasm, even multiple orgasms, did not change with age.

Just as in other body systems, the 'use it or lose it' phenomenon seems to play a role in sexual functioning. The degree that physiological changes are due to age or sexual inactivity is still debatable. Of the eleven elder women studied, three experienced coitus at least twice a week throughout their adult lives. In these women, the vaginal lubrication and expansion were as effective as younger women in the study. Masters and Johnson reported the same disuse phenomena was present in males who had had no sexual interaction for an extended time period.

Although the work of Masters and Johnson greatly expanded knowledge of human sexual response, their work on describing changes in sexual response in older men and women is preliminary. Their data should not be used to generalize about elder sexuality because of their small sample size, scarcity of other corroborative research, effects of a laboratory setting on normal sexual response, and unknown health status of participants. Masters and Johnson (1966, p. 248) assert that their work on elder males "must be accepted in light of an admittedly inadequate study-subject population." They reported extreme difficulty in eliciting active cooperation from elder men, especially those over seventy. With regard to the small sample size of older women, they asserted that their work "will require at least another decade to obtain the cooperation of aging women in numbers sufficient to provide biologic data of statistical significance. Current material is presented to suggest clinical impression rather than to establish biological fact" (p. 223). Despite the preliminary nature of their data, the results of Masters and Johnson's studies have been repeatedly reported as the most definitive study of elder sexual functioning. Until larger and more controlled studies are reported, physiological changes associated with advanced age remain speculative.

Sexual Dysfunction

Sexual dysfunction is a physiological impairment in the sexual response cycle that is an obstacle to achieving satisfactory levels of sexual arousal or orgasm (Hatch 1981). Sexual impairment in the later years is not due to aging, but is associated with factors that occur more frequently with advanced age, such as drug use and chronic disease. Sexual impairment may be due to either physiological or psychological factors; some are easily reversed, others are not.

The most common sexual dysfunction for men is *erectile dysfunction* (commonly called impotence), the loss of ability to experience an erection. However, these males may still have the capacity to reach orgasm. Four factors are needed for potency: a normal male sexual apparatus, adequate circulating testosterone and other hormones, an adequate nerve and blood supply to the penis, and a healthy psychological sexual response. Any one missing factor may result in partial or complete erectile dysfunction (Felstein 1983). Felstein estimates that 15 percent of the male population have potency problems and that percentage rises slowly after seventy. However, another study reported much higher figures. Slagg and colleagues (1983) reported that, upon questioning, one-third of the 1,180 older men attending an outpatient clinic for other purposes admitted to having erectile dysfunction. Although most were able to achieve an erection, the erections were not of sufficient turgidity for intercourse.

It is generally assumed that psychological factors such as anxiety, stress, and depression cause the vast majority of erectile failure. However, among elders, physiological causes and drug reactions are more common causes of impotence. In the study cited above (Slagg et al. 1983), 80 percent of the cases were caused by medication usage or organic problems, whereas only 20 percent of the dysfunctions could be attributed to psychological factors.

Premature ejaculation is another sexual dysfunction that may occur in elder males. It is believed to be psychological in origin. Although more common in young, inexperienced males, premature ejaculation may accompany a new relationship in later life.

Women also suffer from sexual dysfunctions that impair their enjoyment of sexual intercourse. *Dyspareunia* (pain during intercourse) may be due to reduced lubrication and elasticity of the vagina, local infections, or poor hygiene. Dyspareunia may occur during orgasm because of spastic uterine contractions. A related disorder is *vaginismus,* the involuntary constriction of the lower third of the vaginal muscles when intercourse is attempted. Vaginismus may be due to an involuntary protection against painful stimulation associated with intercourse. *Situational orgasmic dysfunction* is the inability to reach orgasm consistently enough to satisfy self and partner. Unlike functional orgasmic dysfunction, situational orgasmic dysfunction infers the woman has achieved orgasms in the past. It is generally believed to be psychologically based. However, the adage, "there is no such thing as a frigid woman, only inept men" may indicate that lack of knowledge and patience of the partner may play a role.

Lack of sexual interest and enjoyment may occur in either sex. It is considered a dysfunction only if it is seen as a problem for the individual or the partner.

Diagnosis of Sexual Dysfunction

Elders are often reluctant to volunteer information regarding sexual behavior to a physician, but are more likely to need help than younger clients. If a physician does not ask about specific sexual problems, only 10–15 percent of adult clients were reported to spontaneously volunteer information or ask questions (Kentsmith and Eaton 1979). It is likely that elders are even less likely to report sexual concerns. They may consider their problems to be due to the normal aging process, minimize the importance of their sexual needs and

desires, or be embarrassed to broach the topic (Salaman and Charytan 1984). When physicians do ask patients if a sexual problem exists, about one-half will volunteer significant concerns (Burnap and Golden 1967). In a more recent study, conducted by Slagg and associates (1983) only six of forty men suffering from impotence raised the problem to their physician. However twenty of the men were interested in receiving treatment for their problem.

Although health professionals believe it is important to address the sexual concerns of elders, most do not have training to deal with them. They may be uncomfortable approaching the topic with a person who is older than themselves or have inadequate knowledge of the sexual needs of the chronically ill. Inasmuch as the first course in sexuality was not offered in medical schools until 1960, such attitude and behavior is understandable (Solnick and Corby 1983).

Just as in other health problems, before a sexual dysfunction can be diagnosed and treated, a physical examination and an extensive medical history are necessary. Laboratory tests to measure blood levels of testosterone and other hormones are important to rule out endocrine problems. The medical history should include family disease history, alcohol and prescription drug intake levels, and a sexual history. A sexual history enables a practitioner to broach the issue of sexuality with the client. It not only assists in the gathering of useful information to enhance diagnosis, but also provides an opportunity to discuss the impact of drugs or illness on sexual function. Parsons (1981) suggests a sexual history include the following:

Potency, including the frequency of erections
Desired level of sexual activity
Satisfaction with frequency and variety of
    sexual activity
Quality of erection, ejaculation, and orgasm
Background and present relationship with
    partner
Level of communication with partner about
    sexual matters

Social situation, including other life stressors

How illness affects sexuality: desire, attitude, and activity

Presence of pain during sexual activity: genital or nongenital

It is often difficult to separate psychological from organic causes of sexual dysfunction. In the case of male erectile dysfunction, psychologically based dysfunction has a sudden onset, is related to specific conditions, and an erection can be attained in early morning, during sleep, and with masturbation. In contrast, the problem is likely to be of organic origin if it progressively worsens and a decrease in erections in the early morning and during sleep is noted. Clinically, organic or psychologic impotence can be distinguished by measuring whether erections occur during sleep since erections during sleep are reported to be universal among normal males (Karacan et al. 1975). Thus, if a male has organic dysfunction, erections will be reduced or absent, whereas in psychologically induced erectile dysfunction, these erections will be present. To measure the number of nocturnal erections and penile turgidity, a patient can be hooked up to a monitor in the laboratory or at home.

For women, it is more difficult to determine whether the loss of sexual desire and function is psychological or physiological. Although clitoral erections occur during sleep in women, its diagnostic potential has not been explored. A pelvic examination can assess the condition of the vaginal wall and the presence of disease or infection that may preclude satisfactory sexual activity. There is very little research on the diagnosis and causes of sexual dysfunctions in women.

Treatment of Sexual Dysfunction

Depending on their origin, sexual dysfunctions can be treated in a variety of ways. If the problem is induced by drug therapy, the physician can prescribe an alternate drug or lower current dosages. When sexual dysfunctions are psychological in origin, the patient and partner are generally referred to a sex therapist. Other treatments include hormone therapy and penile implants. Al-though most of the treatments outlined in this section are focused on restoring erectile function in men, a few address the concerns of women.

It is important to realize that not all elders want their sexual dysfunctions treated. In the study by Slagg and colleagues, almost one-half of the men who reported impotence declined to have the problem examined. These men tended to be older and sicker than the rest of the sample (1983).

Sex Therapy

Most models of sex therapy have grown out of the work by Masters and Johnson (1970) and are based on the assumption that sexual problems arise because normal sexual response is blocked by anxiety or fear of failure. They assert that both partners are responsible for the sexual dysfunction. The couple is seen by a male–female cotherapist team for a two-week period. The treatment includes education and counseling as a couple as well as daily assignments that involve progressive exercises in mutual pleasuring with verbal feedback. The goal of the mutual pleasuring exercises is to learn that sexual contact should not be goal (orgasm) oriented; lovemaking should be pleasurable in itself. Intercourse is banned for a time to reduce performance anxiety. This therapy is the most effective in cases of impotence and premature ejaculation. However, the failure rate for elders is higher than other age groups (Masters and Johnson 1970). Modifications of this model include the use of a single therapist instead of a team, once a week instead of daily sessions, and individual rather than couple counseling.

A different counseling approach may be used when the problem extends to other aspects of the relationship. Long-standing dissatisfaction with both the sexual and nonsexual aspects of the relationship or lack of communication skills indicate a need for more general counseling. In addition, learning to cope with sexual problems created by chronic illness and developing alternative means to express sexuality call for other counseling approaches. No matter what the

A sex therapist can assist older couples in enhancing their sexual interactions.

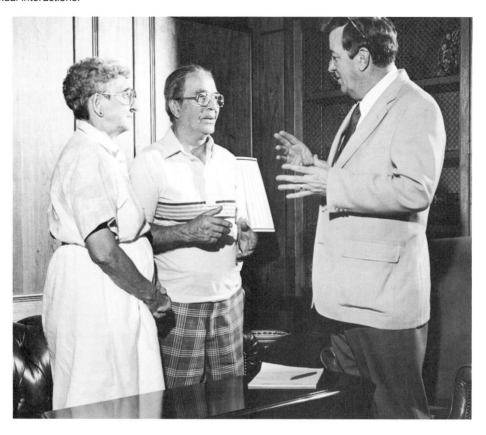

method, the goal of sex therapy should be to increase sexual satisfaction and fulfillment of needs for intimacy, acceptance, and love.

Sexual therapy has also been used to increase sexual satisfaction in elder couples with no sexual dysfunction. Sviland (1975) successfully utilized exercises, education, and psychotherapy approaches with elders. In addition to becoming more sexually liberated, the couples reported increased communication, intimacy, self-esteem and sexual pleasure without guilt.

Penile Implants

If the physician is certain the erectile dysfunction is organically caused, surgery to insert a penile prosthesis may be initiated if the client wants to resume intercourse. Two types of implants are commonly used. One type consists of two semi-rigid plastic rods implanted into the penile shaft, creating a permanent erection (Small 1976). Athletic supporters are recommended so the erection is not detectable in street clothes. Another type is a hydronic device that simulates an erection when fluid is pumped into two cylindrical chambers implanted in the penile shaft (Scott et al. 1973). The pump is activated when a bulb in the scrotum is compressed, causing the cylinders to expand. The erection is released when a valve is pressed, allowing the fluid to flow from the cylinder back into the reservoir. The advantage of the latter is a natural appearance of the penis. However, neither type will restore arousal or orgasm if these capacities are lost.

Hormones and Drugs to Increase Sex Drive and Function

The search for aphrodisiacs is as old as civilization itself. Although a number of substances have been purported to increase sex drive, none have been proven effective in humans. Oysters, Spanish fly, and yohimbine are reported to enhance sexual desire. In fact, Spanish fly (made from a species of European beetle) is a potent and dangerous poison that acts as an irritant as it is being excreted by the urinary tract. Another drug, yohimbine, is synthesized from a tree in West Africa. It is believed to stimulate the lower spinal nerve centers, which control erection. However, its effect on humans has not been fully documented. It seems that the effects of most aphrodisiacs are psychological; that is, the belief of promised virility translates into increased desire. For instance, some substances, such as alcohol or marijuana, reduce inhibitions and enhance sexual enjoyment.

L-dopa increases sexual desire and potency in some male patients who are taking the drug to reduce the effect of Parkinson's disease. The chemical stimulates elevated brain levels of the neurotransmitor dopamine, which is believed to stimulate sexual desire. Although it increases sexual interest in some patients with Parkinson's disease (Brown et al. 1978), there is no clear evidence that the drug increases libido beyond normal levels.

Testosterone therapy for males with low blood testosterone levels is an effective treatment for their lack of sexual desire and function (Spark et al. 1980). Testosterone treatment has no effect upon men with normal testosterone levels. Testosterone injections are not without danger because they may stimulate growth of prostate cancer (Greenblatt and Karpas 1983). Testosterone therapy increases sexual drive in women but dosages must be closely monitored as it causes deepened voice and facial hair growth.

Millions of women are prescribed estrogen during and after menopause and after to treat hot flashes and increase vaginal lubrication. When estrogen is given to women with their ovaries removed, it stimulates vaginal lubrication, sexual interest and enjoyment and orgasmic frequency (Dennerstein and Burrows 1982). However, there is no evidence that it increases sexual interest or enjoyment in women with intact ovaries. Estrogen has a number of side effects. Women receiving estrogen have a higher incidence of headache and depression, which may indirectly influence sexual interest and activity. Further, Masters and Johnson (1966) found that long-term use decreased libido. Since estrogen may play a role in the development of cancer and circulatory problems, its indiscriminate use is cautioned.

The Effect of Chronic Illness on Sexuality

Although frequency of sexual intercourse declines somewhat with advancing age, this decline does not seem to be caused by aging. Rather, the decline in activity is attributed to the rise of chronic conditions and associated drug use among that age group. The presence of chronic illiness may have a powerful impact on sexual interest and ability. Selected chronic illnesses that impact on elders' sexual interest and ability will be presented in this section. Although not discussed, other diseases and conditions such as obesity, muscular atrophy, stroke, respiratory problems, and lower back pain may also affect sexuality.

Heart Disease

It is common for elders who have had a heart attack to be cautious about resuming intercourse because they have the misconception that sexual activity will bring upon another heart attack. Whether emotionally or physiologically based, a number of studies report that 58–75 percent of couples significantly decrease or eliminate intercourse after the husband experiences a heart attack (Bohlen et al. 1984). The most commonly reported reason is decreased function and satisfaction (Mehta and Krop 1979; Sjogren and Fugl-Meyer 1983). It is not clear whether this decrease in erectile function and interest is due to drugs, organic problems, or psychosocial considerations. Among women, heart attacks cause a similarly reduced level of sexual functioning and fear of resumption of sexual activity. In one study, sexual activity ceased in 27 percent and decreased in 44 percent of the women following a heart attack (Papadopoulos et al. 1983).

Researchers believe that the physical demands of intercourse are minimal and sexual activity may be both physically and psychologically beneficial: it reduces tension, aids sleep, increases self-esteem and self-image, and is an enjoyable, low-level physical activity. Hellerstein and Friedman (1970) assert that the physical demands of intercourse are no greater than walking around the block or up a staircase. However, variables such as the strength of the heart, the patient's age, and the status of the central nervous system are important to consider when directing the resumption of sexual activity (Derogatis and King 1981). Typically, it is thought that intercourse can be resumed eight to twelve weeks after the attack. If angina pain occurs during intercourse, physicians generally prescribe nitroglycerine to be taken immediately before sexual intercourse to block possible heart pain. However, since masturbation is less taxing, one investigator suggests that this activity substitute for sexual activity soon after the attack until intercourse can be resumed (Bohlen, et al. 1984).

Lack of communication and inadequate sex education from the physician may contribute to the high incidence of sexual dysfunction after a heart attack. Studies indicate that up to four-fifths of male heart attack patients receive no sexual information from their physicians. In one study of female patients, almost half received no information. When they did discuss sexual matters with their physician, in most instances it occurred because the patient initiated the discussion (Papadopoulus et al. 1983).

Ann Lander's Column

Dear Ann Landers: Three years ago my husband had a heart attack. Now he is afraid of sex—says the exertion might kill him. He doesn't want me to hug or kiss him because he doesn't want to be aroused. Meanwhile, I am climbing the walls. This brother–sister relationship is hell for me. Please advise.—N.Y.

Dear N.Y.: Contact your husband's physician. The man needs to hear from an authority that sexual activity after a heart attack can be physically as well as psychologically beneficial.

In Chico (CA) Enterprise-Record, January 9, 1985. Reprinted with permission of Ann Landers and the Los Angeles Times Syndicate.

Cancer

The effect of cancer upon sexual interest and function depends on the location and extent of the cancer as well as the treatment. Sexual interest and activity may be impaired because of physiological reactions to the cancer or treatment (nausea from chemotherapy, incision pain, and fatigue) or psychological responses such as depression, fear of death or disfigurement, or fear of loss of spouse. Partners of cancer victims may worry whether their partner is well enough for sexual activity or they may be uncomfortable with their partner's altered appearance. Further, the well partner may fear that the cancer is contagious or feel guilty about having sexual interest when the partner is sick or depressed. If one partner is hospitalized, the couple may not have privacy for sexual expression. However, sexual expression is important for cancer victims. Golden (1983) asserts that sexual activity makes cancer victims feel more normal.

Both the cancer patient and partner need support and education to better understand the effect of cancer and its treatment on sexuality. Self-help groups are excellent ways for those with cancer to share information and gain support for sexual concerns. The American Cancer Society has initiated self-help groups for those who have undergone mastectomies or ostomies. These types of cancer treatments particularly impact on elder sexuality and will be discussed under surgery.

Diabetes

Diabetes is probably the most common organic cause of erectile dysfunction and the rate increases with advancing age. This is particularly common among juvenile-onset diabetics. A number of studies report that 30–60 percent of insulin-dependent diabetic males develop erectile dysfunction as their disease progresses (Kolodny et al. 1974). It is generally agreed that the dysfunction is caused by destruction of the nerves that open the penile arteries to permit the blood to enter (Podolsky 1982a). Although erectile function is lost, sensation, orgasm, and ejaculation are unaffected. For diabetic males, the loss of erectile function is more threatening than blindness or the loss of a lower extremity, which may also accompany diabetes (Podolsky 1982b).

Episodes of erectile dysfunction may disappear when the diabetes is controlled. A diabetic should be screened carefully to determine if impotence is drug-induced or due to other physiological or psychological causes. One investigator believes that many diabetics are impotent because they are hypoglycemic (not enough sugar in the blood). He reports that sugar candy taken before sexual activity (he recommends two to three Lifesaver candies) made a significant difference in performance. Of the ten clients he studied, eight were able to resume sexual intercourse after "lifesaver therapy" (Myers 1977). When impotence occurs even when diabetes is controlled, the chance of recovery is unlikely and penile implants may be considered.

Few studies have been conducted on the sexual problems of diabetic women, perhaps because women can still participate in sexual intercourse even when nonorgasmic. One researcher reported no effects of diabetes on women's sexual performance (Ellenberg 1977). Another study compared sexually active diabetic and nondiabetic women between age eighteen and forty-five and found that 34 percent of the diabetic women were nonorgasmic compared to only 6 percent of the healthy women. Many diabetic, nonorgasmic women previously had the capacity for orgasm, but it was gradually lost four to eight years after diabetes was diagnosed. The longer the woman had been diabetic, the less likely she was to be orgasmic. The diabetic women usually maintained sexual interest and activity. However, the majority complained it took longer to become aroused (Kolodny 1971).

Arthritis

Arthritis and related conditions may affect body image, sex drive, sexual competence, and sexual expression (Hamilton 1981). Joint pain and stiffness, deformity, muscle weakness, fatigue, and loss of mobility contribute to sexual problems. Perhaps the greatest effect is that arthritis may make sexual activity painful. The pain may occur in the hips, precluding normal sexual movements, or in the upper extremities, making it difficult to hug, caress, or support body weight. Pain itself is not conducive to erotic feelings. Lack of sexual interest as well as the partner's fear of causing pain can considerably reduce sexual satisfaction for a partner with arthritis.

As in other chronic conditions, elders need education and counseling to cope with the sexual consequences of arthritis. Education should include a discussion of alternative sexual positions to reduce pain, varied forms of lovemaking, the value of a warm bath and analgesics before sexual activity, and plans for sexual activity during times when pain is least. Those with hip replacements need special advice on when intercourse can be resumed and which positions decrease danger of dislocation.

Disabilities need not curtail sexual activity.

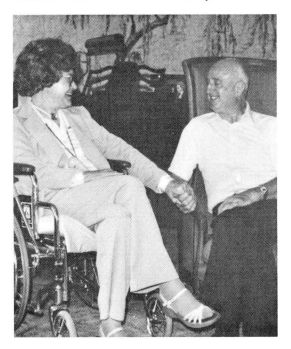

Other Factors Influencing Sexual Function

Sexual function can be profoundly influenced by a number of factors other than chronic illness such as medication and alcohol intake, surgery, prolonged celibacy, testosterone deficiency, or psychosocial variables. This section will discuss the effects of these variables upon sexual interest and activity in the later years.

Prescription Drugs

Medication often influences both sexual desire and sexual response. Some drugs affect the part of the nervous system that controls the sex organs, associated glands, and blood vessels. Others affect the portion of the brain that controls sexual thoughts and desire. Drugs can cause diminished sex drive, abnormal sex response, impotence, ejaculation difficulties, orgasmic dysfunction, and reduced vaginal lubrication. The adverse reaction of a drug upon sexuality depends on the dose, duration of therapy, other drugs taken at the same time, psychological factors, and the state of the circulatory, hormonal, and nervous systems.

Drugs used to treat high blood pressure are the most common causes of drug-induced sexual dysfunction, even at normal therapeutic doses. The most common sexual disorders in males caused by hypertensive drugs are decreased sexual interest, impotence, and impaired ejaculation. In females, decreased sexual interest, reduced vaginal lubrication, and inability to achieve orgasm are most commonly reported (Stevenson and Umstead 1984). Numerous types of hypertensive drugs cause sexual dysfunction. However, the most commonly prescribed hypertensive drug, diuretics, have a low incidence of sexual dysfunction in males although there are reported cases of decreased vaginal lubrication in females (Semmens and Semmens 1978). A relatively new hypertensive drug, prazosin, may have the fewest reported sexual side effects (Stevenson and Umstead 1984).

Psychoactive drugs also cause sexual dysfunction. Large dosages of sedative-hypnotics may affect sexual performance and sexual desire. In women, long-term use of barbiturates commonly causes loss of pleasure in sexual activity and difficulty in attaining orgasm. Antidepressants have been known to cause impotence or to inhibit ejaculation in men, and to cause difficulty in achieving orgasm in women (Partridge 1982). Antipsychotics have been reported to induce impotence, changes in orgasm sensation, and inhibited ejaculation in men, and delayed orgasm and decreased vaginal lubrication in women. Studies report from 10–60 percent of those who take antipsychotics have problems with sexual functioning (Mitchell and Popkin 1983).

Another drug that reduces sexual function is the antihistamine family. They cause drowsiness and decrease sexual desire through the sedative effect. Further, vaginal lubrication may be reduced (Kolodny et al. 1979).

When men are given estrogen therapy to reduce prostate cancer pain, they often experience a gradual reduction of sexual desire. For most men, the frequency of sexual activity drops significantly after estrogen therapy. The incidence of sexual dysfunction in these cases is similar to castration (Bergman et al. 1984).

It is difficult to determine the true incidence of sexual dysfunction resulting from particular drugs because the literature commonly reports only individual case studies. Even when more comprehensive studies are conducted, data conflict and the research design is often poor. Sexual dysfunction is often not defined and other variables affecting sexual interest and activity—the effects of the disease itself, other drugs used, psychological factors unrelated to the drugs, and the presence of preexisting sexual abnormalities—are not controlled (Stevensen and Umstead 1984).

A sexual history conducted before any drug therapy commences with updates throughout treatment will assist the health practitioner to more accurately pinpoint those sexual dysfunctions caused by the drug itself. If a change in sexual activity or interest occurs during treatment, the drug dosage may be altered or another drug may be substituted to allow for maximum symptom control and minimum effects upon sexual function. It is imperative that sexual interest and response be discussed with the client. The client needs to be reassured that, if sexual effects of the drugs occur, they are reversible when dosage is altered or medication is changed. The patient should be encouraged to report such problems as soon as possible. If the patient has a partner, it is important to include the partner in the educational process, especially if the drug may affect sexual interest and function.

Alcohol

Alcohol has a deleterious effect on sexual potency in men and women. The validity of Shakespeare's quote, "(alcohol) provokes the desire, but takes away the performance," is well documented (Farkas and Rosen 1976; Wilson and Lawson 1978). Although low blood levels of alcohol may accelerate sexual arousal by reducing inhibitions, increased blood alcohol levels diminish performance. The reduction of sensitivity varies with the individual. Chronic effects of alcohol severely limit arousal potential in males because alcohol affects the nerve reflex that produces an erection. Thus, alcohol is likely to cause impotence in men (Masters and Johnson 1970). Men who are alcoholic are known to have reduced serum testosterone levels (Williams 1976), which may partially explain their reduced ability and desire. Response to touch may be inhibited, premature ejaculation may occur, and orgasmic function may decline. For women, alcohol reduces the ability to respond to stimulation and to achieve orgasm.

Surgery

Whether surgery causes sexual dysfunction depends upon the extent of nerve destruction in the genital area. Castration, the complete removal of the testes, causes significant impairment of sexual desire and erectile capacity. Further, castrated men commonly reported their partners to be less sexually responsive after the operation, indicating that the change in body image may also have a great effect (Bergman et al. 1984).

Enlargement of the prostate gland is universal among aged men. Some will have to have all or part of the gland removed since the enlargement may interfere with urination. The effect of prostate surgery upon sexual function depends upon the type of surgery performed. In *perineal (or radical)* prostatectomy, the lower abdominal wall is cut to reach the prostate. *Suprapubic* or *retropubic* prostatectomy is accomplished by reaching the prostate under or behind the pubic bone. With *transurethral (TUR)* prostatectomy, the most commonly performed surgery, the prostate is reached through the urethra. In most cases, the ejaculation of semen is not released through the urethra to the outside, but instead flows into the bladder to be excreted during urination (called retrograde ejaculation).

Radical prostatectomy is a notorious cause of erectile dysfunction. In the recent past, most men had erectile problems after that operation.

Chapter 11

Newer methods that attempt to save the major nerves in the area have substantially increased the chances of continued erectile function. Even if erection capacity is lost, penile sensation and ability to reach orgasm will usually be unimpaired, although a decrease in orgasm intensity has been reported (Schover et al. 1984). Suprapubic and retropubic prostatectomies also have a high rate of erectile problems.

In contrast, only 10 percent of TUR prostatectomy patients report decreased erectile ability. However, when cancer is present the incidence may be higher (Shrom et al. 1979).

One contributor to impotence seems to be lack of education regarding the sexual effects of the operation. Zohar and colleagues (1976) reported that five of eight of his patients without education became impotent after TUR surgery while none of seven who received education became impotent.

Another surgery in the genital area that may affect sexual function in males is radical surgery to remove bladder tumors. The percentage of sexual impairment is similar to radical prostatectomy.

Hysterectomies (the removal of the uterus and sometimes ovaries) are one of the most common surgeries performed on adult women. Data on the effect of hysterectomies upon sexual interest and activity are conflicting. Reports indicate that up to 38 percent of women with hysterectomies reported diminished sexual functioning (Dennerstein and Burrows 1982). However, Krueger and colleagues (1979) assert that sexual dysfunction after a hysterectomy is mainly psychological. Dennerstein and Burrows (1982) report that education significantly reduces the negative psychological effects. However, other data indicate the loss of the uterus alters the normal physiology of the sexual response cycle and consequent sexual satisfaction. During arousal, there are fewer vasocongestive changes in the pelvis because of the absence of the uterus. During sexual excitement, the elevation of the uterus is absent and the flexibility of

the vagina may be limited by the inelasticity of the surgical scar. The scar itself may make intercourse uncomfortable if it is irritated by the penis. Sexual tension during the plateau phase may be absent. Since the uterus is a large muscle that contracts during orgasm, many women report orgasms to be less intense (Morgan 1978; Zussman et al. 1981).

Psychological effects are common after a breast removal (mastectomy). The breast is a symbol of femininity in our culture and is a significant part of a woman's sexual identity. The loss of a breast may alter a woman's sex role, sexual image, and sexual relationships. Reduced sexual activity and orgasms are reported consequences of mastectomy (Meyerowitz et al. 1979). However, women over age forty-five rate their sexual adjustment after mastectomy more positively than younger women.

The creation of an artificial opening (stoma) in the abdominal wall is often a consequence of treatment of cancer in the intestinal tract and ulcerative colitis. The stoma allows the rerouting of the digestive system through a new opening because of damage to the intestines and rectum. Physiological effects upon sexual function depend on the extent of the operation and are generally more severe in elder males than elder females (Burnham et al. 1977). Psychological depression and anxiety about stool leakage from the new opening may occur (Orbach and Tallent 1965). Ostomy may also cause marital tension, especially in an already precarious relationship (Burnham et al. 1977). Simmons (1983) suggests a number of ways for women with ostomies to reduce anxiety and enhance sexual interest.

Testosterone Deficiency

The relationship between chronically low testosterone levels and reduced sexual interest and activity is well documented (Cooper et al. 1970). The role of testosterone deficiency in impotency may play a greater role than once assumed. Data

These photos illustrate that sexual attractiveness need not be limited to the young.

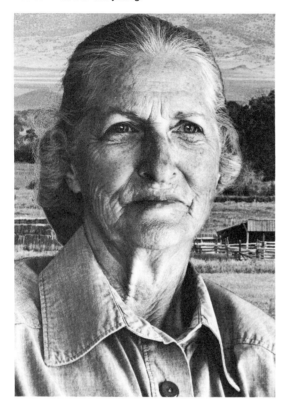

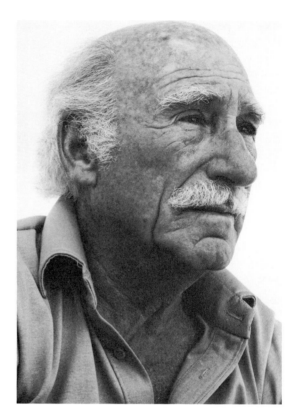

from one study indicate one-third of a sample of 105 impotent men between ages eighteen and seventy-three had some type of endocrine dysfunction that was reversed with hormone therapy (Spark et al. 1980).

Widower's or Widow's Syndrome

If an older man attempts sexual intercourse after being sexually inactive for a year or more, he may be unable to achieve an erection. The initial trauma of impotence may become chronic unless the man has a sensitive partner or therapy is initiated. A similar phenomenon may occur in older women, called the Widow's syndrome (Masters and Johnson 1981). A year or more of abstinence from sexual activity may reduce the elasticity of vaginal walls and reduce the production of vaginal lubrication. Normal vaginal function is

usually reversed within six weeks to three months after resumption of sexual activity. Masturbation reduces the likelihood of these syndromes.

Psychosocial Considerations

Alex Comfort (1972) estimates that 95 percent of the sexual decrements occuring in elders are culturally imposed. Just as other age groups, older men and women are influenced by societal attitudes towards sexuality. In our culture, older men and women are generally not seen as masculine or feminine, but as neuter. When one's sexual identity is not recognized by others, a degree of sexual identity and consequent self-identity is lost. These negative attitudes may also result in a negative self image and loss of sexual interest.

Thus, if an older woman accepts the widely held belief that a youthful and firm body is necessary for sexual attractiveness, she will be less

Chapter 11

likely to initiate or encourage sexual interaction. Similarly, older men are victimized by the emphasis on physical performance. They may focus on the act of ejaculation itself rather than the quality of lovemaking. They may judge their sexual adequacy by comparing the frequency of intercourse, the rapidity in attaining an erection, the firmness of the erection, and the time between erections with their performance during youth. Those men who focus upon their decrements are likely to set up a vicious cycle of impotence that may only be broken by a psychotherapist.

Sex Education

Masters and Johnson (1970) believe ignorance to be the greatest deterrent to sexual function for all ages. This statement seems to be especially applicable to elders who are probably less knowledgeable than any other age group because they had little or no sex education in their earlier years. Although most older people have had a lifetime of sexual experience, attitudes of the older generation reflect a restrictive view of sexuality. Some people believe the primary reason for sexual activity is to bear children and is appropriate only for married persons in their child-bearing years. Self-pleasure or masturbation is unacceptable to many, even though commonly practiced. Such attitudes are clearly detrimental to the full expression of sexuality in the later years, whether alone or as a couple.

Sex education for middle-aged and elder adults is rare, and written and visual teaching materials are sparse. This may be due to the belief that elders have other priorities and are neither sexually active nor interested in learning about sexuality. Others believe that older people already know what they need to know (Smith and Schmall 1983). Another reason for the lack of sex education courses and accompanying materials for elders is the widespread belief that older people do not want to discuss sexual topics. Those who have asked elders have reported otherwise (Feigenbaum et al. 1967; Starr and Weiner 1981; Kaas 1978). One study reported a 90 percent response rate when community elders were issued

written invitations to attend a sex education class in a clinic setting (Salaman and Charytan 1984). The following is only a sample of sexual issues that might be addressed in sex education classes for older people:

Physiological changes accompanying aging that may affect sexual interest and activity
Effects of illness and surgery on sexual interest and activity
Alternative sexual expression, including masturbation
Dealing with sexual repression in our culture
Maintaining sexual identity
Effects of drugs on sexuality
Counteracting myths of sexuality and aging
Communicating with partner about sexual needs
Communicating sexual problems to the health professional

Sex education for elders has been reported to be highly successful in increasing elders' knowledge and changing their sexual attitudes and behaviors. White and Catania (1982) conducted sex education classes for elders and reported a significant increase in sexual knowledge and interest and a more permissive attitude towards sexuality. They reported a 400 percent increase in reported intercourse and masturbation. Whether the increased sexual activity was due to an increased willingness to report or a response to a perceived expectation is not known. West (1983) and Salaman and Charytan (1984) reported similar positive results. Family members and those who work with elders also benefit from education about elder sexuality. White and Catania (1982) reported significant gains in knowledge and sexual permissiveness towards elders as a result of sex education classes for families and nursing home staff.

The attitude of the health professional is an important variable in the educational process for any age group. An older person's willingness to discuss sexual concerns is dependent upon the educator's openness and comfort with the topic. The health professional needs to take educational level

It's Time We Sat Down and Talked About Sex—Again

Bonnie Genevay (1981)

Cast:

Jane, *just now 72*

Abbie, *Jane's sister, 80*

Sharon, *Jane's daughter, fiftyish*

Ted, *Jane's son, in his forties*

Scene: *The family room of Jane's home. A large photograph of her dead husband is on the mantel. The remains of a birthday cake and a centerpiece of flowers grace a lace tablecloth on the table at one end of the room. Abbie sits in a Boston rocker, Jane is on the loveseat, and a couch separates the two women. Sharon enters from the kitchen and sits down heavily on the couch.*

Sharon: Dishes all done, Mother. What a nice birthday party! How does it feel to be seventy-two?

Jane: No different than it felt to be seventy-one, or sixty-one, or fifty-one . . . *(reflectively, looking at the picture on the mantel)* . . . no, I guess that birthday was different because your Dad was so sick that year.

Abbie: *(sighing)* Yes. You aged ten years during that year, Jane. *(pause)* But let's change the subject! Everyone seemed to enjoy themselves today . . . *(clears her throat)* . . . even *that man*—what was his name again?

Jane: *(looking over her glasses first at Abbie, then at Sharon)* Are you talking about Bill Elliot?

Sharon: Mother, I'd rather not talk about anything unpleasant right now—we've had such a nice *family* gathering *(tracing a pattern with her finger on the couch)*. Although I can't imagine that you actually invited him! Everyone was connected to the family in one way or another—except *him*.

Jane: *(voice rising, hands clasping and unclasping in her lap)* Sharon, he *is* connected to the family—through me. First you said you didn't want to talk about Bill, but I notice you *are* talking about him. *(sighing)* We've been putting this conversation off for months. It's time we sat down and talked about . . . my having . . . a friend. I've been feeling very uncomfortable with you lately, and I expect you feel that way too, honey.

Sharon: *(with feeling)* Oh, Mom, I'm so ashamed? How *can* you?

Jane: How can I what?

Abbie: *(getting up from her chair quickly)* Excuse me, I'm just going to put this cake away before it dries out.

Sharon: Aunt Abbie, please stay. I know you don't like that man either!

Abbie: No thank you. I have work to do *(muttering to herself in a stage whisper as she exits)* I'd *never* talk to *my* children about a subject like that. What's gotten into Jane? Our parents never raised us to act that way . . . Jane always was so forward . . .

Sharon: Mom, it's hard for me to say this, but—how do you think we feel—knowing that you and he . . . that he stays overnight, and . . .

Jane: *(interrupting)* Sharon, I really feel quite grownup *(laughing)* at seventy-two, and whatever Bill and I do is our own business! You have no right to criticize my friendship with him!

Sharon: Friendship? *Friendship?* Is that what you call it? Did you think I didn't notice—the morning I popped in accidentally before breakfast—that he was in *Dad's* and your bed? *(with anger)* Do you think I'm blind? After all, I have two teenagers who are up to the *same thing.* What kind of example are you setting for them?

Jane: *(pauses, her voice steely)* I don't have to set an example for your children, Sharon. That's up to you and Fred.

Sharon: *(bitterly)* Fred! Don't bring him into this . . . for all the good *he* does! Mom, you know I love you, but I'm not coming over here any more if you and that lecherous old goat are going to hold hands like a couple of lovesick teenagers.

Jane: *(reaching out and touching Sharon's hand)* Sweetheart, I love you too—very much. I'm sad for you right now, and hurt . . . And *(her voice changes)* so angry I can't think straight! Bill is *not* lecherous, and he's not a goat. And we're both old—is that something we can help?

Sharon: No, of course not. But Mom, he's bald, and he has cataracts, and . . . diabetes . . . and a potbelly! And you're—forgive me for saying it—but you're wrinkled, and gray, and you have arthritis. It's really hard for me to imagine my own mother still . . . *(voice breaking)*

Jane: *(finishes her sentence quickly)* . . . still wanting to love someone?

Sharon: But Mother, he's ten years younger than you are!

Jane: *(in a very low voice)* So?

Sharon: *(staring at picture on mantel, then directly at Jane)* We are a very close family. We all come to see you, and hug you, and phone to see if you're all right . . . what *more* do you need?

Jane: Sharon, are you saying that because I'm old I shouldn't need companionship and affection—except from my family? And that I shouldn't let my grandchildren know I'm still a woman? And it shames you to know I'm attracted to men—especially a man younger than myself? I almost feel as if I don't dare to have a good relationship with Bill because you and Fred are having . . .

Sharon: *(interrupting)* That's off limits, Mom. You make me sound like an overstrict parent—speaking of which, I can well remember when you were so rigid about Ben Nichols! You sat me down and gave me *your* version of "the birds and the bees" for an hour. Just because you didn't like Ben's greasy hair, open shirt, and because he never looked you in the eye. Poor kid!

Jane: Believe me *(laughing)*, I sure feel like the shoe's on the other foot today!

Ted: *(Entering, hugs and kisses Jane)* What're you two laughing about *(tosses his coat on chair)*?

Jane: Sharon and I are having a talk about Bill Elliot and me. What do you think about it, Ted? Does it bother you that Bill and I are close friends?

Ted: Mu-u-uther. I don't want to get in the middle of *this* one! Whatever you do is OK with me.

Sharon: *(stage whisper)* Some help *you* turned out to be.

Ted: I don't care if you have boyfriends, Mom.

Jane: *Boy*friends? Ted, Bill is hardly a boy and I'm not a girl any more. Sorry to be picky, honey. But I'd like you to see me as a very responsible and consenting adult, now that I'm seventy-two! I've been wanting to tell you both about this wonderful book on sex and aging. It talks about *the second language of sex*—you know, being touched, held, appreciated, sharing feelings of tenderness and humor. I wish you kids would read it—oh-oh! I'm sorry. I shouldn't call you kids when I object to being called a girl.

Ted: *(snickers)* Good sex book, huh, Mom? Say, you ought to read the article I just finished on the search for self-fulfillment. It's mostly on the culture, but one guy says it isn't possible to be close to someone unless the relationship is sexual. How about that?

Sharon: It *certainly* depends on your definition of sexuality, Ted. How can you say closeness has to be sexual? That isn't true in *our* family!

Ted: Oh no? I certainly have sexual feelings for my kids, and there's nothing wrong with that. By the way, Mom, Bill told me today he has to have prostate surgery.

Jane: I know. He's really worried about it, I think.

Ted: Speaking of sex Mom, that really finishes a guy off. It's good you two are into this tenderness stuff, because *the other* may be out *(gesturing with his arm and hand across his neck to indicate "cut off")* . . .

Jane: *(interrupting)* . . . you're wrong! Surgery doesn't often stop sexual activity, and I can't believe, Ted, that you believe intercourse is the most important thing between two people who care about each other! I never taught you that.

See, Sharon, it *is* time this family sat down and talked about sex again. We have some catching up to do. *(pauses)* For instance, I've had some strange fears lately—do you care if I tell them?

Ted: Go ahead, Mom.

Abbie: *(entering from kitchen, listening intently, unnoticed by the others)*

Jane: Several times I've had a dream that I was in a nursing home, and I was incontinent. It was so embarrassing to me, having to be changed like a baby, and when I woke up . . . *(pauses and looks at Ted and Sharon)*

Abbie: *(quickly exits, muttering)* Ohmy-gawd, they're at it again! What would the Moral Majority think if they heard all this . . .

Ted: *(simultaneously with Abbie's leaving)* I think I'll go upstairs and watch a little TV.

Sharon: *(in an aside)* Hmph. Real open when it comes to talking about sex, but just let Mom talk about getting sick and dying and you flee like a . . .

Jane: . . . What did you say, dear?

Sharon: Nothing, Mom. What happened when you woke up?

Jane: And then this other fear . . . you'll think I'm awful, honey. But I'm afraid my mind will go, and I'll . . . I'll . . . masturbate in front of people, and embarrass us all. I remember when I used to volunteer at the nursing home and this dear woman—she was actually a friend of my mothers'—was out of her mind a good bit of the time, and she . . .

Ted: *(appears simultaneously with Abbie, who has her coat and hat on—puts his arms around both Jane and Abbie)* Mom,

Sharon—let's go out for Chinese food! I'm buying. We'll pick up Margie and the kids on the way, and . . .

Abbie: *Good* idea.

Discussion Issues

The following issues may arise when this playscript is used for group discussion, and others may be elicited from the family and/or group:

- Agelessness of sexual feelings.

- Scapegoating of a companion/partner by family members.

- Uncomfortableness & value differences regarding discussion of sexuality.

- Acceptability of partners: determined by (1) ageist norms? (2) double-standard of aging? (3) chronological age? (4) degree of health/illness? (5) physical appearance?

- Cross-generational and peer/sibling influence and alliances.

- Adult children's feelings about and perception of parents' sexuality, in relation to their own current life, their sexual satisfaction, and to unfinished, historic family issues.

- Family affection: a substitute for partner intimacy and companionship?

- Sexual responsibility: the necessity for modeling by the grandparent generation?

- Necessity for limit-setting in sexual discussion among family members.

- Role reversal: adult children setting norms for aging parents.

- Productivity/performance ethic in sexuality as a hindrance to older people.

- Sexual components inherent in familial intimacy/lovingness.

- Sexual fears related to illness, functioning, masturbation and mental decline.

and cognitive ability into account. Other factors that influence success are the involvement of elders in the planning, topic selection, publicity, and group facilitation.

Summary

Studies clearly show that sexual interest and activity continue into old age. However, a number of stereotypes about elder sexuality continue to persist. Research on sexuality reflects this bias since studies on elder sexuality are sparse and generally have small sample sizes and other methodological problems. Although a number of activities are important in sexuality, most studies have concentrated on intercourse and masturbation. Preliminary work shows that these behaviors tend to decrease slightly with age. However, frequency of engaging in intercourse among women is highly dependent on the presence of a partner. It is difficult to make generalizations about elder sexuality because there are a number of special populations that have differing interests or frequencies of intercourse such as unmarried women, homosexuals, the institutionalized, and the chronically ill.

Classic work by Masters and Johnson shows some alterations in sexual response with age in both men and women, however, their small sample size precludes generalizations about their findings. Evidence seems to indicate that those who continue sexual activity throughout life have little alteration in sexual response. Sexual dysfunctions are present in both men and women that impair their ability or interest in sexual activity. These include erectile dysfunction, premature ejaculation in men, and dyspareunia, vaginismus, and orgasmic dysfunction in women. These dysfunctions may be caused by drug reactions, psychological effects, or physiological factors and may be treated with sex therapy, penile implants, hormones, or drugs.

A number of chronic illnesses, including arthritis, heart disease, cancer, and diabetes, can affect sexual interest and ability in older people. Testosterone deficiency, prescription drugs, alcohol, prolonged celibacy, or psycho-social factors can influence sexual activity. Although sex education for elders is uncommon, it has been shown to be highly successful.

Activities

1. Ask ten individuals three questions
   a. What is your age?
   b. When does sexual activity cease?
   c. When does sexual interest cease?
   Compare your responses with others in the class. How do the results differ among age groups? What informal conversations did your questions stimulate?
2. Interview five students regarding their estimates of sexual activity between their parents and grandparents. How do they compare to average frequencies discussed in the chapter?
3. Visit a local nursing home and question both an administrator and an aide regarding the sexual life of the residents. Have the administrator describe regulations regarding sexual activity in the home. Is the right to privacy part of the patients' rights? Is sexual activity considered as part of the right to privacy?

Notice the physical layout of the home. How does it discourage or encourage sexual intimacy?
4. Collect cartoons and greeting cards that address sexuality in the later years. Analyze them in terms of the image they project about older people and the myths perpetuated about sex and elders.
5. As a class, perform the play, *It's Time We Sat Down and Talked about Sex—Again* (pp. 308–11). Discuss the questions provided at the end of the script.
6. Develop an instructional program to teach a group of community elders about an aspect of sexuality. Include objectives, methods, teaching materials, content outline, and discussion questions.

Bibliography

Almvig, C. 1982. The invisible minority: Aging and lesbianism. Manuscript.

Barbach, L. G. 1975. *For yourself: The fulfillment of female sexuality.* Doubleday: New York.

Berger, R. M. 1982. *Gay and gray.* Chicago: University of Illinois Press.

Bergman, C., J. E. Damber, B. Littbrand, et al. 1984. Sexual function in prostatic cancer patients treated with radiotherapy, orchiectomy or oestrogens. *Br Jour Urol* 56:64–69.

Bohlen, J. G., J. P. Held, M. O. Sanderson, and R. P. Patterson. 1984. Heart rate, rate-pressure product, and oxygen uptake during four sexual activities. *Arch Intern Med* 144 (Sept):1745–48.

Brown, O. W. E., G. J. Brown, O. Korfman, and B. Quarrington. 1978. Sexual function and affect in parkinsonian men treated with L-Dopa. *Am J Psychiatry* 135:1552–55.

Burnap, D. W., and J. S. Golden. 1967. Sexual problems in medical practice. *Med Educ* 42:673–80.

Burnham, W. R., J. E. Lennard-Jones, and B. N. Brooke. 1977. Sexual problems among married ileostomists. *Gut* 18:673–77.

Butler, R. N., and M. I. Lewis. 1976. *Sex after sixty.* New York: Harper and Row.

Catania, J. C., and C. B. White. 1982. Sexuality in an aged sample: Cognitive determinants of masturbation. *Arch Sex Behav* 11(3):237–45.

Christenson, C., and J. Gagnon. 1965. Sexual behavior in a group of older women. *J Gerontol* 20:351–56.

Comfort, A. 1972. *The joy of sex.* New York: Crown Publishers.

Cooper, A. J., A. A. A. Ismail, C. G. Smith, et al. 1970. Androgen function in "psychogenic" and "constitutional" types of impotence. *Br Med J* 3:17–20.

Dennerstein, L., and G. D. Burrows. 1982. Hormone replacement therapy and sexuality in women. *Clin Endocrinol Metab* 11(3):661–79.

Derogatis, L. R., and K. M. King. 1981. The coital coronary: A reassessment of the concept. *Arch Sex Behav* 10(4):325–35.

Ellenberg, M. 1977. Sexual aspects of the female diabetic. *M Sinai J Med* 44:495–500.

Farkas, G. M., and R. C. Rosen. 1976. Effect of alcohol on elicited male sexual response. *J Stud Alcohol* 37:265–72.

Feigenbaum, E. M., F. M. Lowenthal, and M. L. Trier. 1967. Aged are confused and hungry for sex information. *Geriatric Focus* 5:2.

Felstein, I. 1983. Dysfunction: Origins and therapeutic approaches. In R. Weg ed. *Sexuality in the later years: Roles and behavior.* New York: Academic Press.

Genevay, B. 1981. It's time we sat down and talked about sex—again. *Generations* 6(1):14, 15, 41.

Genevay. B. 1978. Age kills us softly when we deny our sexual identity. In R. L. Solnick, ed. *Sexuality and aging.* Los Angeles: University of Southern California Press.

George, L. K., and S. J. Weiler. 1981. Sexuality in middle and late life. *Arch Gen Psychiatry* 38:919–23.

Golden, M. 1983. Female sexuality and the crisis of mastectomy. *Dan Med Bull* 30, suppl. 2, December:13–16.

Greenblatt, R. B., and A. Karpas. 1983. Hormone therapy for sexual dysfunction. *Postgrad Med* 74(2):78,80,84–89.

Hamilton, A. 1981. Sexual problems in arthritis and related conditions. *Int Rehabil Med* 3:38–42.

Hatch, J. P. 1981. Psychophysiological aspects of sexual dysfunction. *Arch Sex Behav* 10(1):49–64.

Hellerstein, H. K., and E. H. Friedman. 1970. Sexual activity and the postcoronary patient. *Arch Intern Med* 125:987–99.

Kaas, M. J. 1978. Sexual expression of the elderly in nursing homes. *Gerontologist* 18(4):372–78.

Kaplan, H.S. 1979. *Disorders of sexual desire.* New York: Brunner-Mazel.

Karacan, I., F. L. Williams, J. I. Thornby, and P. J. Salis. 1975. Sleep-related tumescence as a function of age. *Am J Psychiatry* 132:932–37.

Kassell, V. 1966. Polygamy after 60. *Geriatrics* 21:214–18.

Kentsmith, D. K., and M. T. Eaton. 1979. *Treating sexual problems in medical practice.* New York: Arco.

Kimmel, D. 1978. Adult development and aging: A gay perspective. *J Soc Issues* 34:113–30.

Kinsey, A. C., W. B. Pomeroy, C. R. Martin, and P. Gebhard. 1953. *Sexual behavior in the human female.* Philadelphia: W. B. Saunders.

Kinsey, A. C., W. B. Pomeroy, and C. R. Martin. 1948. *Sexual behavior in the human male.* Philadelphia: W. B. Saunders.

Kolodny, R. C. 1971. Sexual dysfunction in diabetic females. *Diabetes* 18:858–66.

Kolodny, R. C., C. B. Kahn, H. H. Goldstein, and D. M. Barnett. 1974. Sexual dysfunction in diabetic men. *Diabetes* 23:306–9.

Kolodny, R. C., W. H. Masters, V. E. Johnson, and M.A. Biggs. 1979. *Textbook of human sexuality for nurses.* Boston: Little, Brown.

Krueger, J., J. Hassell, D. Goggins, et al. 1979. Relationship between nurse counseling and sexual adjustment after hysterectomy. *Nurs Res* 28:145–50.

Kuhn, M. 1977. Lecture to Dallas county employees of social service agencies that provide services to the aged. Dallas.

Marshall, D. S. 1971. Sexual behavior in Mangaia. In Marshall, D. S., and R. C. Suggs, eds. *Human sexual behavior: Variations in the ethnographic spectrum.* New York: Basic Books.

Martin, C. E. 1981. Factors affecting sexual functioning in 60–79 year-old married males. *Arch Sex Behav* 10(5):399–420.

Maslow, A. H. 1972. The plateau experience: A. H. Maslow and others. *J Transpersonal Psychol* 4:107–20.

Masters, W. H., and V. E. Johnson. 1966. *Human sexual response.* Boston: Little, Brown.

Masters, W. H., and V. E. Johnson. 1970. *Human sexual inadequacy.* Boston: Little, Brown.

Masters, W. H., and V. E. Johnson. 1981. Sex and the aging process. *J Am Geriatr Soc* 29(9):385–90.

Mehta, J., and H. Krop. 1979. The effect of myocardial infarction on sexual functioning. *Sex Disab* 2:115–21.

Merriam, A. P. 1971. Aspects of sexual behavior among the Bali. In Marshall, D. S., and R. C. Suggs, eds. *Human sexual behavior: Variations in the ethnographic spectrum*. New York: Basic Books.

Meyerowitz, B. D., F. C. Sparks, and I. K. Spears. 1979. Adjuvent chemotherapy for breast carcinoma: Psychosocial implications. *Cancer* 43:1613–18.

Mitchell, J., and M. Popkin. 1983. The pathophysiology of sexual dysfunction associated with antipsychotic drug therapy. *Arch Sex Behav* 12(2):173–83.

Morgan, S. 1978. Sexuality after hysterectomy and castration. *Women Health* 3:5–10.

Myers, S. A. 1977. Diabetes management by the patient and the nurse practitioner. *Nurs Clin North Am* 12:415–26.

Orbach, C. E., and N. Tallent. 1965. Modification of perceived body and of body concepts. *Arch Gen Psychiatry* 12:126–35.

Papadopoulos, C., C. Beaumont, S. I. Shelley, and P. Larrimore. 1983. Myocardial infarction and sexual activity of the female patient. *Arch Intern Med* 143(8):1528–30.

Parsons, V. 1981. Assessment of older clients' sexual health. In Irene Burnside, ed. *Nursing and the aged*. New York: McGraw Hill.

Partridge, R. V. 1982. Sexuality and drugs. In E. M. Lion, ed. *Human sexuality in nursing process*. New York: John Wiley and Sons.

Peplau, L. A. 1981. What homosexuals want. *Psychology Today* March. 28–38.

Pfeiffer, E., A. Verwoerdt, and H. S. Wang. 1968. Sexual behavior in aged men and women: Observations on 254 community volunteers. *Arch Gen Psychiatry* 19:753–58.

Pfeiffer, E., A. Verwoerdt, and G. C. Davis. 1972. Sexual behavior in middle life. *Am J Psychiatry* 128(10) 1262–67.

Pocs, O., A. Godow, W. L. Tolone, and R. H. Walsh. 1977. Is there sex after 40? *Psychology Today* June: 54–56,87.

Podolsky, S. 1982a. Diagnosis and treatment of sexual dysfunction in the male diabetic. *Med Clin North Am* 66(6):1389–96.

Podolsky, S. 1982b. Sexual dysfunction in diabetic men. *Pract Diabetol* 1(1):1–5.

Raphael, S., and M. Robinson. 1981. Lesbians and gay men in later life. *Generations* 6(1):16–18.

Salaman, M. J., and P. Charytan 1984. A sexuality workshop program for the elderly. *Clin Gerontol* 2(4):25–34.

Schover, L. R., A. C. von Eschenbach, D. B. Smith, and J. Gonzalez. 1984. Sexual rehabilitation of urologic cancer patients: A practical approach. *Cancer* 34(2):66–74.

Schrom, S., H. Lief, and A. Wein. 1979. Clinical profile of experience with 130 consecutive cases of impotent males. *Urology* 13:511–15.

Scott, F. B., W. B. Bradley, and G. W. Temm. 1973. Management of erectile impotence: Use of implantable inflatable prosthesis. *Urology* 2:80–82.

Semmens, J. P., and F. J. Semmens. 1978. Inadequate vaginal lubrication. *Med Aspects Hum Sex* 12:58–71.

Silverstone, B., and L. Wynter. 1975. The effect of introducing a heterosexual living space. *Gerontologist* 15:83–87.

Simmons, K. N. 1983. Sexuality and the female ostomate. *Am J Nurs* March: 409–11.

Sjogren, K., and A. R. Fugl-Meyer. 1983. Some factors influencing quality of sexual life after myocardial infarction. *Int Rehab Med* 5:197–201.

Slagg, M. F., J. E. Morley, M. K. Elson, et al. 1983. Impotence in medical clinic outpatients. *JAMA* 249:1736–40.

Small, M. P. 1976. Small-Carrian penile prosthesis. *Mayo Clin Proc* 51:336–38.

Smith, M. M., and V. L. Schmall. 1983. Knowledge and attitudes toward sexuality and sex education of a select group of older people. *Gerontol Geriatr Educ* 3(4):259–69.

Solnick, R. E., and N. Corby. 1983. Human sexuality and aging. In D. S. Woodruff and J. E. Birren, eds. *Aging: Scientific perspectives and social issues*. Monterey, Calif.: Brooks/Cole.

Sontag, S. 1972. The double standard of aging. *Saturday Review* Sept 23.

Spark, R. F., R. A. White, and P. B. Connolly. 1980. Impotence is not always psychogenic. *JAMA* 243(8):750–55.

Starr, B. D., and M. B. Weiner. 1981. *The Starr-Weiner report on sex and sexuality in the mature years.* San Francisco: McGraw Hill.

Stevenson, J. G., and G. S. Umstead. 1984. Sexual dysfunction due to antihypertensive agents. *Drug Intell Clin Pharm* 18:113–21.

Sviland, M. A. 1975. Helping elderly couples become sexually liberated: Psychosocial issues. *Couns Psychol* 5:67–72.

Thomas, L. E. 1982. Sexuality and aging: Essential vitamin or popcorn? *Gerontologist* 22(3):240–43.

U.S. Bureau of the Census. 1982. Marital Status and Living Arrangements. *Current Population Reports,* March, 1981. Series P-20, No. 372, June.

U.S. Senate, Special Committee on Aging and American Association of Retired Persons. *Aging America: Trends and projections, 1984.*

Wasow, M., and M. E. Loeb. 1979. Sexuality in nursing homes. *J Am Geriatr Soc* 27:73–79.

White, C. B. 1982. Sexual interest, attitudes, knowledge and sexual history in relation to sexual behavior in the institutionalized aged. *Arch Sex Behav* 11(1):11–22.

White, C. B., and J. A. Catania. 1982. Psychoeducational intervention for sexuality with the aged, family members of the aged, and people who work with the aged. *Int J Aging Hum Dev* 15(2):121–38.

Williams, K. H. 1976. An overview of sexual problems in alcoholism. In Newman, J., ed. *Sexual counseling for persons with alcohol problems.* Pittsburgh: University of Pittsburgh Press.

Wilson, G. T., and D. M. Lawson. 1976. Effects of alcohol on sexual arousal in women. *J Abnorm Psychol* 85:489–97.

Winn, R. S., and N. Newton. 1982. Sexuality in aging: A study of 106 cultures. *Arch Sex Beh* 11(4):283–98.

Zohar, J., D. Meirag, B. Maoz, and N. Durst. 1976. Factors influencing sexual activity after prostatectomy: A prospective study. *Jour Urol* 116:332–34.

Zussman, L., S. Zussman, R. Sunley, and E. Bjornson. 1981. Sexual responses after hysterectomy-oophorectomy: Recent studies and reconsideration of psychogenesis. *Am J Obstet Gynecol* 140:725–29.

12 Medical Care

You, the individual, can do more for your own health and well-being than any doctor, any hospital, any drug, any exotic medicinal device.
Joseph Califano

Introduction

The American medical system has evolved into two separate sub-systems: acute and long-term care. Acute medical care is geared towards short-term, episodic treatment of illness or injury and is generally provided by physicians in hospitals and outpatient clinics. Traditionally, this aspect of the health care system has accounted for the majority of expenditures for personnel, equipment, and facilities. In contrast, the long-term care system includes nursing homes, mental institutions, and a vast array of health and social services available in the community. Because the two systems developed separately, there is little synchrony of care between the two; each system depends on different methods of funding, administration, and eligibility criteria. The acute system is heavily financed by federal and private health insurance while funding for long term care is extremely variable and depends on changing federal and state legislation and appropriations.

This chapter will focus on the acute care system, mainly the services of physicians and hospitals. The utilization and financing of medical care by older people, barriers of the system that reduce its effectiveness in serving elders, and a number of directions for change will be addressed. Chapter 13 will discuss institutions and community services that comprise long-term care in our country. Mental health services encompass both acute and long term care and were discussed earlier in Chapter 8.

Older people frequent hospitals more than any other age group.

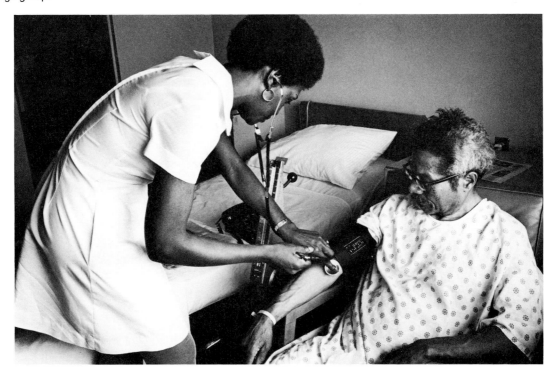

Physician and Hospital Utilization

Compared to other age groups, elders use a disproportionate amount of physician services. Although they comprise 12 percent of the total population in our country, they account for 20 percent of the office visits (Koch and Knapp 1987). On the average, persons sixty-five and older visit a physician six times for every five visits by the general population. In 1983, about 80 percent of the older population saw a physician at least once. About 25 percent saw a physician between five and twelve times, and almost 7 percent visited a physician thirteen or more times (National Center for Health Statistics 1983). Since the enactment of Medicare and Medicaid, both the average number of physician contacts and the percentage of those sixty-five and older who visit physicians has increased significantly, especially among the poor (Wilson and White 1977).

Elders utilize hospitals at a significantly higher rate than younger groups, and account for about 40 percent of all utilized bed days. Twenty percent of those age sixty-five and older are admitted to a hospital each year and one-fourth of those return twice or more within the same year (Brody 1985). The average length of hospital stay also increases with advancing age. In 1985, patients between the ages of fifteen and forty-four stayed an average of almost five days, those forty-five–sixty-four stayed seven days, and those sixty-five and older stayed almost nine days (National Center for Health Statistics 1986). Those eighty-five and older use 50 percent more days of care than the sixty-five and older group (National Center for Health Statistics 1985).

Elders utilize physician and hospital services more than younger groups for a number of reasons. First, they have a higher need due to the higher prevalence of chronic illness in the older age groups. Because the older population is growing, especially among the old-old, utilization will continue to rise. Further, the extensive coverage provided by Medicare and Medicaid to hospitals has facilitated more intensive use. Finally, the lack of Medicare reimbursement for home health services has forced inappropriate and excessive use of hospitals by sick elders.

Use of physician and hospital services among elders varies greatly. A small number of elders utilize a large porportion of medical services. Many elders do not use physicians or hospitals; about 20 percent have not seen a physician in the last two years and 80 percent have not been in a hospital in the last year. At the other end of the continuum, those elders in the last year of life use the most services. Lubitz and Prihoda (1983) documented that about 30 percent of Medicare monies are spent by the 5 percent of enrollees who are in their last year of life. Half of those in the last year of life had bills of $5,000 or more.

Other factors besides the presence of illness influence an elder's use of medical services. Perceived health status, health beliefs, socioeconomic status, ethnicity, degree of isolation, and availability of medical care are only a few influences. One study reported the reasons commonly given by elders for not seeing a physician when needed were cost concerns, travel difficulties, belief that symptoms were due to age, and appointment difficulties. Another study reported that those with lower income, lower morale, and a high number of functional impairments were less likely to see a physician (Branch and Nemeth 1985). In contrast, worries about health and the perception that poor health is interfering with desired activities have been reported to increase the number of physician visits. Repeated office visits often occur because the physician directs the patient to return (Stoller 1982).

Elders who seldom consult with physicians may be in better health than those who visit more often. There is evidence that those who do not utilize acute care services are at no greater risk of poor health or disease than those elders who visit a physician more often (Shapiro and Roos

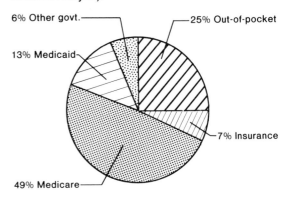

Figure 12.1 Health care expenditures. (Source: Health Care Financing Administration, Office of Financial and Actuarial Analysis).

1985). One British study of nonutilizers reported them to be in better health than those who used physician services (Williams and Barley 1985).

Financing Medical Services

Those sixty-five and older rely primarily on federal insurance programs to finance the majority of their health care needs (see figure 12.1). Federal support for personal health expenditures for elders comes from two main sources: Medicare and Medicaid. Medicare has by far the largest monetary commitment (49 percent of personal health expenditures for elders) followed by Medicaid (13 percent) (Waldo and Lazenby 1984). Together these two public programs finance almost two-thirds of the personal health expenditures of the nation's elderly. The Veteran's Administration and Supplementary Health Insurance also provide some support for elders in financing health care.

Medicare

Medicare, Title XVIII of the Social Security Act, was initiated in 1966 to provide a range of selected medical benefits for those sixty-five and older who qualify for Social Security, regardless of income. In 1972 and 1973, legislation was expanded to cover those sixty-five and older who previously did not qualify for Social Security and certain disabled people. In 1984, about 95 percent of the nation's elders were covered by Medicare.

Medicare insurance coverage is divided into two parts: Part A and Part B. Part A is directed primarily towards hospital care, but in some instances will reimburse skilled services of home-health, hospice care, and limited stays in a skilled nursing facility following hospitalization. Chapter 13 will detail benefits and restrictions of Medicare regarding long-term care services. Part A is financed by a special hospital insurance payroll tax levied on employers, employees, and the self-employed. Part B is a medical insurance that reimburses 80 percent of reasonable charges for medically necessary physician services, medical devices, diagnostic tests, and outpatient hospital and lab services after meeting a yearly deductible. Part B is voluntary; that is, individuals who want this coverage must pay a monthly premium. Part B is financed through the general revenues of the Federal Government and through the monthly premium payment of those who enroll.

Neither Part A nor Part B offers coverage for all needed medical services. Further, neither part reimburses fully for any benefit. Additionally, both parts have deductibles (a set price a beneficiary must pay for each type of service each year before Medicare pays) and copayments (percentage of charge paid for by the patient for each service). Although Medicare paid an average of 49 percent of elders' personal health care expenditures in 1984, the benefits varied for each according to the service: it covered 78 percent of hospital costs, 58 percent of physician visits, 2.1 percent of home-health services, and 20 percent of other medical services (Waldo and Lazenby 1984).

Method of Reimbursement

Medicare has two methods whereby a physician may bill for services. A physician may *accept assignment* on each covered medical service. This means that the physician agrees to accept Medicare's determination of reasonable charge for that

procedure as full payment. If the yearly deductible is met, Medicare pays 80 percent of the reasonable charge directly to the physician. The physician may then bill the patient for the remaining 20 percent copayment. If a physician does not accept assignment, he or she charges the patient an additional cost over and above the 20 percent copayment. For instance, Medicare agrees that $100 is a reasonable charge for a particular medical procedure. If the physician accepts assignment, Medicare pays the physician $80 and the patient pays the $20 copayment. If the physician does not accept assignment, the patient may be charged $140 for the same medical procedure. Medicare will still only reimburse the physician $80, but the patient then must pay $60. In many cases, the patient must pay the physician the entire charge and wait for partial reimbursement from Medicare at a later date. A recent study by the Health Care Financing Administration (1986) reported that only 27.9 percent of physicians in our country accept assignment. In response to pressure from Medicare consumers, Massachusetts passed a law that all physicians in that state must accept assignment. In other words, physicians are prohibited from charging Medicare patients more than Medicare's reasonable charge.

The government has implemented a new and controversial method to reimburse hospitals for Medicare patients. In the past, Medicare payments to hospitals were called retrospective, that is, the bills were paid after the service was rendered (on a fee-for-service basis). This type of reimbursement structure encourages more treatment since it places few limits on the quantity of medical procedures provided. Part B still utilizes the fee-for-service, or retrospective payment system. This system gives physicians incentive to use more medical resources as they care for Medicare patients.

In an attempt to reduce costs, Congress amended the reimbursement process for hospital care (Part A) in 1983. Instead of a fee-for-service, hospitals are now reimbursed before

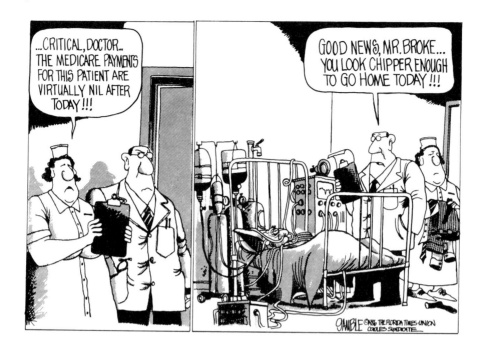

treatment begins (prospective). The government reimburses the hospital a fixed fee based on the patient's diagnosis, not the length of treatment or nature of procedures. This new system, called Diagnostic Related Groups (DRGs), classifies diseases into 470 categories and places a non-negotiable fee for each group that is calculated to be the average cost incurred for treatment of patients with similar conditions. Upon hospitalization of the Medicare patient, hospitals are paid a flat fee considered as full payment according to the diagnosis. If the hospital can treat an elder for less, a profit is made on that patient; if a patient needs more care, the hospital loses money on that patient. The intent of the legislation is to reward hospitals for managing resources well and keeping costs down by decreasing hospital stay, diagnostic testing, medical supplies, and therapy.

There are a number of problems with the DRG system of payment. The most widely publicized criticism is the phenomenon in which hospitals attempt to make a profit by releasing Medicare patients prematurely, termed "quicker but sicker." Often, this means increased return hospital visits, greater risk for the patient, and ultimately higher costs, because of inadequate services at home to assist in recuperation. Discharge of Medicare patients to nursing homes has significantly increased since the DRG legislation. Not only has the demand for these services exceeded the supply, but many facilities are unable to deal with these very ill patients and Medicare coverage for aftercare at home is limited. As a result, many obtain sub-optimal care after hospitalization while others receive none (Kotelchuck 1986).

Since DRGs do not take the various degrees of illness severity into account, it is feared that hospitals may begin to restrict their services to those potential patients who are not as sick and reject those who will consume more resources or have long stays. Also, complications that arise during treatment that were not part of the original diagnosis upon admission, but require more services or an increased length of stay, are not reimbursed. There is evidence that physicians and hospitals are beating the system by manipulating the principal diagnosis to get a higher payment. Another fear is that hospitals may eliminate those needed services that are less profitable.

A report of the Health Care Financing Administration (1986) indicated that, of over two thousand hospitals surveyed in eighteen states, the average profit for each hospital in 1984 was one million dollars, with a 15 percent profit margin. Eighty-two percent of the hospitals surveyed earned profits. Further, the change in reimbursement procedure has significantly reduced the average length of hospital stay for Medicare recipients in the United States. Reduction in hospital stay and cost may be harmful to patients if they are released while still ill. However, costs do need to be contained. Many believe shorter stays are better because the incidence of hospital-induced illness increases with length of stay. It remains to be seen whether the benefits outweigh the risks. See next page for two perspectives on DRGs.

Limitations of Medicare

Medicare has been criticized on a number of counts other than the DRG system. Although its enactment has increased access to health care for older people, restrictions on benefits have created gaps in availability of many needed services. For instance, Medicare focuses primarily on the provision of acute care, rather than maintenance of the multiple, chronic illnesses common among older people. Further, Medicare does not pay for drugs purchased when not hospitalized, dental care and dentures, routine physical examinations, vision or hearing exams and appliances, routine foot care, orthopedic shoes, custodial care (personal assistance with grooming, cooking, or bathing), and many others. Medicare's failure to provide preventive care was criticized eloquently at the White House Conference on Aging (1981): "A program offends common sense when it saves

seventy-five dollars by denying an elderly individual eyeglasses, but reimburses that same individual thousands of dollars after a fall or accident caused by poor vision."

Copayments, deductibles and benefit restrictions make Medicare complex. Because Medicare has two parts, there are two sets of coverage, fees, and appeal processes. The act of filing a claim is beyond the ability of some older people, especially the sick and uneducated.

Medicare is a very expensive program, costing the nation almost fifty-nine billion dollars in 1984 (Waldo and Lazenby 1984). It is generally agreed that the costs for Part A (hospital services) will deplete the Hospital Insurance Trust fund in the 1990s. Further, it is questionable whether these increasing federal contributions are reducing elder's health expenditures. Medicare was originally implemented because elders were paying about 15 percent of their income for health care, necessarily reducing money left for food, shelter, and other basic needs. Ironically, twenty years after Medicare implementation elders can still expect to pay about 15 percent of their income for medical expenses.

Medicare is ineffectual at serving minority populations because many minority persons die before they are old enough to qualify for Medicare. It has been suggested by many advocates that the age of eligibility for specific minority groups be reduced.

Medicare has also been criticized because it encourages excessive expenditures by reimbursing expensive hospitalization, but not home-health care. As a result, if home-health care cannot be financed by personal funds, inappropriate and more expensive hospitalization or nursing home care is chosen because it is reimbursed by Medicare. This practice increases the national Medicare bill and encourages excessive dependency in elders. These issues will be explored more fully in Chapter 13.

Two Perspectives on DRGS

"Premature Discharge, Premature Death" (Kotelchuck, 1986)

Citizen Betty Kratt's testimony before the Senate's Special Committee on Aging, Sept. 26, 1985, was one of many statements of bereaved family members which called attention to the tragic pitfalls of the Prospective Payment System. Her words, which follow, offer a glimpse at a system which has victimized patients when they were least able to defend themselves.

"My mother was 85 years old when she died early this year. She had been ill with kidney failure, high blood pressure, heart condition, blindness and lack of hearing. I entered her into the hospital January 9, 1985, with a heart attack and kidney failure. The hospital took good care of her, except for her meals. She was so weak and unable to feed herself. She was on oxygen 24 hours a day and her heart was so bad her skin color had turned blue. During her hospital stay, my mother required around-the-clock oxygen, she had a catheter, IV tubes and a feeding tube.

Then, on January 29, 1985, I received a call from the hospital stating that my mother would have to go to a nursing home because she no longer needed their acute level of care. On January 31, they sent for an ambulance and transferred her to a nursing home. This was done against Dr. Kellawan's orders and while he was out of town. I was not told anything at all at the time that I could appeal to the hospital to not send her out. I did everything I could to prevent them from moving her, but they told me that Medicare would not let her stay any longer and they were losing money on her. To make matters worse, the hospital informed the nursing home that she was able to feed and bathe herself and also had bathroom privileges. This was absolutely not true. She could not move at all.

My mother passed away on February 13, 1985, just 14 days after entering the nursing home. A day or so after her death, I received a letter at my home from the hospital saying that if I did not agree with my mother's discharge, I could send in a written appeal."

"More Is Not Always Better" (Excerpted from Levin, 1986)

Does doing less necessarily cause harm? . . . Progressive concerns about health care during the 1960s and 1970s principally focused on achieving equitable access for all citizens. Activists struggling toward the goal of expanding access continue to proclaim that health care is a "right" not a privilege—and indeed it is. But advocates for equity appear to assume that medical services have intrinsic value and that better access, almost by definition, produces better health. Many also assume that a known standard of care exists and that practitioners always agree on what constitutes optimal treatment. Unfortunately, none of these assumptions is true.

The pages of medical journals have always been ruffled by questions and controversies about the safety, efficiency and utility of various medical practices. And it's no secret that practice decisions and treatment modalities are influenced at least as much by education, specialty training and a practitioner's environment as by scientific rationale. Moreover, diagnostic and therapeutic practices sometimes continue to be used long after their efficacy or safety has been disproven. . . .

During the 1980s another question is being asked with increasing frequency. Can the United States afford to spend 11 percent of its gross national product on health care? Most critics say no, emphasizing that the United States spends a larger share of its GNP on health than any other industrial country. (In true conservative fashion, they fail to mention that the United States, unlike every other industrialized nation but South Africa, lacks a program of national health care entitlement). Others argue that we can and should commit to spending these dollars to ensure adequate health services and cite a bloated defense budget as a more appropriate area of cost containment. . . .

Consumer groups and others argue that DRGs have harmed the health of older Americans, but are they guilty of the "less is bad assumption"? In addition, practitioners warn that any restriction on their ability to do whatever is "needed" for a given patient violates their oath and is likely to result in harm. Have they also fallen victim to the "more is better assumption"? I think so.

In medicine, as in other human services, the possibility exists that doing less may sometimes produce a better result. History repeatedly tells us that the more technical and invasive human activity becomes, the greater the risk of harm rather than benefit. The past promise of nuclear energy, for example, has emerged as a threat to our present well-being. Much of medical practice has not been shown to be efficacious and/or safe when scientific standards of proof are applied. To assume that limiting such practices will necessarily be harmful ignores that reality.

Now an endangered species, retrospective payment was often accused of encouraging unnecessary medical services—tests, surgical procedures and hospital stays—all of which put people at risk and were often economically wasteful. The goal of "first do no harm," an important standard to apply when assessing medical practices, should also be applied to monitoring our new, more stringent cost-containment program.

Everyone must keep in mind the obvious question as the content of medical practice changes. Does it do more good than harm? Most of all, we need to stop assuming that doing more necessarily improves the quality of our lives and that doing less necessarily diminishes it.

Reprinted with permission from Health Policy Advisory Center, 17 Murray Street, New York, N.Y.

Medical Care

Medicaid

Medicaid, Title XIX of the Social Security Act, was legislated at the same time as Medicare to provide protection against the high costs of hospital, nursing home, and physician care for the poor, the blind, and the disabled. Medicaid was designed as a catch-all program to handle the expense of medical and rehabilitation services not covered by Medicare for poor elders and to provide medical assistance to those needy groups of other ages. Medicaid (called MediCal in California) is financed jointly by the state and federal government, but is administered by each state. The level of eligibility is based on monthly income and assets. Both eligibility and extent of coverage vary from state to state. Some states provide coverage for all below the poverty level, while others have more stringent requirements. In all states, however, an individual qualifies for Medicaid only when personal resources are drained. Most states use fixed fee schedules to reimburse medical procedures. Those physicians who agree to participate must accept the state's Medicaid reimbursement as full payment and cannot bill the patient for any additional expenses.

In 1984, about 12 percent of those on Medicare also received Medicaid benefits. For eligible elders, Medicaid finances the yearly deductibles, copayments, and monthly premiums of Medicare. Additionally, Medicaid finances many other costs not covered by Medicare. For instance, all states must finance in- and outpatient hospital care, physician services, lab and X-ray diagnosis, skilled home-care nursing services, and some home health services. In addition, some states provide private duty nursing, dental care, physical therapy, drugs, dentures, glasses, and hearing aids.

Private Insurance

Many elders, generally those with more education and income, supplement Medicare coverage with individually purchased private health insurance policies. However, these policies do not significantly reduce the national cost of medical expenses since only 7 percent of total health expenditures for elders are paid by private health insurance coverage (figure 12.1) (Waldo and Lazenby 1984). Most private policies concentrate on reimbursement of hospitalization costs, picking up a portion of what Medicare does not. Although there is variability among policies, they generally pay for some or all of Medicare deductibles or co-payments. A very few will pay for services not covered by Medicare.

Catastrophic or major medical expense policies help cover the high cost of serious injury or illness, including some services not covered by Medicare. However, many of these policies have large premiums, large deductibles, or do not fully cover Medicare deductibles or copayments.

Some limited scope policies pay fixed amounts to patients in nursing homes, hospitals, or those with specific diseases. However, these policies can be very misleading and almost always pay a fixed amount that does not rise to meet increasing health care costs. Additionally, nursing home policies generally finance medical care in a skilled nursing facility only, rather than the custodial institutional care most commonly needed.

There are a number of problems with supplementary health insurance policies for elders. There is some question whether the extent of coverage is adequate, whether there is duplicate coverage, and whether they provide a good rate of return for the premium paid. Further, the policies are very complicated and most elders should have trained assistance in choosing among them. In many cases, these policies are purchased without adequate information of benefits and restrictions.

Many states have encouraged private insurers to develop supplementary health insurance policies that adequately cover long-term care. Some states have set standards and/or mandated specific coverage. These state laws are intended to protect consumers against inadequate coverage. However, as the insurance is expensive, the federal government needs to play a role in increasing long-term care costs. Elder advocacy groups are exerting pressure for increased federal involvement.

Veteran's Administration

The Veteran's Administration (VA), an independent agency of the federal government, operates the largest centrally directed hospital and medical services in the United States. There are four overlapping groups of veterans eligible to receive VA medical care: veterans with service-connected disabilities, recipients of VA pensions, veterans sixty-five and older, and medically indigent veterans. Veterans with service-connected disabilities receive priority when seeking hospital care. As long as there is room in the hospital, veterans with non-service-related disabilities receive care after stating that they cannot pay for care elsewhere. All veterans over sixty-five are considered to be disabled, making the VA a major health care resource for that group. In 1983, twenty-eight million veterans, or 12 percent of the population were eligible to receive at least a portion of their medical care in a VA medical facility (Veteran's Administration 1984a).

There is at least one VA hospital in every state except Alaska and Hawaii. In 1983, the VA had 172 medical centers with extended care, surgical, and psychiatric services. There were almost three hundred outpatient and satellite clinics providing physician service in ambulatory settings to reduce the need for hospitalization. These clinics treated veterans with or without service-related disability. One hundred of the centers had nursing homes and a few had board and care facilities. The staffing in the majority of VA hospitals is provided by medical schools. More recently, schools of nursing, dentistry, rehabilitation medicine, and social work have developed affiliations with the VA hospitals (Veteran's Administration 1984b).

The major challenge currently facing the VA system is to accommodate for increased utilization of their medical services due to the rapid aging of the veteran population. It is estimated that by 1990, 25 percent of the veterans will be over sixty-five, and by 2000, one-third will be over sixty-five, placing a tremendous burden upon the Veteran's Administration health care system (Veteran's Administration 1984b). As many as two-thirds of the men over age sixty-five during the next twenty years will be veterans and eligible for this service.

National Health Insurance Proposals

Widespread concern that an increasing amount of people cannot afford medical care is not new. Over the years a number of proposals have been presented to attempt to provide national health insurance for all citizens. Proposals have varied from partial health insurance to pay for catastrophic illness to comprehensive insurance.

Proposals to increase federal involvement in medical care predictably generate much controversy. Historically, the proposals are not adopted because of the strong, well-financed and consistent opposition from organized medicine, especially the American Medical Association. The AMA opposes national health insurance because more federal control of health care will likely decrease physicians' profits and control. Both hospital and physician groups have indicated that they do not want significant changes in the present system, unless there is a reduction of governmental regulations. Despite this philosophy, a great number of people in the United States assert that health care is a right of every citizen and that it is the government's responsibility to ensure that no one is denied medical care because of a lack of funds.

Federal financing of the medical needs of its citizens would require an overhaul of the current system of medical delivery as we know it today. Further, if the comprehensive medical needs of those in our country, including elders, are to be met, the current financing system needs to be modified. The bottom line is, how much are federal policy makers willing to spend for health care, what types of health care should be provided, and how can the cost of health care be balanced with other demands on the federal budget?

Barriers to Effective Delivery of Medical Care

Physicians have a realm of diagnostic tests, drugs, surgical treatments, and modern equipment at their disposal and research continues to increase knowledge of the causes and treatments of many diseases. Despite these 20th century improvements, the medical care system has failed to meet the special needs of the age group that uses its services the most—the old. There are a number of reasons for this: the high cost of care, over-specialization, and lack of coordination with community resources impair the system's ability to provide quality, comprehensive care to elders. Additionally, the lack of practitioners with geriatric training, poor physician-patient relationships, and lack of interdisciplinary team approaches further reduce the quality of care. This section will highlight some of the characteristics of the medical system that serve as barriers to effective care for older people.

High Cost of Care

The cost of medical care in the United States is rising at an astronomical rate—faster than any other commodity. Since 1965, expenditures for health care have increased at an average annual rate of almost 13 percent, significantly more than the rate of inflation. Health care costs have risen to such a level that some individuals must choose between the necessities of life and medical care. The Senate Labor Committee reports that illness and medical costs are the number one cause of bankruptcies in our country.

Hospitalization expenses account for the largest single expense in the national health bill and that figure continues to rise. Inflation and an increased population of older people who use hospitals are two of the reasons for the increase. However, the major contributor to skyrocketing costs of hospital care is the financing of unnecessary hospital beds, unnecessary equipment and diagnostic procedures, and unnecessary hospitalization. People commonly say, "I didn't have to

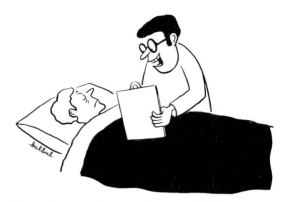

"*Have I got good news for you. Medicare covers 50%. —Now all you owe is $28,432.52.*"

pay for most of my care because it was covered by my insurance." However, consumers pay directly by increased out-of-pocket expenses and insurance premiums and indirectly through increased federal taxes and rising costs of goods because of higher health insurance premiums paid for employees by industry.

It is clear that elders use far more health services than the rest of the population. Those sixty-five and older are responsible for one-third of the nation's health expenditures and over 50 percent of government expenditures on health care, even though they account for about 12 percent of the total population. In 1984, the average expenditure in the United States for each elder for personal health services was $4,202. Despite the benefits of Medicare and Medicaid, older persons continue to pay about one-fourth of their total health care bill out of their own pockets—an average of $1,059 in 1984 (Waldo and Lazenby 1984).

Ironically as elders' medical needs increase with age, they become less able to pay for health care because of reduced income. Elders spend more on out-of-pocket medical expenses than younger groups, yet the median income of elder individuals and families is little more than one-half that of the younger age group. Those who are very old, who live alone or are part of a minority group are more likely to be both poorer and sicker.

Hospital Horror Stories

(Adapted from Carlson, 1984)

In response to an appeal, the American Association for Retired Persons received over one thousand letters with complaints from elders regarding exorbitant hospital fees and questionable charges. Hospital bills in the hundreds of thousands of dollars were received by some respondents, many of whom reported they were not consulted about the necessity and cost of the treatment procedures for which they were charged. A sixty-five-year-old widow received a 120 page hospital bill for $238,000 after her husband spent a little over three months in intensive care. Another elder woman, depending entirely on Social Security payments of $475/month, received a bill for over $250,000 after her husband's five and a half-month hospitalization. Although Medicare and other insurance covered all but $14,000, the woman was responsible for that bill—in $25 a month payments—plus a bill from the physician who did not accept Medicare assignment and required additional payment.

Another woman reported that she received an $895 bill for physician visits at the hospital that were brief and perfunctory, usually from the doorway, but occasionally included a handshake.

Even more startling were the reports of inflated charges for medication and diagnostic tests during hospitalization. A sixty-seven year old woman was charged for a pregnancy test (unneeded and unrequested) and another was charged $75 for a small pillow to rest her foot after bunion surgery. Drugs and lab test fees were commonly reported to be grossly inflated when compared to the prices at local drug stores and commercial laboratories. For instance, a man was charged $1,276 for a blood compatability test which normally costs about $25. In another case, a woman received a hospital bill for her husband's care that included seventy-five unauthorized X-rays taken over an eighty-seven day period.

Much of the problem of costs is due to the fact that physicians often do not concern themselves about costs of care. It is easier to order tests than to ask questions or confer with the patient and family on the proposed direction of care. Many physicians believe that no cost should be spared to keep one alive. Family members often hesitate to ask for the justification and cost of diagnostic procedures and treatment when told of their necessity by the physician because they want to do everything possible for a loved one.

Traditional Medical Model

Medical care in our country is most skilled in the treatment of acute, short-term, curable disease. This emphasis can be traced historically to the discovery that microorganisms cause infectious illnesses and the subsequent discovery that these can be countered by antibiotics. In the traditional medical model, physicians analyze symptoms, diagnose a specific disease, provide treatment (generally a drug or surgery), and cure the disease. This model presupposes that illness has a specific organic basis that has one cause (e.g., a virus or bacteria).

The traditional medical model is more effective in treating accident victims or those with acute illnesses who can be restored to previous levels of health than in treating the more progressive chronic conditions common among elders. We are increasingly aware that elders' health problems require more complex, multi-disciplinary approaches than the simplistic disease model can address. Even in the best conditions, chronic illness will not be cured. The goal in many cases is symptom relief and slowed deterioration.

This model does not account for the myriad of environmental variables influencing the development and course of a disease, such as marginal nutrition deficiencies, stress, psychosocial problems, or negative health behaviors. Successful treatment of a chronic illness must incorporate a number of strategies that may or may not include drug therapy. Physicians need to assess the benefits and risks of medication, surgery, or other invasive methods and expand their mode of treatment to include health behavior change or psychological counseling. In contrast to the traditional disease model of care, effective management of chronic illness requires long-term treatment and an understanding of the psychosocial and economic forces impinging on the individual.

Because they were educated under this traditional medical model, physicians are biased toward interventionist drug and surgical treatments and the treatment of acute illnesses. Thus, physicians may find the treatment of the chronic conditions of older people unsatisfying. This frustration may result because the patient is not ultimately restored to a healthy condition. Physicians may look at their inability to cure elders or the death of older people in their care as personal failures in healing.

Inadequate Patient/Physician Relationship

Patients' disenchantment with physicians may be the most common criticism of medical care today. Patients commonly complain of long waits, cursory visits, and inadequate explanations of diagnosis and treatments. Additionally, many criticize physicians for their impersonal manner, authoritative stance, and lack of empathy. Many consumers are dissatisfied with physicians' over-reliance on drugs and surgery to treat illness. The recent increase in malpractice litigations is more likely a reflection of dissatisfaction with the patient-physician relationship than physician incompetence.

Despite the fact that elders generally have more health problems than younger groups and the diagnosis and treatment of chronic illness is more complex, the average physician visit is shorter for patients over sixty-five than those age forty-five–sixty-four, especially for comprehensive and consultive visits (Keeler et al. 1982). The length of visits is woefully inadequate for meeting elders' complex needs. Elders need longer visits because they may have educational or sensory deficits that impair communication, often have multiple, coexisting illnesses, or may need to discuss treatments they are receiving from other practitioners. Further, elders may not report all symptoms so extra time is needed for probing. A number of studies show that 40–50 percent of elders' health problems are unknown to their physician. While cardiac, pulmonary, and major nervous system disorders were commonly diagnosed, incontinence, mobility problems, feet problems, depression, sensory decrements, alcoholism, and social needs were rarely noticed (Stultz 1984).

A study by Green and colleagues (1986) reported that physicians relate differently to their old and young patients. The physician discussed more medical problems and fewer psychosocial concerns (such as family, financial concerns) with their elder patients. Further the physicians were more egalitarian, patient, and respectful to younger patients. Elders had more difficulty getting the physicians to address their concerns and answer their questions.

The widespread lack of compliance with prescribed treatment strategies is partly attributed to a poor patient/physician relationship. When the importance of the regimen is not clearly discussed, compliance is decreased. One study of elders found that half of them deviated from the prescribed therapy, most commonly because they did not understand the regimen (Libow and Sherman 1981). However, even when the patient asks questions, the physician may not provide clear explanations or the explanations may be too brief. Conversely, patient satisfaction with physicians increases with the amount of information given to them. It is estimated that increased compliance and patient satisfaction can be accomplished with about five minutes more time in each physician visit (Bertakis 1977).

The blame for poor patient/physician relationships should not rest solely on the physician. Both physician and patient perpetuate the view that the physician is infallible and possesses a large body of knowledge too complex for the average person to understand. The physician has expertise, medicine, and advice to dispense and passive acceptance of what the doctor ordered is encouraged. In addition, the public overestimates the effectiveness of prescription drugs and high-tech medical practices.

The healing powers of the physician are not as great as many patients believe. Results of studies such as the classic one conducted by Berman (1976) engender public doubt on the effectiveness of physicians. He showed no significant increase in death rate when physicians went on strike in New York and San Francisco, and only 15 percent of hospital beds were filled. Estimates vary, but from 70 to 90 percent of all illnesses that people bring to physicians are self-limiting or beyond the medical profession's capacity to cure. If the physician makes the patient feel better, it is due to patient reassurance, palliative medicine, and an occasional operation. Many studies indicate that physician intervention has done little to prolong life and eradicate the source of health problems.

Fortunately, many American health care consumers are becoming less inclined to leave decisions about their health care to their physicians. Instead, they are taking responsibility for their own health and being more assertive with their physician in order to receive quality health care. This attitude is changing the physician's role from one of dominance to a team member. However, the increase in personal responsibility and assertiveness does not seem to be occurring as quickly among the older age group.

Lack of Geriatrics Training

Shifting demographics continue to increase the need for medical care for elders. Consequently, more physicians need to be educated about chronic illnesses and the special needs of elders. A 1982 study by the American Medical Association revealed that only seven hundred physicians in the United States have a primary interest in geriatrics. This number is inadequate to effectively treat today's elder population and train future physicians. It is estimated that 7,000–10,000 physicians skilled in dealing with the special health care problems of elders will be needed by 1990 (Kane et al. 1980). Although experts debate whether geriatric specialists are needed or whether all primary care physicians should have knowledge in geriatrics, it is apparent that there are far too few physicians educated about the health needs of the elderly.

The great dearth of physicians trained in geriatrics puts the elderly at a disadvantage. Some of their health problems may be overlooked, others may be misinterpreted and mistreated. Various popular forms of treatment may be inappropriate for elders. Also, the considerations of the multiple causes and treatment of diseases primarily affecting the aged need more than passing attention. A negative attitude towards the treatment of health problems among older people is not uncommon and precludes effective prevention, treatment, and rehabilitation strategies. Some physicians believe there is little or nothing they can do for the health of older people, and many believe that there is little older persons are able to do themselves to improve their health status.

Despite the urgent need, specific training in geriatrics is not common in medical schools. Medical school texts and curricula focus predominantly on acute illness and surgery, not on prevention or treatment of chronic illness. Internships generally occur in hospitals, not in long-term care institutions or community-based clinics. However, there are bright spots. Findings from a study conducted in 1985 report that one-third of the medical schools in our country had clinical geriatric programs in all three departments: internal medicine, family practice, and psychiatry, and half had geriatrics in at least one of those departments. Only 6 percent of the responding schools had no clinical geriatrics programs at all. Despite the increased geriatric focus in medical schools, only 3 percent of these geriatric programs were required: the vast majority of courses were only elective (Beeson 1985). An Association of American Medical Colleges survey found that only 2.5 percent of 1982 medical school graduates took adequate geriatrics electives (Johnson 1985). Further, there is a severe shortage of academic geriatricians qualified to teach future medical students and conduct research in geriatrics (Kane et al. 1980).

Recruitment of students into geriatrics programs is hampered because there is less prestige associated with working with older people and many believe it to be less rewarding. Perhaps the presence of positive role models on the medical school faculty might increase interest in geriatrics.

Overspecialization and Fragmentation of Services

With the increase in medical technology and medical knowledge, many physicians have elected to specialize in one area of medicine to better keep abreast of technological advancement. Whereas elders may have previously relied on one family physician who provided comprehensive medical care, most older people outlive their family physician and must enter a system full of "ologists" (figure 12.2). Because elders generally manifest multiple, coexisting physical conditions, they need to visit various specialists to diagnose and treat a different health problem. Treatments may be difficult to coordinate and may even be incompatible, increasing the chance of drug interactions.

Unfortunately, when an elder sees a number of specialists, no one is responsible for coordinating care as specialists seldom act as a team.

Another barrier to comprehensive care for older people is a lack of connections among various physicians and health and social services in the community. Although we commonly talk of the health care system, it is more aptly described as a "nonsystem" or even an "antisystem" because of a lack of coordination. Needed services are in different locations and treatment, rehabilitation, prevention and support services are separated. Further, medical, health, and social services differ with regard to eligibility requirements, administration, and financing mechanisms. This occurs because legislation does not promote interaction or continuity of care among medical, health, and social service providers. The increase of for-profit medical and health facilities and community-based health agencies may further decrease cooperation as these compete with one another for clients. Finally, there are gaps in needed services and care in many communities.

Obtaining proper care for multiple health problems and coordinating medical services and treatment are formidable tasks at any age, but the problem is particularly evident among the old. Effective use of the current health care system requires mobility, strength, competitiveness, money, and a keen awareness of ways to gain access to the splintered services—characteristics not possessed by most elders (Michelmore 1975).

The interdisciplinary team approach is an excellent way to ensure comprehensive care especially for older people. Each member contributes specialized knowledge and skills to attend to their diverse needs and reduce the problem of fragmentation of services. The team approach to geriatric care is illustrated on page 332. Even though comprehensive medical care under one roof is uncommon, medical and allied health and social service personnel can integrate care by providing appropriate linkages to other services.

Figure 12.2   Physician Specialties*

Allergist—Inhalant and food allergies

Anesthesiology, administration of anesthesia

Cardiology—heart

Dermatology—skin

Endocrinology—glands and hormones

Gastroenterology—GI tract and liver

Gynecology—female reproductive system

Hematology—blood

Nephrology—kidneys

Neurology—nervous system

Opthamology—eye diseases and surgery

Oncology—tumors and cancer

Orthopaedics—skeletal system

Otolaryngology—ear, nose, and throat

Physiatry—diagnosis and rehabilitation of movement problems

Proctology—colon and rectum

Psychiatry—mental disorders

Pulmonary specialty—lungs

Radiology—diagnosis and treatment with radiation

Rheumatology—joints

Surgery—surgical operations, some specialize on particular body systems

Urology—urinary and genital tract

*The specialties of genetics, family medicine, and internal medicine are used much like the family general practitioners. They provide comprehensive medical care and usually serve as an entry point into the medical system. When needed, these physicians refer their patients to other specialists.

The Geriatric Team-Case Approach

(Adapted from Charatan et al. 1985.)

Mrs. H. W., seventy-eight years old, was admitted to a hospital emergency room. She had been found lying on her bathroom floor by a neighbor. The patient was disheveled, confused, and disoriented. A physical examination revealed shortening and external rotation of the left leg. X-rays showed a fracture in the left hip. There was no evidence of a recent stroke.

Hip surgery was considered urgent, but the patient was incompetent to give consent. The patient had no personal effects to help in contacting relatives. She stated that her husband was dead and she had no children. Whether she had relatives was unclear. The patient's neighbor was contacted. She knew the patient only vaguely and regarded her as strange and a recluse. She had entered the patient's home because of the constant whining of the patient's dog. The patient's consent for surgery was completed by a surgeon and administrator following evaluation by a psychiatrist.

Following hip surgery, the patient's mental status further deteriorated, with agitation requiring psychotropic medication that calmed the patient. Nasogastric feeding tube was necessary and a catheter was inserted. A pressure sore developed on the left heel. Medications added included procainamide for arrhythmias and antibiotics for a urinary tract infection. The nursing notes portrayed a demented, sick, old woman.

On the eighth day, the patient's eighty-four-year-old sister visited. She was apparently shocked by her sister's condition, but little was thought of this because she was also regarded as somewhat demented. She met with the social worker to whom she gave personal documents and effects from the patient's home that included spectacles and a nonfunctioning hearing aid. Arrangements were made for the patient's transfer to a nursing home.

The nursing home evaluation was initially based on the acute hospital's representation of the patient. Days later, the nursing home social worker contacted the patient's home physician who surprisingly stated that Mrs. H. W. had been healthy and lucid, but that her husband had died five months earlier. This new information was presented to the nursing home patient care team of nurses and recreational therapist. The attending physician was unimpressed when contacted by telephone. The head nurse, in contrast, was most impressed and called a family meeting with the patient's sister, which the physician reluctantly attended. After this meeting, the physician was antagonized when the nurse suggested the psychotropic medications were exacerbating the patient's problems by producing lethargy, which necessitated heavy nursing care. The physician was concerned with skin breakdown and insisted the catheter treatment be continued. No rehabilitation therapy was possible.

One week during a team meeting, the recreational therapist mentioned a case report she had read recently regarding the interaction of psychotropics and procainamide in producing reversible dementia.

Suddenly interested and not threatened, the physician discontinued the medications. The nursing staff, with renewed enthusiasm, offered to include the patient in their pressure sore protocol that included removing the catheter. The physician agreed to this. A nursing aide whose mother had a hearing aid similar to that of the patient thought to insert a new battery. The dietician suggested a higher nutrient intake and the others concurred.

Two weeks later, the patient, fully coherent, lucid, bespectacled and communicating normally, was progressing with increasing enthusiam in a rehabilitation program and was talking openly, for the first time, of her distress and depression at her late husband's death. Four weeks later, Mrs. H. W. returned to her spotless and obviously well-managed home.

Adapted from Charatan, et al. (1985). Used by permission of McGraw-Hill Book Company.

Inaccessiblity of Services

The traditional medical care system depends on an individual's decision to seek a physician and the motivation and ability to travel to the site of care. Medical self-neglect is often caused by an inability to get to medical resources (Gretz and Peth 1974). The lack of outreach services is a major shortcoming in the health care of elders since many lack transportation or have mobility decrements. This is a real concern for elders because major functional disabilities occur in nearly 20 percent of those age seventy-five–eighty-four and 30 percent of those eighty-five and over (U.S. Dept. of Health and Human Services 1981). Some older people cannot use public transportation, cannot walk easily, and some lack the strength to sit through long waiting periods in the waiting room or even to leave their homes. Adequate transportation services and outreach to elders who are unable to travel are needed. Not only should access to primary care be provided, but a mechanism is needed to enable elders to have continual access during treatment, rehabilitation, and long-term maintenance. For the homebound, outreach services can go into the person's home to assist in identification of the health problem and link elders with needed resources.

Unnecessary Diagnostic Tests

More than twelve billion medical tests are performed in the United States each year, an average of more than forty tests per person. Tests are ordered by physicians to establish the correct diagnosis so that treatment can be rapidly initiated. When direct and indirect costs are considered, the total bill comes to approximately $160 billion a year, or about $600 per person (Pinckney 1984). Historically, physicians relied predominantly on their trained observations to diagnose illnesses. With the proliferation of high-technology diagnostic equipment, both physicians and the public are putting their trust in expensive, often dangerous diagnostic tests of questionable accuracy. Elders may be subject to even more diagnostic tests than the rest of the population because of their high number of hospital and doctor visits. Further, elders are at higher risk of adverse effects of laboratory tests.

A number of studies have documented that some laboratory tests are unnecessary or ineffective. For instance, an estimated 30 percent of all X-rays, mainly those of the chest and skull are unnecessary (Office of Technological Assessment 1982). The new testing procedures for osteoporosis are expensive and of questionable value in diagnosing osteoporosis. Goldman (1984) analyzed autopsy data and reported that the rate of

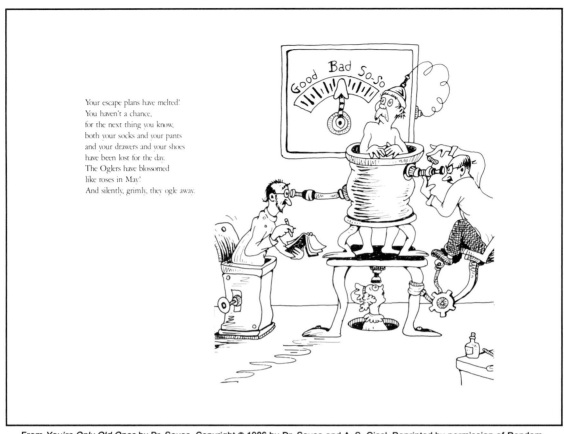

Your escape plans have melted!
You haven't a chance,
for the next thing you know,
both your socks and your pants
and your drawers and your shoes
have been lost for the day.
The Oglers have blossomed
like roses in May!
And silently, grimly, they ogle away.

From *You're Only Old Once* by Dr. Seuss. Copyright © 1986 by Dr. Seuss and A. S. Giesl. Reprinted by permission of Random House, Inc.

missed diagnosis in the 1980s is the same as in 1960—about 25 percent—despite the advent of high technology equipment such as ultrasound, cat scan, and nuclear medicine. In many cases, laboratory tests do not need to be done because the findings will not alter the proposed treatment.

Not only are some diagnostic tests expensive, unnecessary, and inaccurate, they may be misinterpreted or not interpreted at all. One study reported that when a group of radiologists were shown the same X-ray film, 25 percent of the radiologists' interpretations differed from the rest. When re-reading the same film, almost one-third disagreed with their former finding. Other studies indicate that from 20 to 50 percent of lung cancers visible on X-rays were not spotted by radiologists. Even after physicians receive laboratory results, they may not be interpreted.

It is estimated that 25 to 50 percent of abnormal test results are not followed up by physicians (Pinckney, 1984).

Finally, diagnostic tests can be outright harmful for the patient. One pilot study (Schroeder et al. 1978) found that complications occurred in 14 percent of all hospitalized patients undergoing moderate diagnostic risk procedures; three-fourths of these required further hospitalization or additional therapy. Even the process of taking blood for diagnostic tests may result in anemia or the need for transfusions among hospital patients. Patients in intensive care had an average of two pints of blood drawn during their hospital stay and 17 percent had losses from blood-taking significant enough to create a need for transfusions (Smollar and Krushkall 1986).

Chapter 12

The Grey Panthers actively lobby for laws that increase the quality of life for older people.

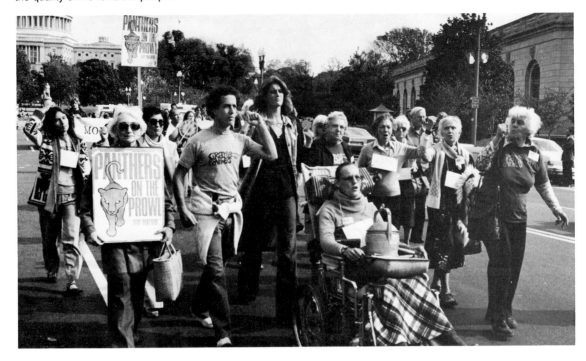

Despite their problems, useless diagnostic tests are still commonly ordered. There are many reasons for this. Physicians often comply with patients' requests for tests because the public places more confidence in technological tests than a physician's trained observations. Physicians may also order tests because they are reimbursed more for a diagnostic test than for the time it would take to diagnose the patient. Some diagnostic tests can be profitable for physicians when they can be accomplished in the physician's office for a fraction of the cost billed to insurance plans. One study found that physicians whose fees are based on the services they provide order 50 percent more electrocardiograms and 40 percent more chest X-rays than doctors, whose patients pay a pre-set fee for medical care (Epstein et al. 1986). Finally, with the increase in malpractice litigations, physicians may wish to protect themselves by ordering every possible test. The likelihood of being sued for not ordering a necessary test is much greater than being sued for unnecessary testing. A survey by the American Medical Association reported that at least three out of four doctors admitted having ordered tests for the sole purpose of having a better defense should a patient bring a suit against them (Sobel 1986).

The elder consumer and family members, if available, can play a significant role in reducing unnecessary medical tests. The physician should be asked a number of questions before the patient consents to a medical test: Why is the test needed? Will the results affect the treatment strategy? Are there enough symptoms to warrant a test? Is the test safe? Is a test the most cost-effective way to gather information? An interpretation of test results should always be requested. In some cases, retesting or a second opinion is helpful. An excellent resource for health consumers regarding specific diagnostic tests is *The People's Book of Medical Tests* by D. S. Sobel and T. Ferguson (1985).

Unnecessary Surgery

Of the twenty-five million annual surgeries performed in North America, an estimated 20 percent, or five million, may be unnecessary (Denney 1979). Although surgery may be necessary, even life-saving in some cases, it carries high risks. Elders are especially vulnerable to the risks of unnecessary surgery because they are more prone to adverse effects of immobility caused by longer bed rest, anesthesia complications, infection, adverse drug reactions and surgical complications. A number of surgical procedures commonly performed on elders are of questionable value in treating illness and may be unnecessary and harmful.

Hysterectomy, the removal of the uterus, is one of the most common elective surgical procedures in North America. However, the medical necessity of such surgery is questionable. Doctors in Britain perform only half as many operations as North American physicians (McPherson et al. 1982). It is thought that many physicians perform hysterectomies on women after menopause because they regard the uterus as a useless organ with the potential to develop cancer. Many physicians also remove healthy ovaries when removing the uterus (radical hysterectomy) to prevent ovarian cancer. Removal of the ovaries and uterus increases the likelihood of heart disease, osteoporosis, loss of libido and prolonged depression.

Until recently, a malignant breast lump always resulted in a radical mastectomy—the surgical removal of the tumor, breast(s), lymph nodes under the arms, and the pectoral muscles. While radical mastectomy is the most common, less invasive techniques are as effective and less disfiguring. Less radical therapy has been shown to be as effective as radical mastectomy (Fisher et al. 1985).

Almost 30 percent of all prostatectomies (surgical removal of the prostate gland) are thought to be unnecessary. Prostatectomy can carry complications of sterility or erectile dysfunction along with associated psychological changes. In many cases, less drastic surgical procedures are better choices.

Coronary artery bypass surgery is the most common surgical treatment for coronary artery disease. This surgery involves grafting veins from the legs to bypass obstructions in the coronary artery. This surgery may be effective in reducing pain and mortality in those with incapacitating angina or serious blockages (a small minority of those currently receiving such surgery). However, this is a dangerous and costly procedure that does not cure or retard the underlying disease. For the majority of patients with heart disease, artery bypass offers no significant advantage over drug treatment. Further, mortality rate may be as high as 5.5 percent during and after coronary bypass surgery (Christian and staff 1980).

Pacemaker implantation surgery is another expensive, often unnecessary procedure. The Special Committee on Aging of the United States Senate (1986) estimated that almost half the 130,000 pacemaker operations in America were unnecessary.

Carotid endarterectomy is performed on more than 100,000 patients each year, half of which do not have symptoms. A recent study reported that even though the operation is conducted to prevent strokes, the procedure itself places patients at higher risk of heart attacks and strokes. Further, because half of those who undergo the operation are already at low risk, the need for surgery is questioned (Chambers and Norris 1986).

About 200,000 back operations are performed each year in North America. Although surgery may be helpful in treating back problems caused by spinal abnormalities, it is ineffective for back pain due to muscle strain, the most common cause of back pain. Alternative treatments such as medication, heat, whirlpool baths, exercises, relaxation techniques, and behavior modification are the most effective treatments for back pain caused by muscle strains.

To avoid unnecessary surgery, elders and their families should be encouraged to get a second opinion when surgery is recommended. In addition, elders should question the physician about alternative treatments and their survival rate without surgical intervention. They should ask about the risks and benefits of surgery and determine if the least invasive method has been selected. If surgery is necessary, information on the surgeon's complication rate and experience in performing that surgery on elders should be requested.

Iatrogenic Illnesses

When diagnostic tests, medical treatments, or the hospital environment make sick people sicker, the person is said to have an iatrogenic illness. Although aging itself is not a risk factor for iatrogenic illness, the accompaniments of aging—multiple diseases, high drug use, age-associated decrements, and higher rates of hospitalization—create a higher risk for iatrogenic illness among that group (Steel 1984). Diagnostic tests, inaccurate diagnoses, overuse of interventive therapies, patient neglect, and overprescription of medication contribute to the high rate of iatrogenic illnesses in elders. The costs are more than monetary and may include lengthened hospital stay, physiological complications, depression, deterioration, and even death in some instances.

Iatrogenic illnesses are most common in the hospital setting because of the procedures that may accompany hospitalization and the presence of virulent microorganisms in the hospital environment. Gillick and colleagues (1982) examined a large sample of patients and found that 41 percent of the elder patients reported symptoms such as confusion, anorexia (loss of appetite), falling, and incontinence that were unrelated to their diagnosis upon admission. Over half the time, these symptoms were related to the use of psychotropic drugs, restraints, feeding tube, or catheter. Another study reported that 36 percent of all elder patients admitted to one teaching hospital suffered an iatrogenic illness, and in 9 percent, the incident threatened life or caused disability (Steel et al. 1981).

A cardinal principle of geriatric medicine, especially when the course of a patient turns suddenly for the worse, is to ask first, "What have I done to the patient?" rather than "What has the environment done?"

William Hazzard (1985)

Directions for Change

The medical care delivery system in the United States is technologically one of the best in the world. However, skyrocketing costs for health care, the rise in malpractice suits and the increased criticism of American physicians and hospitals point to a need for reform. The previous section discussed reasons why the current system is ill-equipped to deal with the complexity of chronic illness in the aged.

A number of strategies to improve health care delivery to elders have come about in response to the criticism and are listed below.

1. An expanded definition of health care that takes into account psychological, social, cultural, and physiological factors in the prevention and treatment of illness.
2. Decreased reliance on drug therapy and invasive diagnostic and surgical treatment and increased emphasis on lifestyle modification and other alternative treatment approaches.
3. Increased emphasis on prevention of disease and health promotion, including patient education in the medical setting, as well as health education and health behavior change programs at sites convenient for elders.

4. Increased use of case management, using a team of medical specialists, health and allied social service personnel to facilitate comprehensive, continuous care.

5. Development of comprehensive care that incorporates medical and social services, if not under one roof, then with effective linkages.

6. Increased training in geriatrics in medical schools and more opportunity for continuing education for current physicians regarding the special problems and needs of elders.

7. Expanded access to medical care services by making health care affordable and with a minimum of bureaucratic red tape.

8. Provision of low-cost transportation, neighborhood clinics, and outreach services into individual homes to provide diagnostic, treatment, and health maintenance services; outreach services also need to find individuals who may not otherwise seek care.

9. Involvement of elders in the planning and operation of those services geared to their use to optimize the types and modes of services offered.

10. Provision of support services to families involved in the care of their older members.

11. Increased responsibility and control of the patient for personal medical care choices.

12. Expansion of the use of patient advocates trained to help elders who cannot traverse the medical system alone.

This section will focus on only a few of the many trends that are changing the face of the medical system in the United States.

Health Promotion

Although it is widely accepted that preventing an illness is preferable to treating it after it happens, disease prevention is not a priority in the health care system. Because there is a high prevalence of disease in older persons, the potential to prevent these diseases is great. A broader implementation of preventive health care has the potential to prevent or postpone the onset or decrease the severity of illness in elders. There are many levels of prevention. Primary prevention is keeping a disease from occurring and includes immunization and promoting positive health behaviors through education. Among elders, influenza immunizations, education, and encouragement of physical fitness, accident prevention, and proper nutriton are beneficial. Secondary prevention refers to the early detection of common health problems so treatment can begin early to minimize the effects of disease. Screening for breast cancer, colorectal cancer, glaucoma, visual and hearing decrements, and hypertension are the most helpful for the older population. Secondary prevention may include yearly physical examinations by a physician, health screenings at community locations, or home assessment by health workers. Screening is especially effective for certain high-risk groups of elders such as those living alone, the recently bereaved, the mentally impaired, and the physically disabled (Fry 1985).

Physicians and elders may be discouraged from initiating preventive activities because there is little to no financial support from governmental or private sector health insurance for preventive activities. Some private companies have found that programs to promote health in the workplace are cost-effective because participants have lower absenteeism, use fewer medical services, and ultimately reduce employer costs. Likewise expenditures for medical services might be reduced among elders if Medicare reimbursed for preventive activities.

> Our fascination with the more glamorous "pound of cure" has tended to dazzle us into ignoring the more effective "ounce of prevention."
>
> Jimmy Carter

The goal of health promotion programs is to assist the public to facilitate changes in behaviors that enhance health. Health promotion programs generally focus on education and accompanying techniques to improve diet, lose weight, implement an exercise program, cease smoking, reduce alcohol consumption, reduce the potential for accidents, or cope with stress. Alteration in health behaviors brought about by health promotion activities can have a great impact on the development and progression of many of the chronic illnesses common among older people. Epidemiologists report that the greatest impact on chronic illness can be made through life-style changes rather than technological interventions, such as drugs or surgery. The American Medical Association reports that as many as 80 percent of the diseases that plague Americans are related to lifestyle. For instance, the incidence of heart disease is thought to be declining because of increased public awareness regarding factors affecting its development and consequent change in health behavior to reduce risk factors.

Studies conducted on young and middle-aged adults report that health promotion can reduce health care costs, increase health and productivity, and decrease absenteeism. One study reported that education about self-care (by individual consultations and educational materials) decreased health care utilization by 14 percent as compared to a control group (Vickery et al 1983). Further, among working adults, a physical activity/educational program in the workplace reduced the number of disability days and caused a 37.5 percent decrease in major medical

Although lifestyle modifications are known to prevent or slow the progression of many chronic conditions, little is known about the effectiveness of health promotion activities in altering negative behaviors among elders. The lack of research on elders may reflect the professional bias that it is futile to attempt to change the behaviors of elders since they have so little time left to live or their health habits are too ingrained to change. How-

ever, one preliminary study with elders who attended a lecture series on clinical medicine documented an increase in health knowledge, reported quality of life, improved health behaviors, and self-confidence. However, no alteration in health status or utilization of health services was noted (Nelson et al. 1984). It is obvious that more research is necessary to determine which, if any, health promotion strategies improve elders' health status.

Experts in health promotion recognize that many health behaviors associated with disease are under the control of the individual and can be modified. However, there are many health behaviors that are not under personal control, but are due to societal factors. For this reason, professionals are cautioned to be aware of the victim-blaming mentality in which clients are blamed for their health problems because of negative personal health behaviors that are beyond individual control (Minkler and Pasick 1986). For instance, it is not reasonable to recommend that an elder get more physical exercise by taking long walks if she or he lives in a crime-ridden neighborhood nor is recommending a special diet that is expensive for an individual depending on food stamps.

Because of the many socially induced variables that affect personal health, some health professionals consider health promotion to include the mobilization of individuals to become active in political change that will improve health care for a far greater number of people. For instance, elders may become active in efforts to change local laws regarding smoking in public places, advocate for more stringent nursing home regulations or national health insurance. In this way, professionals involved in health promotion activities can work on two fronts—not only encouraging individual health behavior change, but also reducing political, social, and other environmental influences that ultimately impinge on health status (Minkler and Pasick 1986). Green and colleagues (1980) provide a broad definition of health promotion to include "any combination of health education and related organizational, political, and economic interventions designed to facilitate behavioral and environmental changes conducive to health."

Consumer Health Movement

Dissatisfaction with the system of medical care is rampant in our country. High costs, the mixed success of many traditional medical practices, and inadequate physician/patient relationships, have driven an increasing number of consumers to learn more about health matters and to become more assertive in directing their medical care. The myriad of health-related articles in newspapers and magazines and self-help books attest to the increasing responsibility individuals are shouldering for their own well-being. Consumers need information to make educated choices about their health care, to avoid quackery, and to select low-cost, effective health care products and services. The consumer health movement involves the education of individuals about their rights and responsibilities so they can maximize their health care.

Elder consumers need to be educated about the medical care system, how to seek retribution for poor medical care, and current understandable information regarding personal health issues. Further, they often need training in being assertive with their physician to ensure optimum treatment.

Although Western medicine generally recognizes the patient's right to make personal decisions regarding medical care, not all possess the ability to act on their own behalf, especially if weakened by illness. Advocacy is "action designed to help the powerless acquire and use power and to make social systems more responsive to their needs" (Rogers 1980). Patient advocates are a product of the consumer health movement. These advocates assist elders—especially the uneducated, poor, or ethnic minorities—become informed and take responsibility for their health care. Patient advocates are generally nurses or trained laypersons (often elders themselves) who educate, support, and assist clients in making important health care decisions as they travel through the complex health care system. Advocates may educate clients on their disease, drugs or surgery, assist in decision-making regarding diagnostic testing and treatment modalities. Many also accompany a patient to the physician to ensure information is understood and questions are adequately answered. If not informed by the physician, they also find and coordinate needed health care services. Because advocates generally follow an individual throughout the course of treatment, they are in a prime position to deal with the psychosocial issues surrounding the illness. The federal government has formalized patient advocacy in nursing homes by promoting the development of ombudsman programs throughout the nation. This will be discussed in more depth in the next chapter.

The following is a case history that exemplifies the power of advocates in enhancing the health of elders.

An advocate began working with a seventy-five year old man who lived alone and had moderate mobility problems. After a home visit, the advocate determined that the man was not eating adequately and arranged transportation to and from a daily meal at a congregate meal site. Additionally, the man frequently complained of foot problems, but said he had not brought them to the attention of his physician. The advocate arranged a visit to a podiatrist and accompanied the elder on the visit. The problems were minor, but the care provided significantly improved the man's ability to walk. The advocate also found that the man was not following the restricted diet for diabetes. The advocate discussed the nature of the disease and the importance of the special diet and assisted the man in planning and shopping for foods he enjoyed. The advocate also taught him to do a simple urine test to monitor his diabetes.

Alternative Healing Approaches

Many alternative treatment approaches have been around for centuries. Although most alternative methods are decried as unscientific by some, a number are becoming more accepted among the public and the scientific community. Elders may be more likely to use alternative methods of healing because they do not have the same faith in science as younger groups. They tend to be less educated and may be more likely to adhere to their ethnic healing practices. However, over-reliance on alternative treatment modalities may cause elders to delay seeking needed care. On the other hand, because health is affected by psychological and social factors, these alternative modalities may be well-suited to many of their problems as modern medicine is often ineffective in treating the diseases of elders. Many alternative treatments are less invasive than drugs or surgery and even if they do no good, at least they do no harm. A brief overview of the most common alternative treatments will be discussed below. Some are recognized by traditional medical practitioners and others are not.

Chiropractors manipulate the spine and other bones to relieve pressure on nerves and cure disease. Chiropractors believe partially dislocated vertebrae emit heat from pressure on the nerves and these pressures are the cause of discomfort. Although physicians believe their claims are unscientific, many Americans are very satisfied with the treatment they have received from Doctors of Chiropractic.

Doctors of Osteopathy also utilize spinal manipulation to treat several health problems. Osteopaths are licensed on the same basis as M.D.s to practice medicine, perform surgery, and prescribe drugs. These doctors emphasize the relationship between body structure and function and tend to be general practitioners, rather than specialists. In the past few decades, osteopaths have received increasing responsibilities and privileges.

Acupuncture is an ancient Chinese technique to reduce pain by inserting long thin needles in specific points in the body. The Chinese have

Acupuncture is an alternative to drugs for reducing pain.

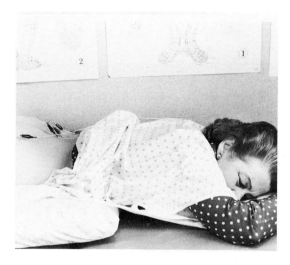

been able to perform major surgery without anesthesia using acupuncture. Acupuncture has been used successfully in dental surgery, skin grafts, and tumor biopsies in the United States. Acupuncture may be especially useful for elders since it reduces surgical complications caused by anesthesia use. There is still much to be learned about how and why acupuncture works. The major danger with this treatment is that uncertified persons may practice it. Acupressure utilizes the same theories as acupuncture, except pressure is applied to the points where needles might be inserted.

Other alternative healing strategies are practiced among particular sub-groups with varying degrees of success. Naturopathy relies entirely on natural methods to cure illness. Massage, physical exercise, health-food diets, vitamins, fasting, vegetarianism, vibration, sunshine, heat, and rest may be used. This method of healing avoids invasive drug and surgical treatments and considers disease to be a result of a violation of nature's law. The premise of homeopathy is that an imbalance in the vital force is the cause of illness and that herbal extracts serve to allow the person to heal him or herself. Hypnotherapy is the use of hypnosis to place the individual in a very relaxed state. The individual is put into a trance and the hypnotist uses the power of suggestion to alter behaviors or perceptions. Hypnosis has been used to reduce pain in childbirth and dentistry and to treat emotional problems, headaches, and to aid in weight loss or other behavioral modification. Faith healing, which involves prayer and often laying on of hands, is based on the belief that some healers can remove disease by appealing to God.

A Service Alternative: The Health Maintenance Organization

Traditional medical services charge an individual for each medical service provided; the more goods and services provided, the higher the total bill. Instead of paying physicians a fee for each service rendered, patients who enroll in a Health Maintenance Organization (HMO) pay a fixed monthly premium that covers all medical services they require. A group practice HMO is the most common. In this case, a group of physicians, employed by the organization, serves patients at one location. A few HMOs without a central location utilize fee-for-service physicians who work out of their own offices on a prepaid basis for HMO participants. In any case, the Health Maintenance Organization also arranges with a local hospital to provide inpatient care and contracts outside specialists as needed. The plan assumes the financial risk for keeping costs within the total premiums they receive. HMO physicians have a strong incentive to keep services to a minimum, so preventive measures and avoidance of unnecessary diagnostic tests, drugs, surgery, or hospitalization are stressed.

Very few elders belonged to an HMO in the past. Medicare beneficiaries could not join because the monthly fee was not reimbursed by Medicare. However, the 1982 Tax Act authorized Medicare to pay prepaid benefits to any HMO that enrolls Medicare patients and by 1987, about 867,000 older people were enrolled. Medicare pays an amount equal to 95 percent of the average cost of treating a Medicare patient, taking age, sex, and institutional status into consideration. Both hospital use and total health care cost of those enrolled in HMOs are significantly less than private practitioners (Luft 1981).

An even broader program, a social/health maintenance organization (SHMO), has been developed by Brandeis University and has been implemented at four sites in the nation. Their services include medical services as well as a broad range of home-health and other services aimed at keeping people out of hospitals and nursing homes (Demkovich 1985). These will likely become more popular in the future, especially among elders, because of the emphasis on rehabilitation, continuity of care, and reducing unnecessary hospitalization or nursing home placement.

Summary

Although elders utilize physician and hospital services more than any other age group, these services have not been geared to their special needs. Elders finance the majority of their health care through governmental health insurance policies—Medicare and Medicaid. Medicare is available to all elders over age sixty-five and mainly finances physicians and hospital costs. Medicaid is a health insurance for the poor, blind, and disabled of all ages and provides broad coverage for those poor enough to qualify.

There are a number of barriers in the current medical care system that reduce its effectiveness in meeting the needs of older people. These include: high cost, poor physician/patient relationship, traditional medical model, lack of training in geriatrics, fragmentation and overspecialization of services, inaccessibility, unnecessary procedures, and iatrogenic illnesses. Because of these barriers to effective health care delivery, a number of trends have emerged that are changing the face of medical care in this country, such as increased attention to prevention, health promotion, and consumer rights. Further, alternatives to traditional medicine are gaining credibility. Finally, health maintenance organizations are becoming an option for elders.

Activities

1. Question a social worker at your county welfare department, the president of an elder activist group, the planner at your local Area Agency on Aging, and a member of the local health department to determine their perception of the medical needs of elders in your community.

2. Collect advertisements and articles on alternative healing techniques. To what age group are these articles geared? Discuss their credibility.

3. Informally survey the physicians in your community by telephone to determine if they accept Medicaid. How many accept Medicare assignment? Do those who accept Medicaid have a limit on how many patients they will take?

4. What current legislation is pending in your state that would affect medical care of elders? Write a letter to your representative outlining the reasons it should or should not be passed.

5. Research the health care system of another developed country. What might be the advantages and drawbacks of such a system in our country? What special considerations does the system have for its elders? Do you think this system would be more or less effective in meeting the needs of our country's elders?

6. As part of a class project, debate the statement: "Medical care is the right of all individuals in our country, regardless of ability to pay."

7. Find out if your community offers the following health services to elders:

   free or reduced rate medical care
   mass screening programs
   health promotion programs
   medical outreach into elders' homes or
       neighborhood sites
   transportation to medical care
   other medical services

8. Many hospitals are reaching out to serve the special needs of elders. Find out what special services are offered to elders by the hospital(s) in your community.

9. Using the two perspectives on DRGs and other information, hold a class debate on the topics: DRGs will improve the health of elders in our country.

10. Devise an ideal federal health insurance package for elders that would alleviate the problems with the current system. Is your proposed system cost-effective?

Bibliography

Beeson, P. B. 1985. Institute of medicine report on aging and medical education. *Bull NY Acad Med* 61(6): 478–83.

Berman, E. 1976. *The solid gold stethoscope.* New York: MacMillan.

Bertakis, K. D. 1977. The communication of information from physician to patient: A method for increasing patient retention and satisfaction. *J Fam Practice* 5:217–22.

Bowne, D. W., M. L. Russell, J. L. Morgan, et al. 1984. Reduced disability and health care costs in an industrial fitness program. *J Occup Med* 26:809–16.

Branch, L. G., and K. T. Nemeth. 1985. When elders fail to visit physicians. *Medical Care* 23(11): 1265–75.

Brody, S. J. 1985. Formal health support systems. In Andres, R., E. L. Bierman, and W. R. Hazzard, eds. *Principles of geriatric medicine.* San Francisco: McGraw-Hill. 187–198.

Carlson, E. 1984. Hospital horror. *Modern Maturity,* October–November: 108–10; 112–14.

Chambers, B. R., and J. W. Norris. 1986. Outcome in patients with asymptomatic neck bruits. *N Engl J Med* 315(14): 860–865.

Charatan, F. B., C. J. Foley, and L. S. Libow. 1985. The team approach to geriatric medicine. In Andres, R., E. L. Birren, and W. R. Hazzard, eds. *Principles of geriatric medicine.* San Francisco: McGraw-Hill. 170–71.

Christian, R. and staff. 1980. *Prevention guide to surgery and its alternatives.* Emmaus, Pa.: Rodale Press.

Demkovich, L. 1985. Are HMOs what the doctor ordered? *Modern Maturity* December 1984–January 1985: 120–24, 126–27.

Denney, M. K. 1979. *Second opinion.* New York: Grosset and Dunlap.

Epstein, A. M., C. B. Begg, and B. J. McNeil. 1986. The use of ambulatory testing in prepaid and fee-for-service group practices. *N Engl J Med* 314 (17): 1089–94.

Fisher, B., M. Bauer, and R. Margolese. 1985. Five year results of a randomised clinical trial comparing total mastectomy and segmental mastectomy with or without radiation in the treatment of breast cancer. *N Engl J Med* 312: 665–73.

Fry, P. S. 1985. *Depression, stress, and adaptations in the elderly.* Rockville, Md.: Aspen Systems Corp.

Gillick, M. R., N. A. Serrell, and L. S. Gillick. 1982. Adverse consequences of hospitalization in the elderly. *Soc Sci Med* 16: 1033–8.

Goldman, L. 1984. Diagnostic advances vs. the value of the autopsy 1912–1980. *Arch Pathol Lab Med* 108: 501–5.

Green, L., M. Kreuter, S. G. Deeds, and K. B. Partridge. 1980. *Health education planning: A diagnostic approach.* Palo Alto, Calif.: Mayfield.

Green, M. G., R. Adelman, R. Charon, and S. Hoffman. 1986. Ageism in the medical encounter: an exploratory study of the doctor-elderly patient relationship. *Lang and Commun* 6:113–124.

Gretz, F. K., and P. R. Peth. 1974. An outreach program of medical care for aged high-rise residents. *Gerontologist* 14(5): 404–07.

Hazzard, W. R. 1985. The practice of geriatric medicine. In Andres, R., E. L. Bierman, and W. R. Hazzard, eds. *Principles of geriatric medicine.* San Francisco: McGraw Hill. 3–5.

Health Care Financing Administration. 1986. The financial impact of the prospective payment system (PPS) on Medicare participating hospitals—1984. (ACN-09-62021). Washington, D.C.: Dept. Health and Human Services.

JAMA. 1985. Medical schools face challenge of preparing physicians to care for a fast-growing elderly population. March 1. 253(9): 1225–7; 1231.

Johnson, J. E. 1985. Geriatrics and medical education-initiatives of the Association of American Medical Colleges. *Bull NY Acad Med* 61(6): 484–91.

Kane, R. L., D. H. Solomon, J. C. Beck, et al. 1980. Geriatrics in the United States: Manpower projections and training considerations. Rand Corp. Publication Number R-2543 HJK. Santa Monica, Calif.: Rand Corp.

Keeler, E. B., O. H. Solomon, J. C. Beck, et al. 1982. Effect of patient age on duration of medical encounters with physicians. *Medical Care* 20: 1101–08.

Koch, H., and D. A. Knapp. 1987. Highlights of drug utilization in office practice: National Ambulatory Medical Care Survey, 1985. *Advance Data from Vital and Health Statistics* No. 134, May 19, 1987. Hyattsville, Md.: U.S. Public Health Service.

Kotelchuck, R. 1986. And what about the patients? Prospective payment's impact on quality of care. *Health/Pac Bulletin* 17(2):13–17.

Levin, A. A. 1986. More is not always better. *Health/Pac Bulletin* 17(2): 21.

Libow, L., and F. Sherman. 1981. *The core of geriatric medicine.* St Louis: C. V. Mosby.

Lubitz, J., and R. Prihoda. 1983. *Use and costs of medical services in the last years of life: Health, United States. 1983.* DHHS Publication Number (PHS) 84–1232. National Center for Health Statistics, Public Health Service, Washington, D.C.: U.S. Government Printing Office.

Luft, H. 1981. *Health maintenance organizations: Dimensions of performance.* New York: John Wiley.

McPherson, K., J. E. Wennberg, O. B. Hovind, P. Clifford. 1981. Small-area variations in the use of common surgical procedures: An interdisciplinary comparison of New England, England and Norway. *N Engl J Med* 307(21) 1310–14.

Michelmore, P. 1975. A modern geriatric health care system: Coordinated endeavor of patient care and physician training. *Geriatrics* 30(2):147–55.

Minkler, M., and R. J. Pasick. 1986. Health promotion and the elderly: A critical perspective on the past and future. In Dychtwald, K., ed. *Wellness and health promotion for the elderly.* Rockville, Md.: Aspen Systems Corp.

National Center for Health Statistics. 1983. Physicians visits: Volume and interval since last visit: United States, 1980. *Vital and Health Statistics,* Series 10, No. 144. Hyattsville, Md.: U.S. Public Health Service.

National Center for Health Statistics. 1986. 1985 Summary: National hospital discharge survey. *Advance Data from Vital and Health Statistics* No. 127. DHHS Pub. No. (PHS) 86–1250. Hyattsville, Md.: Public Health Service.

National Center for Health Statistics. 1985. 1984 Summary: National hospital discharge survey. *Advance Data from Vital and Health Statistics.* September 27, 1985. No. 112. Hyattsville, Md.: U.S. Public Health Service.

Nelson, E. C., G. McHugo, P. Schnurr, et al. 1984. Medical self-care education for elders: A controlled trial to evaluate impact. *Am J Public Health* 74(12) 1357–62.

Office of Technological Assessment. 1982. The implications of cost-effectiveness analysis of medical technology. Background Paper #5: Four common X-ray procedures; problems for economic evaluation. Washington, D.C.: Office of Technological Assessment, April.

Pinckney, E. 1984. Diagnostic tests. *Health Facts* 9(67): 3–4.

Rogers, J. C. 1980. Advocacy: The key to assessing the older client. *J Gerontol Nurs* 6(1): 33–36.

Schroeder, S. A., K. I. Marton, and B. L. Strom. 1978. Frequency and morbidity of invasive procedures. Report of a pilot study from two teaching hospitals. *Arch Intern Med* 138: 1809–11.

Shapiro, E., and N. P. Roos. 1985. Elderly non-users of health services. *Medical Care* 23(3): 247–57.

Smoller, B. R., and M. S. Kruskall. 1986. Phlebotomy for diagnostic laboratory tests in adults: Pattern of use and effect on transfusion requirements. *N Engl J Med* 314(19): 1233–35.

Sobel, D. S. 1986. When not to take medical tests. *American Health* November: 54–57, 59–60.

Special Committee on Aging. U.S. Senate 1986. *Pacemakers revisited: A saga of benign neglect.* Hearing of 99th Congress. May 10, 1985. Serial H 99–4. S. Hrg. 99–608. Washington, D.C.: U.S. Govt. Printing Office.

Steel, K., R. M. Gertman, C. Crescenzi, et al. 1981. Iatrogenic illness on a general medical service at a university hospital. *N Engl J Med* 304: 638–42.

Steel, K. 1984. Iatrogenic disease on a medical service. *J Am Geriatr Soc* 32(6): 445–49.

Stoller, E. P. 1982. Patterns of physician utilization by the elderly: A multivariate analysis. *Medical Care* 20(11): 1080–89.

Stultz, B. M. 1984. Preventive health care for the elderly. *West J Med* 141(6): 832–45.

U.S. Department of Health and Human Services. 1981. *A chartbook of the Federal Council on Aging. 1981.* DHHS Pub. No. (OHDS)81–20704. Washington, D.C.: U.S. Government Printing Office.

Veteran's Administration. 1984a. *Annual report. 1983.* Washington, D.C.: U.S. Government Printing Office.

Veteran's Administration. 1984b. *Caring for the older veteran.* Washington, D.C.: U.S. Government Printing Office.

Vickery, D. M., H. Kalmer, D. Lowry, et al. 1983. Effect of a self-care education program on medical visits. *JAMA* 250: 2952–56.

Waldo, D., and H. Lazenby, 1984. Demographic characteristics and health care use and expenditures by the aged in the United States: 1977–1984. *Health Care Financ Rev* 6(1).

White House Conference on Aging: Technical Committee on Health Services. *1981 Executive Summary.* Washington, D.C.

Williams, E. S., and N. H. Barley. 1985. Old people not known to the general practitioner: Low risk group. *Br Med J* 291: 251–54.

Wilson, R. W. and E. J. White, 1977. Changes in morbidity, disability and utilization differentials between the poor and the non-poor, data from the Health Interview Survey, 1964 and 1973. *Medical Care* 15: 636–46.

13 Long-Term Care

Everyone who is born holds dual citizenship, in the kingdom of the well and in the kingdom of the sick. Although we all prefer to use only the good passport, sooner or later each of us is obliged, at least for a spell, to identify ourselves as citizens of that other place.

Susan Sontag (1978)

Introduction

Long-term care includes a wide range of health and social services provided in institutional, community, or home settings to promote the maximum level of physical, psychological, and social functioning. Both long-term care facilities and home-care programs are developing rapidly. They serve millions of Americans who are physically and mentally disabled from birth defects, accidents, or chronic diseases that interfere with normal activities of daily living.

This chapter will explore both home-health care and long-term care institutions. The history of long-term care, types, costs, quality of care, and the benefits and drawbacks of both home care and institutionalization will be discussed. Various funding mechanisms will be addressed. Factors to consider in planning for long-term care will be considered as well as special concerns of the families of frail elders.

Only about five percent of the elder population resides in long term care facilities.

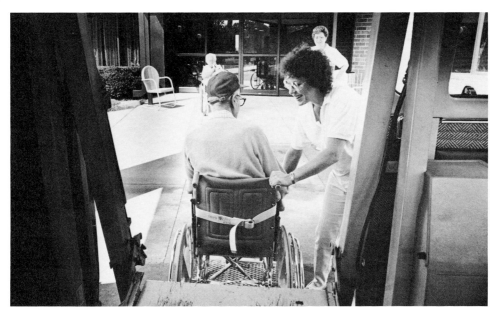

The Need

All age groups utilize long-term care services, but those over sixty-five are the prime recipients. Elders have more impairments and assorted medical conditions than any other age group. It is estimated that 2.8 million people aged sixty-five and older need the help of another person to carry out everyday activities. The need for help increases sharply with age; fewer than one in ten of those age sixty-five to seventy-four need help, but four of ten of those eighty-five and older need assistance (Feller 1983).

The need for long-term care is increasing drastically in our country and is directly related to the rapid increase in the sixty-five-and-older population. The group of highest users for long-term care, age seventy-five and older, is increasing the most dramatically. By 1990, it is estimated that ten to eleven million elders will need some type of long-term care (Wetle and Pearson 1986). Some estimate that by the year 2020, our country will need twice the services presently available.

In addition to changing demographics, a number of changes in social values and living patterns are causing a shift from family-oriented care toward a greater need for formal services in our country. Statistics reveal that those who live alone are at the highest risk for dependency on long-term care. The number of older people living alone is increasing. In 1950, less than 15 percent of elders lived alone, but by 1980, that figure doubled. The high divorce rate is increasingly responsible for the number of elders who will live alone. The increased percentage of women in the labor force reduces the number of wives and daughters available at home to care for frail family members. Additionally, the trend toward small families is reducing the number of adult children able to care for a disabled parent. Finally, advances in medical care enable those with chronic diseases to live longer, but many spend a greater length of time in a disabled state.

Financing Long-Term Care

Federal and state funding have made both institutional and home-care services more available to elders, the poor, and the chronically ill. The major sources of public funds for these services will be discussed below.

The Social Security Act of 1935 guaranteed a monthly income to eligible elders and the disabled. Financed through equal contribution of employer and employee wages, it provides a low-cost, federally sponsored insurance to partially provide for participants and their surviving spouses in old age. If Social Security benefits are less than that needed to survive, public assistance is available from Supplemental Security Income programs (SSI). Eligibility for public assistance is based on income and assets. Both Social Security and SSI programs provide elders with a guaranteed monthly income to allow them to choose to either remain in their own home or move into more sheltered settings.

In 1965, Medicare legislation (Title XVIII) was added to the Social Security Act. Medicare allows anyone age sixty-five and older, regardless of income, to use public funds to purchase selected health services. Medicare was intended mainly to support hospitalization and physician visits rather than extended long-term care. However, Medicare does fund limited skilled home-health services after hospitalization using the rationale that extended care in the home is less expensive than hospitalization.

As noted in the previous chapter, Medicare services are divided into two parts. Part A finances hospital care and skilled health services of a home-health agency following hospitalization. Benefits under Part A for nursing home care are very limited. The homes must be certified by Medicare, benefits cover only the first one hundred days of care, and patients must have been hospitalized previously with a condition requiring skilled nursing care. Because of these limitations, only 1 percent of Medicare dollars are spent on nursing home care (Waldo and Lazenby 1984). Part B reimburses a portion of a doctor's services, diagnostic tests, some drugs, and skilled health care in the home without any prior hospitalization requirement. However, Part B of Medicare also places many restrictions on home-health benefits. Home-health care reimbursement is restricted to the provision of skilled nursing services to homebound patients as prescribed by a physician as part of treatment plan. Unfortunately it does not cover services related to assisting with activities of daily living that permit individuals to remain in their own homes (e.g., bathing, dressing, housekeeping).

Medicaid legislation (Title XIX of the Social Security Act) provides medical and rehabilitation services to the poor, aged, blind, and disabled, and to poor families with dependent children. Medicaid is much less restrictive in financing long-term care than Medicare. To qualify, individuals must prove they have little to no assets. Eligible individuals can receive a wide range of both health and personal care services and do not need to be homebound. Medicaid also provides long-term, unlimited nursing home care without requiring previous hospitalization. However, the services must be authorized by a physician and the patient treatment plan must be reviewed every sixty days. Medicaid is the principal public mechanism for funding nursing home care; almost half the nursing home residents have Medicaid as their sole source of payment and 68 percent of Medicaid dollars are spent on nursing home care (Waldo and Lazenby 1984).

The Older Americans Act (OAA) was passed in 1965 to improve the lives of elders by providing monies for a broad range of health and social services as well as support for gerontological research and education. Although funding for this program is limited compared to Medicare and Medicaid, it enabled the development of a network of services for elders and a number of innovative programs to maximize their independence. The original act has been amended a number of times and programs have grown significantly. Departments of Aging in each state oversee a network of Area Agencies on Aging.

Each Area Agency on Aging plans and coordinates programs to benefit elders in its region. A large portion of the OAA allocations are used for in-home supportive services, nutrition and transportation services, legal services, and information and referral. In addition, each Area Agency on Aging is mandated to offer a nursing home ombudsman program to advocate for those in nursing and board and care homes in their areas.

Title XX of the Social Security Act, implemented in 1975, significantly expanded the availability of home-health care services for the poor. Under Title XX the Federal government matches the state's contribution to fund social services for low income individuals. Each state must assess its needs and resources and develop the social services it needs. Ten percent of Title XX funds is spent on in-home services, mainly for homemaker and home-health aide services.

The Veteran's Administration provides institutional care for those who have served in the military. The administration also pays for home-health assistance to disabled veterans with service-connected disabilities. Several VA hospitals have established their own programs to deliver home-health care services.

For those not sufficiently poor for Medicaid or Title XX monies, savings or private insurance are generally the only funding option for home-health or institutional care. About 40 percent of those in nursing homes pay their own way. Those sixty-five and older may purchase insurance to supplement Medicare coverage. However, supplementary health insurance generally restricts coverage to skilled nursing services, not the more commonly needed intermediate or board and care homes. Home-care services in some communities charge on a sliding scale based on the ability to pay.

Home-Health Services

Home-health care includes a wide range of services provided in the home or community to impaired individuals and their families to enable disabled individuals to remain at home as long as possible. Home-health care generally includes the following: medical, dental, and nursing services, nutrition services, rehabilitation services (physical, speech, and occupational therapy), personal care services (bathing, toileting, dressing), and homemaker services. Additionally, transportation, lab services, and medical equipment and supplies are sometimes included in home-health care. The primary target groups for home-health services are those recuperating from hospitalization, the chronically ill who can benefit from rehabilitation and health maintenance, the acutely ill who can be managed at home with help, and the dying. The decision to utilize home care is influenced by a number of variables: the elders' needs and desires, available support services in the community, and the elder's financial situation, among others.

History of Home-Health Services

Home-health care is not a new idea in our country. In the late 1700s, home-health care was popular since hospitals were feared because of high mortality rates due to poor sanitation and rudimentary medical techniques. In the late 1800s, the public health movement accompanied the development of home-health care as an organized component of the health delivery system (Ward 1983). Voluntary agencies, such as the Visiting Nurse Association, were formed to provide home nursing care. Health departments also began to offer nursing services to the poor.

By the early part of the twentieth century, improvement in sanitation procedures, infection control, and medical techniques made hospitals more popular. However, hospitals became overcrowded as those with chronic conditions entered and remained there. This forced hospitals to release patients, especially the poor, to free more hospital beds. Because of this increased demand, visiting and public health nurse services flourished as well as novel programs integrating homemaking, transportation, and health care services.

Home-health care continued to increase throughout the early twentieth century. After World War II, insurance companies began to include home nursing services in their benefit packages. In the early 1960s the federal government allocated grants to public agencies to develop hospital-based home-health services. The enactment of Medicare and Medicaid provided further encouragement for the development of home-health services.

Because of an increase in funding sources, a rise in the number of elders who need such services and the skyrocketing costs of institutionalization, the market for home-care products and services is growing. It is currently the fastest growing segment of the health care system, increasing at a rate of 20 percent a year (Barhydt-Wezenaar 1986).

Benefits and Limitations of Home Care

Home care for elders is generally far superior to the routine, impersonal care received in an institution. When the elder is able to be at home, the family and other social networks remain intact. Further, the individual and family can select particular services that meet their needs without financing unnecessary care. The availability of home-care services may postpone or even eliminate the need for a nursing home. Aside from humanitarian reasons, home-health care is less expensive than care in an institutional setting, especially if twenty-four-hour health care is not needed. One pilot study compared the costs of treating patients with senile dementia at home with those treated in a nursing home. The average cost for home care was half that of a nursing home—$11,735 vs. $22,458 per year (Hu et al. 1986). Although home-health care is comprehensive, inexpensive, and accessible in theory, in practice, the services often fall short of these goals.

A major limitation to home-health care is the unavailability of many home-health services. Despite the rapid growth in home-health care, most communities, especially rural areas, have only a few types of home-health services. Those that are available are of uneven quality because few states have minimum training standards and there is no governmental mechanism to oversee them. When services are present, they are often underdeveloped and fragmented. They usually focus on a specific health need or professional specialization instead of meeting the various needs of the client. As a result, when many different services are utilized, none has full responsibility for the client. This fragmentation makes it difficult for elders—especially those with disabilities and language difficulties—to consolidate home-care services to meet their needs. Further, elders may be unaware of home-care services, even when available. One study reported that almost half of an elder sample questioned was not aware of available home-health care services (Holmes et al. 1981).

Another barrier to home-health care service availability is its cost to the client. Whether or not an elder is eligible for governmental financial support can be a significant factor in deciding between home care or institutionalization. Despite the fact that home care generally costs less than institutional care, the out-of-pocket expenses for the individual choosing home care are significantly higher because eligibility standards and reimbursement criteria differ among services. Most have strict income eligibility standards and some do not reimburse those with long-standing chronic illness. In many cases, reimbursement criteria make it less expensive to enter an institution than use home-health services. For instance, although the very poor can receive home-health services through Medicaid, the near poor, those who are ineligible for federal reimbursement and unable to afford home care, may be prematurely institutionalized. A significant number of those in institutional settings do not need that level of care and are there because health services allowing them to stay at home do not exist in their communities or are not reimbursable.

The implementation of the Diagnostic Related Groups (DRG) system as payment for hospitalized Medicare patients has greatly increased the need for home-health care since many Medicare patients are released from the hospital who are still in a debilitated state. Despite these increased demands, a study by the American Association of Retired Persons Public Policy

Institute revealed that home-health payments have dropped considerably since the implementation of DRGs, because of a tighter eligibility for home-health care. This has created a serious gap in needed services as many patients enter a no care zone—qualifying neither for institutional or home-health care services (Brickfield 1986–87).

Because of limited availability and accessibility, very few elders actually utilize home-health care services. Until these drawbacks are remedied, home-health care will not be a reasonable option for many elders. Results from a national survey revealed that in a six-month period in 1985: 15 percent used a senior center, 8 percent of the elders surveyed ate meals at a senior center, 1 percent used homemaking services, 3 percent used visiting nurses, 2 percent used home-health aides, and less than 1 percent utilized adult day care centers (Stone 1986). Although these figures are low, the extent of unmet need for various services is not known.

Types of Home-Health Services

The following paragraphs outline the types of home-health services available. Despite the broad range of services listed, most communities offer few of these services. Instead, most elders must rely on their families or friends for long-term care or enter a nursing home to receive the services they need.

Physician Services

The physician is responsible to prescribe treatment needed at home for recovery and maintenance, which may include medication, therapy, or skilled care. The family or home-health agency staff generally implement the plan and periodically inform the physician about the health status of the patient.

Physicians are seldom willing to make house calls, preferring to treat patients in the office or emergency room. Because it is often difficult for a frail elder to visit the physician, some large cities have physician organizations that make house calls. In addition, some states enable physician

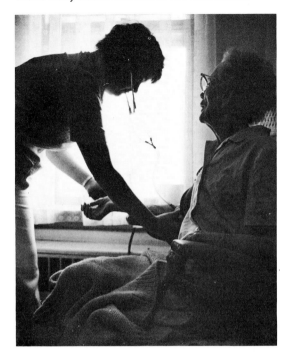

Visiting nurses provide necessary medical care which allows many elders to remain in their own homes.

assistants and nurse practitioners to make home visits and perform some diagnostic and therapeutic procedures formerly accomplished by physicians.

Nursing Services

Nursing services are commonly provided by registered nurses (RN) or licensed vocational nurses (LVN) from visiting nurse associations, public health departments, or home-health agencies. Nurses working under the auspices of health departments provide free services, mainly to poor and inner city elders. Other agencies adjust fees based on the client's income or may be reimbursed by Medicare or Medicaid. The provision of skilled nursing care service is a requirement for all home-health agencies certified by Medicare.

Nurses commonly visit sick individuals in their homes to evaluate their condition and determine the type of nursing care required to carry out the prescribed medical treatment plan. They also provide direct patient care, monitor treatment and serve as a referral source to other social and medical supports as needed. They provide health education and instruct the patient and family on basic home-care techniques such as changing sterile dressings, catheter care, and insulin injections.

Visiting Dentists

Although not yet common, some dentists make house calls to homebound elders. Dentists may perform routine preventive mouth care, treat dental problems, or fit dentures. Although this service is not covered by Medicare, in some states Medicaid pays the fee to those who qualify.

Physical, Speech, and Occupational Therapists

A physical therapist is needed when some use of the limbs or muscles is lost because of illness or accident. A speech therapist helps a patient who has suffered an illness or injury affecting speech to relearn and maintain this skill. An occupational therapist is used when illness or injury has affected the ability to perform routine functions. Activities and devices are also introducd to maintain or restore skills needed to function independently. For elders, stroke is the most common medical crisis that utilizes these therapists.

Individuals may receive physical, speech, or occupational therapy at home if it is part of their prescribed treatment plan. After assessing the client, therapists develop a treatment schedule and routinely visit in the home or a community setting until therapy is no longer needed. Therapists may also instruct the patient and family on rehabilitation activities that can be accomplished between visits.

Homemaker/Home-Health Aide Services

Homemaker/home-health aide services may be the most important services to postpone or prevent institutionalization. *Homemaker aides* perform a full range of homemaking activities—light

Most older women care for their spouses at home without the assistance of formal support services.

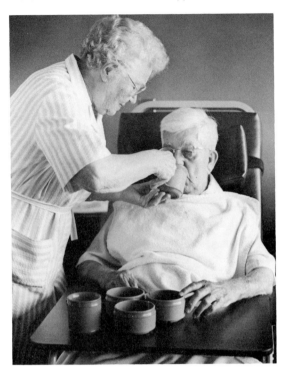

housekeeping, laundry, shopping, and meal preparation. *Home-health aides* provide for personal care, such as assisting with bathing, grooming, or therapy. In many cases, a paraprofessional performs both housekeeping and personal care activities.

The service of a home-health aide is reimbursed by Medicare, but homemaker services are not. Further, Medicare has very stringent criteria for eligibility and extent of health aide benefit. For those poor enough to qualify, homemaker and home-health aide services are available through local Departments of Social Services (funded by Title XX). For those who do not qualify for Medicaid or Medicare, some agencies funded by the Older American's Act charge for these services on a sliding scale based on income. However, the need for both homemaker and home-health aides currently far exceeds the supply.

Monitoring Services

Elders living alone may utilize monitoring services to decrease their isolation and fear of lack of help in a medical crisis. Monitoring services maintain regular contact with elders living alone in a variety of ways. Perhaps the most effective programs are those that make personal contact with needy elders. For instance, the Friendly Visitor Program provides individuals to visit isolated or homebound elders in their homes once or twice a week. The visitors are trained to recognize health problems and serve as an information and referral source for local services. These visitors may be paid or volunteer and are often old themselves.

In some communities, other personnel, such as mail carriers, are trained to check up on homebound elders on their routes. Telephone reassurance programs locate homebound elders in the community and enlist volunteers to make a phone call at a pre-arranged time each day. If the caller receives no answer after several calls within an hour, either a friend, neighbor, police officer, or nurse is dispatched to the home to check if the elder has had an accident or needs help.

Some hospitals have developed a monitoring system that attaches to a standard telephone and provides immediate access to emergency help at any time of the day or night. The emergency system works as long as the person stays within two hundred feet of the telephone. An elder wears a portable help button at all times. If the wearer has an emergency, he or she pushes the button, which automatically alerts the hospital by phone. Hospital personnel then call the elder to determine the problem. If there is no answer, the hospital either contacts a neighbor who has previously agreed to be called to help or dispatches an ambulance.

Nutrition Services

Nutrition services, both home-delivered and congregate meal programs, are an important support for those who cannot shop, prepare meals, or who have special dietary requirements. Home-delivered meals, usually called "Meals on Wheels," provide homebound elders one hot meal a day, five days a week. Sometimes the service provides a cold meal at the same time to be refrigerated for the evening. For those who are ambulatory, congregate meal programs serve a hot lunch and an opportunity to socialize at selected community sites five days a week. Transportaton to and from the site is included. Additionally, the sites are often used for education, outreach, health screening, and social activities. The Older Americans Act funds the majority of these nutrition programs. Some communities have developed additional funding mechanisms through the United Way, senior organizations, and city funds.

For those needing tube feeding, Home-Health Care of America provides a home-care program. This program is reimbursed by Medicare and costs significantly less than hospitalization.

Day Care Centers

Day care centers provide supervision, care, and companionship for elders who cannot be left to themselves during the day. This service is especially helpful for families who care for a dependent adult but must work during the day. Adult day care is increasingly becoming the preferred option for the treatment of mentaly ill elders. Meals and transportation to and from the site are usually included. In addition, some centers, called adult day health centers, offer nursing and rehabilitation services as needed. Sometimes adult day care centers or day hospitals are located in a wing of a nursing home or hospital. Services are offered during business hours. The service is reimbursable through Medicaid, but for those who do not qualify, many centers adjust cost according to ability to pay.

Hospice Care

Hospice care was developed as a more humane alternative to dying in a hospital. A team of medical and social service personnel and trained volunteers provide physical and psychological care to the dying person and family. Some services may be provided in a special hospital wing, but most

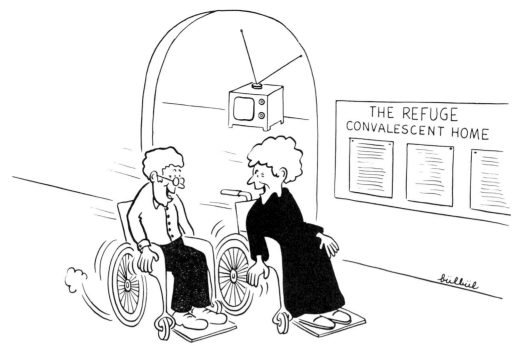

"We've locked the Director in the broom closet . . . we're busting out of the joint tonight."

consist of support offered to the terminally ill and family at home. Hospice services will be discussed in more detail in the following chapter.

Comprehensive Community-Based Care

Comprehensive community care facilities offer an extensive evaluation by a multi-disciplinary team. They develop a treatment plan, arrange for needed health and social support systems and periodically evaluate the client to determine changing needs. Sometimes the program has its own medical and social support staff, but more often the program arranges needed care through other providers in the community.

These services are most often found in large population centers. One well-publicized program of this type is the Minneapolis Age and Opportunity Center, a nonprofit organization owned and administered by elders. Services may be offered on location or in close cooperation with other agencies. Services include home-delivered meals,

chaplain contacts, dietary counseling and referral, legal and employment services, telephone reassurance programs, emergency food supply, volunteer visitors, pharmacy, individual and group counseling, health screening, and homemaker and home-health care services. The center is financed through both public grants and private contributions.

Some communities are experimenting with other models of coordinated services. Case management services do not provide direct care, rather they utilize multi-disciplinary assessment teams to design a plan of care, arrange contact with the necessary services, and conduct periodic followups to continually adapt service delivery to meet the client's needs. One program in California, the Multipurpose Senior Services Project, is designed to serve elders who are at a high risk of institutionalization and eligible for Medicaid. These types of programs enable elders who would otherwise be institutionalized to remain in the community (Nocks et al. 1986). Although these pilot programs are highly successful, very few communities can offer such assistance.

Family Providers of Home Care

Families, not formal services, provide from 80 to 90 percent of home care to frail elders, often at great emotional and financial cost. The care includes medically related care, personal care, household maintenance, transportation and shopping needed by older persons. Family members choose to care for elder relatives at home because of a bond with the loved one and an aversion to institutionalization.

Most caregivers in the United States are women (72 percent). The largest group of caregivers are daughters (29 percent). Wives comprise about 23 percent of caregivers. More wives than husbands care for their frail spouses. Husbands comprise about half the number of caregivers as wives. This difference may be due to men's shorter life expectance, the likelihood that they are older than their spouse, or their reluctance or inability to assume the caretaker role. The average age of caregivers is 57. A significant number of the caregivers are vulnerable themselves. One-third are over 65, indicating that the young-old are caring for the old-old. One-third are poor or near poor and one-third report themselves to be in fair to poor health (U.S. House of Representatives, Select Committee on Aging 1987). The story on page 356 illustrates one woman's experience as a caregiver.

The most important consideration in determining whether a frail elder can remain at home is the presence of a close family member or friend. Further, is that person able to perform the physically and emotionally taxing role of the caretaker? Caregiver effectiveness depends on a number of factors: the patient's degree of disability and dependence, the caregiver's own health and mobility, and the availability of effective emotional, social, and psychological support (formal and informal). The caregiver's other roles and responsibilities in the family and community and the degree to which the caregiver can obtain

relief can also affect the ability to serve a frail elder. Older caregivers may have more time to devote to patient care and often structure their lives around the patient's schedule. However, many older caregivers face high levels of stress because they are themselves impaired and commonly face failing health, declining energy, and often strained finances (Goldstein et al. 1981).

A common problem for caregivers is the accompanying confinement within their homes and restriction from outside activities. In many cases, caregiver become as housebound as the family member they serve. Caregiving functions demand increasing time and energy, often without relief. Isolation from friends, other family members, and even the patient occurs, especially if the disability is severe. Often caregiving is hard physical work, particularly if one must move the patient or if the patient is violent. Disruption of sleep during the night is common. Finally, watching a loved one slowly deteriorate is painful. Despite these drawbacks, it is apparent that many kin are willing to pay the price as evidenced by the high numbers of elders being cared for in their homes.

Given the multiple stresses placed upon those caring for an invalid at home, it is not surprising that many families find it difficult to cope. Those who care for disabled elders at home need education and support. Caregivers should be thoroughly educated about the patient's illness or disability, its danger signs, use of special equipment, transport techniques, rehabilitation strategies, and how to administer medications. They also need to become aware of the availability of community resources and funding mechanisms to meet current and future needs of the patient and family. Further, caregivers need an opportunity to air feelings of resentment, anger, or hopelessness. It is important that caregivers obtain periodic respite from the stress of constant care provision. Such education and support helps caregivers to better care for the disabled patient, reduce premature institutionalization, and maintain their own physical and mental health. Unfortunately, in many cases, this type of support is sorely lacking.

Till Death Do Us Part

"My life is rotten—just rotten." These are the words of a sixty-five-year-old woman who cared for her invalid, brain-damaged husband, fifteen years older than she, a stroke victim, for fourteen years before finally committing him to a nursing home. Her account, along with that of others interviewed, is frightening. There are probably half a million more such stories to be told—stories of back-breaking lifting, urine-soaked sheets, eight-hour enema stints to relieve blocked intestinal tracts, and interrupted sleep. Another woman said, "I think incontinency is what makes women give up. I think we can stand anything but this getting up at night and changing beds. I don't know a single woman (in this situation) who sleeps through the night."

Traditionally women are the care-givers. We learn our nurturing roles as daughters, wives, and mothers. Those women interviewed often state that while a doctor will help a man find assistance in caring for an invalid, brain-damaged wife, he will send a husband in the same condition home to his wife with such words as, "Isn't he lucky to have a wonderful woman like you to take care of him!" The role of the medical profession in perpetuating this situation needs some scrutiny.

Medical science is prolonging life and it is the wives, who are usually younger than the men they marry, who are carrying the tremendous burden of caring for their older husbands, victims of stroke, Parkinson's, and Alzheimer's disease among others.

Assuming that wives should carry the total burden of long-term care in the home, no matter what the toll on their own health and economic status, without regard for their own futures, is a concept that should be laid aside once and for all. Changes in social policy related to long-term care are definitely needed. . . The vow " 'till death do us part" is a promise, not a life sentence. There is a need to organize, advocate, and educate so that women can have rights as well as duties, and a life of fulfillment for their own remaining years.

Excerpted from Older Women's League (1982). Reprinted courtesy of the Older Women's League.

Two main types of services have been implemented to meet the needs of the caregiver: support groups and respite care. Support groups provide emotional and practical support to caregivers and allow them to share experiences, develop coping strategies, enhance knowledge about disease and treatment, and gain access to community resources. Some groups become political advocates to bring about legislative change and development of respite care programs in the community. A professional facilitator may or may not be present.

Respite care is similar to babysitting in that it offers temporary, infrequent care or supervision of frail and disabled adults to provide relief for caregivers. Such care may occur in an institution, such as a wing of a hospital or a nursing home, or may be provided by a worker who comes into the home. Respite care can prevent institutionalization by temporarily relieving the intolerable level of stress experienced by the caregiver. Adult day care facilities and homemaker/home-health aides may also serve as respite care.

Despite the amount of money the government saves when family members assume primary care of a sick elder, only a handful of model programs pay the caregiver. Further, in California, one of the most liberal states in regard to social service provision, Medicaid denies payment for any homemaking or personal care services if an "able and available" spouse is present in the home.

Long-Term Care Institutions

More than 1.5 million elders are institutionalized (Manton and Liu, 1984). Although some are in mental institutions and homes for the aged, most are in nursing homes. In 1985, there were over 19,000 nursing and personal care homes with over one and one-half million beds (Hing 1987). Even though only 5 percent of the elder population are in nursing homes at any one point in time, the probability an elder will spend time there is much higher: about one in five elders will spend some time in a nursing home before death (Kane and Kane 1980). It is projected that by the year 2000, this figure will swell to over two million and by 2050, the institutionalized elder population is expected to more than double that figure (figure 13.1). Within the last thirty years, the number of long-term care facilities has more than tripled because of tremendous increases in the older, disabled population and the advent of federal reimbursement for institutional care, mainly Medicaid. Within the last ten years alone, the number of homes has increased 22 percent and the number of beds has increased 38 percent (Hing 1987).

Nursing homes in the United States have a bad reputation. They are considered to be places where frail, dying, slightly crazy people shuffle aimlessly down dimly lit halls. Institutions are seen as a last resort—a place to go to die. The deplorable quality of care in nursing homes is commonly reported, generally with accompanying examples of neglect or abuse of patients.

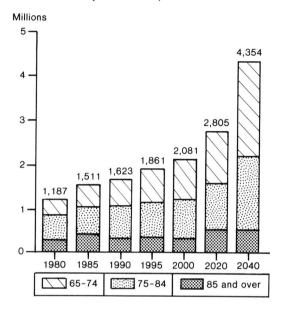

Figure 13.1 Nursing home populations. (Source: Manton and Liu. The Future Growth of the Long-Term Care Population: Projections Based on the 1977 National Nursing Home Survey and the 1982 Long-Term Care Survey. March 1984).

Because of its reputation, most families are hesitant to place a loved one in an institution. Even when the nursing home is of good quality, institutionalization is usually accompanied by trauma for both the elder and family. Despite their tarnished image, nursing homes are an important component of long-term care since they are the only alternative when home-care services are not suitable or available.

History of Nursing Home Care

Early long-term care institutions in our country were almhouses built in the 1600s to house the poor, sick, and old who had no relatives to provide for them. Almhouse residents were expected to work for low wages to partially defray the cost of their care and the remainder of their expenses were the responsibility of the towns in which they were located.

In the early 1900s, privately endowed foundations and philanthropists began to fund boarding homes for elders that replaced many of the almhouses. At first, these boarding facilities offered only custodial care, but as the residents became older and sicker, the homes began to provide nursing care. The passage of the Social Security Act of 1935 resulted in a tremendous increase in the number of nursing and board and care homes since more elders were able to afford them. In the 1950s, the government authorized a number of grants and loans for the construction of long-term care institutions. This legislation was prompted by the shortage of hospital beds as patients with chronic illnesses were taking up beds needed for acute care.

In response to an increased concern over rising health care costs for the old and poor, two pieces of important legislation were added to the Social Security Act. The enactment of Medicare and Medicaid helped elders finance nursing home care and spurred the development of profit-making nursing homes previously managed by religious and philanthropic organizations. These federal programs set national standards for staffing, physical facility, and services provided by the institutions that they will reimburse.

Types of Nursing Homes and Sheltered Care

Both Medicare and Medicaid require nursing homes to meet certain standards in order to be certified and reimbursed. Nursing homes have two levels of care: skilled and intermediate care. Skilled nursing facilities are an alternative to hospitalization for elders who need continuing medical management and skilled nursing care, but not the constant physician supervision of a hospital. A skilled nursing home provides care by nurses under orders from a physician. Most people in skilled nursing facilities are confined to bed and cannot help themselves. Skilled nursing homes are reimbursible under both Medicare and Medicaid. Reimbursable services of a skilled facility include physician fees and nursing care as well as rehabilitative, pharmaceutical, nutrition, laboratory, and radiologic services. Skilled nursing homes are required to have periodic physician visits and a required number of nurses on staff.

An intermediate care facility is certified under Medicaid, but not Medicare. These facilities are primarily for those who are unable to live independently, but do not need twenty-four-hour nursing home care or supervision. Typically, the persons in these homes have greater mobility and are not confined to bed. Intermediate care facilities offer personal care and help with daily activities, along with less intensive nursing home care than a skilled nursing facility.

Board and care facilities, sometimes called homes for the aged, are the most common long-term facility. They are designed for individuals who are fairly independent, but need help in some personal care and daily living activities. The residents are generally capable of completing most activities of daily living, but are not able or do not wish to have the burden of homemaking or house and lawn maintenance. These homes ideally provide for social needs in a safe, secure living arrangement. Medical care and supervision are not available and residents generally arrange their own medical care. In most states, these homes need to be licensed if they serve more than three or four persons.

Multi-level care homes (also called continuing care or life care) offer several levels of care from independent living facilities to skilled nursing home care in one setting. Generally, an elder signs a contract that obliges the home to provide the level of care needed for the rest of the person's life. This type of arrangement eliminates the problems of seeking out and financing health services and provides one with the security of lifelong care. The services provided usually include living space, one or two meals a day, twenty-four-hour emergency call service, laundry and housekeeping service, recreational facilities, transportation, and a variety of health and social services as needed. The sicker one becomes, the more medical supervision is available. Such facilities are effective because they save an elder the stress of relocation as health conditions worsen.

Ideally, the long-term care facility should be matched with services needed to maximize independence so that the cost of unneeded care can be avoided. Unfortunately, a number of studies indicate that many institutionalized elders are inappropriately placed and some do not need such extensive care. This misplacement can reduce independence and cause depression or frustration. However, continued relocation with each change in health condition may not benefit the patient. Facilities with multiple levels of care will help to resolve this problem.

Nursing Home Costs

Nursing home costs are skyrocketing and causing a substantial drain on both the federal budget and personal finances. On the average, skilled nursing homes cost private patients $61 a day (over $22,000 a year). The average cost of intermediate care is $48 a day and board and care, $31 a day. These figures do not include any added services not covered by the per diem rate (Strahan 1987). There is no relief in sight because increasing numbers of elders need nursing home care every year. Almost one-half of all residents in nursing homes use Medicaid as their primary source of payment. Despite the substantial contribution of public funds, elders still pay a significant portion of nursing home fees out of their pocket. About 40 percent pay nursing home bills with their personal savings. On the average, nursing home expenses accounted for 42 percent of out-of-pocket expenses spent by elders on medical care in 1984 (Waldo and Lazenby 1984).

Experts assert that nursing home costs impoverish the vast majority of older persons within two years after entry. A study by Blue Cross and Blue Shield Insurance Company of Massachusetts reported that two-thirds of single adults and one-third of married people will be forced into poverty within thirteen weeks of nursing home admission. Unfortunately, many elders do not know that Medicare and private insurance only pay for skilled nursing homes and do not cover extended nursing home stays (*AARP News Bulletin* 1985).

Although Medicaid pays for nursing homes, only the poor are eligible. A spend down phenomenon is often necessary when an elder is institutionalized. *Spend down* is when the individual must deplete almost all personal financial resources to qualify for Medicaid assistance. This process creates an economic catastrophe for the spouse as the family savings are depleted to pay for the institutionalized partner.

Nursing Home Population

The risk of institutionalization increases steadily with advancing age. While only one percent of those age sixty-five to seventy-four are in nursing homes, 22 percent of those eighty-five and older are institutionalized. The average age of nursing home residents is eighty-two. However, not all those in nursing homes are old: about 1.2 percent are under sixty-five (Hing 1987). The average length of stay is 2.6 years. A little over one-third of those institutionalized stay six months or less, while almost two-thirds stay for a year or more (U.S. Department of Health and Human Services 1981).

Most elders are admitted to nursing homes because of poor physical health (78 percent), but some are institutionalized for mental illness (7 percent), mental retardation (4 percent), or for social, economic, or other reasons (11 percent). Those admitted into a nursing home have an average of four chronic conditions per resident. The most prevalent are atherosclerosis, heart trouble, dementia, arthritis, and rheumatism (U.S. Department of Health and Human Services 1981). Not surprisingly, most elders admitted to nursing homes have a number of functional dependencies. It is likely that these dependencies were the reason for admittance. Ninety-one percent of the residents needed assistance in bathing, 78 percent in dressing, 63 percent in using the toilet, 63 percent in transferring from bed to chair. Fifty-five percent were incontinent (bowel and/or

Spousal Impoverishment

Caution: If you are the spouse of a nursing home patient, Medicaid can be hazardous to *your* health.

Grace Halperin (a member of the Older Women's League in Northside Chicago) is a typical victim of the punitive and short-sighted Medicaid system. In order to secure needed care for her institutionalized, dying husband, and to avoid being left in abject poverty herself, Halperin was forced to file for legal separation.

"I felt angry and resentful. Our resources were dwindling away. It's a hard and cruel experience. I wanted to care for him, to stick it out. But the toll on physical, emotional and financial health is terrible. There has to be better way," Halperin said.

As often happens, her husband Lee's monthly retirement of $1,110 covered only half his nursing home charges. She had to use their stocks and securities to pay the bills. Within eighteen months, half their life's savings were gone, and no end was in sight. Lee told her to "do what I had to do," Halperin remembers. The legal separation assigned their remaining assets to her and made him eligible for Medicaid.

Lee died three months later, but for Grace the guilt and trauma linger. "Even though I knew I had to go through with the separation, even though he wanted me to, I'm still not sure I did it in the best way. I still feel as if I put something over on him."

Like the Halperins, millions of couples plan carefully throughout their lives together, setting aside savings and making investments to see them through old age as independently and comfortably as possible. Too few realize how very fragile a nest egg can be if one spouse must be institutionalized and forced to turn to Medicaid, the only government program that covers long-term care.

It is not easy to qualify for such aid. Under current federal and state regulations, an older couple must first virtually exhaust their combined assets (excluding their house and a car) before the applicant can be eligible for Medicaid. The resources and assets of the well spouse are deemed to be available to pay for the nursing home care of the institutionalized spouse. The couple must "spend down" their resources by paying for nursing home care or other medical expenses until their remaining resources are below the levels set for Medicaid eligibility.

Once the couple has qualified for Medicaid coverage of the sick spouse, any ongoing income is considered the separate property of each spouse, depending on whose name is on the pension or social security check, stock dividend, etc. The noninstitutionalized spouse can keep for her own support a minimum amount of income that is in her own name. However, all of the income of the institutionalized spouse (except for twenty-five dollars) is available for nursing home costs. In cases where the institutionalized spouse is a husband who has been the primary income earner during the marriage, the pension, dividends and other income are likely to be in his name and must be used to pay Medicaid for his nursing home care. This leaves the wife with little or no income to support herself during his institutionalization or after his death.

bladder) and 40 percent needed assistance in eating. The average number of dependencies per resident was four (Hing 1987).

The chance of being institutionalized is increased with lack of a spouse. Eighty-four percent of all residents have none as they are either widowed, divorced, separated, or never married. Seventy-five percent of nursing home residents are female. The overrepresentation of women in nursing homes is partially due to their longer life expectancy and the greater tendency among women without spouses and in poor health to enter nursing homes. In contrast, frail elder men are more likely to have a wife to care for them because of their shorter life expectancy and tendency to marry younger women. Although most residents have living children (63 percent), whether they live close, or are physically able to care for a frail parent is not known. It is likely that the children are themselves old, perhaps in their sixties or seventies, and are not physically able to provide the level of care needed (Hing 1987).

Minorities are underrepresented in nursing home populations. Although the proportion of the ethnic population in these homes varies geographically, nationally 93 percent of the residents are white, 6 percent are black (Hing 1987). One explanation for the disparity is that black populations are congregated in the South where few elders of any ethnicity are institutionalized. Another reason is that minority groups may have greater kinship networks that minimize the need for institutionalization. They may also have a strong cultural bias against institutionalization.

Many minority elders have a shorter life expectancy and never reach the age of admission to a nursing home. Finally, racial discrimination and the high cost of nursing home care have kept out many minorities who need such care. In some states, elder blacks are more likely to reside in mental hospitals while their white counterparts are placed in nursing homes (Kart and Beckham 1976).

Limitations of Institutional Care

Institutional care has significant advantages. The patient has access to twenty-four-hour supervision and services. The staff has extensive opportunities to collect information on the patient's behavior, enhancing the opportunity to make effective treatment decisions. Coordination of care is facilitated because many services are under one roof. Furthermore, the group-living environment provides elders with opportunities for social interaction. Finally, institutionalization reduces the burden of care felt by relatives.

However, in many institutions these advantages are not realized. Rather, the limitations of institutionalization stand out more clearly. The best nursing homes offer adequate care; in the worst, the conditions are deplorable. Perhaps the most extensively documented study on nursing home quality was conducted in 1974 by the U.S. Senate Special Committee on Aging. Other nursing home critics have since written about nursing home inadequacies (e.g., Mendelson 1974; Tobin and Lieberman 1976; Gubrium 1975; Bennet 1980; Moss and Halamandaris 1977). These inadequacies include high cost, poorly trained staff, little physician-patient interaction, over-reliance on drug treatments, and an environment that promotes further dependence.

The Federal government mandates standards for staffing, services, and the physical facility of nursing homes and some states have imposed further regulations. However, it is difficult to measure and regulate quality of care, staff sensitivity, and patient rights. In many instances, regulations are not strictly enforced until a family member files a complaint. When a nursing home is cited for lack of conformance to regulations, its license is generally not even revoked temporarily because the need for nursing home beds is so great in most communities. Stricter standards for nursing home quality are difficult to legislate because of strong lobbying by the nursing home industry.

Multiple deficiencies in nursing home care point to the need for broad nursing home reform. Institutionalized elders may not be able to choose their doctor and when physicians do visit it is often cursory since they may be less motivated to spend time diagnosing or treating someone with multiple, chronic problems. An unfortunate condition is that physicians seldom visit patients as often as needed, partly because of the reimbursement requirements of Medicare and Medicaid. Diagnosis and treatment of vision, hearing, dental, or foot problems is rare. Drug misuse in institutions is widespread. Physicians may prescribe drugs when another therapy would be more appropriate. Laxatives and sedatives may be prescribed indiscriminately. Major tranquilizers may be over-used to manage disruptive patients. Although a monthly drug review is required, the reviewing pharmacist may also be the drug supplier, creating a conflict of interest.

Perhaps the most serious problem with nursing homes is the difficulty in recruiting, training, and retaining qualified, sensitive staff. Nurses may not be attracted to nursing home work because of low pay and the low value placed on the very old and sick. Even when nurses are employed there, they may have predominantly administrative duties and little direct patient care. Instead, untrained and poorly paid nurse's aides provide most direct patient care. The work of nurse's aides is frustrating especially when given responsibility for more patients than they can handle effectively. Because they are overworked, nursing aides are often more concerned with finishing the necessary "bed and body" work than spending time to encourage independence in their patients. The excessive care provided to many residents undermines their ability and confidence to care for themselves, causing more disability than is necessary. For instance, aides may insist on feeding elders or using wheelchairs to transport them because it is quicker and easier than allowing patients to do it themselves. Because of time constraints, opportunities to offer emotional or social support are extremely limited. Staff commonly talk to residents like children or talk about them with each other as if the resident were not there. At any one time, many nurse's aide positions are vacant because of the high turnover.

Governmental regulations specify that nursing homes consult with a dietician to ensure that meals meet the Recommended Dietary Allowances for vitamins and minerals. However, there is some debate whether the RDA is adequate for meeting the nutritional needs of elders, especially those with multiple chronic illnesses. Further, the RDA guidelines do not include fiber, which has been documented to prevent constipation and other health problems. Meal planners often substitute heavily processed foods for fresh fruits, vegetables, seafood, and meats that are more expensive and harder to prepare in large quantities. Often no effort is made to make food look or taste appetizing. Meals are generally scheduled according to staff convenience rather than the resident's desire. Many institutions provide no food for patients from 5:30 P.M. until breakfast the next morning.

Institutional environments generally exacerbate existing sensory deficits. Lack of sensory stimulation caused by the sameness of rooms and corriders can cause orientation problems. Glare,

What Are You Thinking When Looking at Me?

What do you see, nurses, what do you
see?
What are you thinking when looking at me?
A crabby old woman, not very wise,
Uncertain of habit, with far-away eyes?
Who dribbles her food and makes no reply
When you say in a loud voice—
"I do wish you'd try."

Who seems not to notice the things that
you do,
And forever is losing a stocking or
shoe . . .
Who unresisting is not, lets you do as you
will,
With bathing and feeding, the long day to
fill,
Is that what you're thinking, is that what
you see?
Then open your eyes nurse, you're not
looking at me!

I'll tell you who I am as I sit here so still,
As I do at your bidding, as I eat at your will,

I'm a small child of ten with a father and
mother
Brothers and sisters who love one another.
A girl of sixteen with wings on her feet,
Dreaming that soon now a lover she'll
meet;
A bride soon at twenty—my heart gives a
leap,
Remembering the vows I promised to
keep.

At twenty-five now I have young of my
own,
Who need me to build a secure happy
home.

A woman of thirty, my young now grow
fast,
Bound to each other with ties that should
last.

At forty, my young sons have grown and
have gone,
But my man's still beside me to see I don't
mourn.

At fifty, once more babies play around my
knee,
Again we know children, my loved one and
me.
Dark days are upon me, my husband is
dead,
I look at the future, I shudder with
dread . . .
My young ones are rearing young of their
own,
And I think of the years and the love I've
known.

I'm an old woman now and nature is
cruel—
'Tis her jest to make old age look like a
fool.
The body is crumbling, grace and vigor
depart.
There is now a stone where I once had a
heart.

But inside this old carcass, a young girl still
dwells,
And now and aging my battered heart
swells.
I remember the joys, I remember the pain,
And I'm loving and living life over again.
I think of the years, all too few, gone too
fast,
And accept the stark fact that nothing can
last.

So open your eyes nurse. Open and see!
Not a crabby old woman. Look closer—
See Me!

The above poem is believed to have been written by Phyllis McCormack, a nurse employed in a hospital in Scotland (Stilwell 1977).

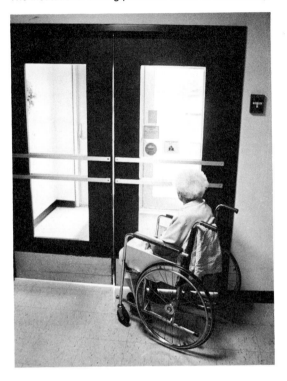

The institutional setting promotes a loss of individuality.

2. Daily activities are carried out in the immediate company of a large number of others, all of whom are treated alike and required to do the same thing.
3. The day's activities are tightly scheduled with each leading at a prearranged time to the next; the sequence of events is imposed by those in authority.
4. Activities are carried out for the sake of the institution, not of those residing there.

A number of factors contribute to the self-mortification of nursing home residents. Upon entering an institution, such self-identity is lost because most new residents can bring little clothing or personal items with them. Institutionalization detaches an individual from previous lifestyle, friends, and society at large. Institutionalized elders are often unable to enter or leave a facility at will, visiting hours may be restricted, phones may be inaccessible, and residents may lack access to newspapers or radios. Privacy is rare in institutions. Facts about the patient are listed on medical charts for anyone to peruse. Personal acts—such as dressing, bathing, toileting, and catheter care—become public. Elders can seldom find a place or time to be alone because doors are usually left open and staff enter and leave at will. Privacy during visits with relatives or friends is difficult.

Because nursing home residents are extremely dependent on staff, they may hesitate to assert themselves for fear of retribution. Institutions remove an elder's freedom of personal choice. Social activities, mealtimes, waking and retiring, toileting, even naps are arranged without the resident's input. Individuals seldom have sufficient living space to move about freely and privacy may be further compromised by a lack of barriers between the beds. Because of their proximity, elders must associate with each other, even with those who are irrational and confused.

Our country is one of the few in the world in which a profit is made by caring for sick old people. More than three-fourths of all nursing

caused by enameled walls, waxed floors, and fluorescent lights, reduces vision. Background noise, such as grocery store music and institutional clatter, can make hearing even more difficult for the hearing impaired.

Institutional living, no matter what its type or quality, creates an impersonal and impersonalizing environment. Goffman in his book, *Asylums* (1961), asserts that many types of total institutions (e.g., prisons, mental institutions, nursing homes, army barracks, monastaries) contribute to the "mortification of self," or profound loss of individuality of those residing there. A total institution has the following characteristics:

1. All aspects of resident life (sleep, work, and play) are conducted in the same place under the same authority.

Chapter 13

homes are profit-making (Strahan 1987). Some critics believe profit-making nursing homes have a conflict of interest since providing quality care costs money and reduces profits. Data from the National Center of Health Statistics (Strahan 1987) indicate that profit-making homes employed significantly less administrative, medical, therapeutic, and nursing staff than did voluntary non-profit and governmental institutions. However, the daily rate for private pay patients in skilled and residential homes was somewhat lower in the for-profit institutions. Recent studies have shown that profit-making homes provide inferior care to nonprofit institutions. Elwell (1984) reviewed over four hundred skilled nursing homes in New York and assessed staffing and resource distribution. He reported that the nonprofit homes allocated more money per patient day for goods and services and offered more staff hours per patient per day than for-profit facilities.

Nursing Home Advocacy

Because nursing home policies and procedures often conflict with those of good patient care, federal and state legislation has been implemented to protect those in nursing homes. In 1974, Congress mandated that residents of nursing facilities who are reimbursed by Medicare and Medicaid have certain rights protected by law (see next page). Some states and individual nursing homes have expanded these rights. Each state has guidelines regarding the steps an individual can take to report to the proper state authorities if a patient's rights have been violated.

The federal ombudsman program, mandated under the Older Americans Act, requires states to establish investigative units to assure that nursing homes provide good patient care and ensure patients' rights. In addition, ombudsman programs in each state have been established to respond to complaints on behalf of nursing home residents. Ombudsmen are trained to respond to specific complaints, document significant problems in the home, advocate for improvement of quality of care, and facilitate constructive working

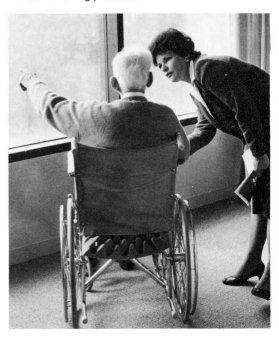

Nursing home ombudsmen advocate for institutionalized elders by responding to complaints and documenting problems.

relationship among staff, administration, patient, and the family. The program authorizes ombudsmen to serve those in skilled and intermediate care facilities and boarding homes. Most programs use trained volunteers who are themselves elderly.

Some nursing homes have residents' councils that enable residents to discuss problems encountered with the administration or staff. Unfortunately, these councils may be used to make small decisions—such as what movies to see—instead of dealing with the larger issues of good patient care and patient rights. Some institutions have grievance boards within the homes to enable patients, family, staff, and administrators to air their differences and arrive at workable compromises without outside intervention.

In addition to the formal ombudsman program, members of the community may act singly or as a group to improve nursing home care in

Patient Bill of Rights

Under Federal regulations, nursing homes must have written policies covering the rights of patients. These rights must be posted where residents and visitors can easily see them. A patient bill of rights ensures that each person admitted to a facility will have his/her rights protected. Flagrant violations of these rights should be reported to the proper state authorities.

A Patient:

1. is fully informed, as evidenced by the resident's written acknowledgment of these rights and of all rules and regulations governing the exercise of these rights.

2. is fully informed of services available in the facility and of related charges for services not covered under Medicare/Medicaid, or not covered by the facility's basic daily rate.

3. is fully informed of his/her medical condition unless the physician notes in the medical record that it is not in the patient's interest to be told, and is afforded the opportunity to participate in the planning of his/her medical treatment and to refuse to participate in experimental research.

4. is transferred or discharged only for medical reasons, or for his/her welfare or that of other residents, and is given reasonable advance notice to ensure orderly transfer or discharge.

5. is encouraged and assisted, through his/her period of stay to exercise his/her rights as a resident and as a free citizen. To this end, he/she may voice grievances and recommend changes in policies and services to facility staff and/or outside representatives of his/her choice without fear of coercion, discrimination, or reprisal.

6. may manage his/her personal financial affairs, or is given at least a quarterly accounting of financial transactions made on his/her behalf if the facility accepts the responsibility to safeguard the funds.

7. is free from mental and physical abuse, and free from chemical and physical restraints except as authorized in writing by a physician for a specified and limited period of time or when necessary to protect patients from injury to themselves or others.

8. is assured confidential treatment of his/her personal and medical records and may approve or refuse their release to any individual outside facility.

9. is treated with consideration, respect, and full recognition of his/her dignity and individuality, including privacy in treatment and in care of his/her personal needs.

10. is not required to perform services for the facility that are not included for therapeutic purposes in this plan of care.

11. may associate and communicate privately with persons of his/her choice, and send and receive his/her personal mail unopened.

12. may meet with, and participate in activities of social, religious, and community groups at his/her

13. may retain and use his/her personal clothing and possessions as space permits, unless to do so would infringe upon rights of other patients, or constitute a hazard of safety.

14. is assured privacy for visits by his/her spouse; if both are inpatients in the facility, they are permitted to share a room.

SOURCE: Suggested by the Health Care Financing Administration, U.S. Department of Health and Human Services, Washington, D.C.

their locale. Some individuals make unannounced visits to nursing homes to ensure conformity to the Patient's Bill of Rights and report any suspected abuse, neglect, or mistreatment. Community groups, such as Boy or Girl Scouts, Soroptimists, or Candy Stripers volunteer to visit nursing home residents. The presence of many visitors in the home reduces patient maltreatment. Butler and Lewis (1982) urge the formation of a national federation of friends and relatives of nursing home residents to monitor and lobby to improve nursing homes. A number of local and regional groups have been set up for this purpose.

Families of the Institutionalized

Contrary to popular belief, the majority of frail elders are not dumped into nursing homes by uncaring kin. A number of elders are institutionalized because they have no family to care for them. When families are present, nursing home placement is generally a last resort when patient care becomes too draining or increased medical support becomes necessary. Spouses and children of the institutionalized commonly need emotional support to cope with feelings of guilt and personal failure at abandoning a loved one, especially if the decision was made without the elder's consent.

A member of the nursing home staff is in a good position to provide education and support to family members to help them adapt to the many stresses and problems inherent with institutionalization. However, institutions seldom offer such services. When they do occur, support may take a number of forms. A group of family members who intend to place an elder in a nursing home might congregate for education and support before placement or during the first few weeks of institutionalization. Groups such as these commonly address feelings about placement, institutional routines, preparing an elder for institutionalization, nursing home adjustment, and rehabilitation and treatment. Groups composed of spouses of residents are especially helpful and needed. Periodic meetings between staff and family can serve to update the treatment plan, clarify institutional policies, and resolve complaints. Periodic newsletters or lecture/discussions on topics of interest to nursing staff and families can maintain family involvement in care. At times, professional counseling or an ombudsman may be brought in to resolve problems between the nursing home staff and the resident or family.

Planning for Long-Term Care

To effectively plan for the long-term care needs of a frail elder, whether it be in an institution or at home, a thorough assessment is necessary. Ideally, a team of medical and social service professionals evaluate the individual's level of functioning and need for supportive services and a treatment plan is developed. Preferably, the assessment should take place in the elder's home to determine whether a disability (e.g, inability to bathe oneself) is due to physical decrements or environmental barriers. The components of a successful assessment are outlined below.

Physical assessment: Evaluate mental function, projected course of illness, ability to complete tasks of daily living, presence of chronic or acute illness, rehabilitation potential, and presence of hearing, mobility, speech, and visual decrements.

Environmental assessment: Observe furniture placement, lighting, presence of support bars, stairways, throw rugs, presence of a telephone, refrigerator and stove, and other factors that affect ability to function independently. Check the proximity of grocery stores and medical facilities and availability of transportation.

Socioeconomic consideratons: Establish income, savings, and eligibility for federal and state funding programs. Additionally, cultural considerations, presence of neighbors and other social supports should be ascertained.

Family resources: Determine availability of a willing and able caretaker and level of care he/she can provide. Also, establish resources needed to assist the caretaker.

Patient's desires and goals: Discuss the services the patient thinks are necessary, the conditions under which institutionalization would be desired, views toward home care, and the role the patient wishes the family to play.

Availability of community resources: Ascertain what health and social services are in the area. Eligibility of the elder for services and alternative financing mechanisms should be explored.

When an elder leaves the hospital, Medicare requires a discharge plan to ensure continuing care. The individual's level of functioning, medical treatment plan, availability of home-care services and family and community supports are taken into consideration. A nurse or social worker, patient and family members, and the physician are ideally involved in devising the discharge plan. Since the advent of DRG's, hospital stays are shorter, making discharge planning imperative because patients may be unable to care for themselves at discharge. The quality of discharge planning and the availability of support services in the community are the main factors affecting whether an elder becomes institutionalized after hospitalization.

For those frail elders who have long-term care needs, but have not been hospitalized, their physician should conduct a medical evaluation and work with a home-health agency to devise a treatment plan. A number of communities have implemented case-management services to determine whether institutionalization or home health care services will best suit the patient. As in discharge planning, the evaluation team, the frail elder, and the family should cooperate in the final decision between home care and institutionalization. Without professional guidance, the elder and family will have much difficulty in piecing together needed services. They also run the risk of making the wrong choice out of ignorance of other options.

When given a choice, most individuals prefer to remain in their own homes as long as possible. People recover more quickly and comfortably in familiar surroundings. Additionally, care at home can be tailored to an individual's need and lifestyle. However, home is not always the best choice. If an individual needs more care than the family or community can provide, institutionalization may be the only option. Further, elders may dislike their current living situation and prefer to move to a safe, sheltered environment. Some elders would rather move into an institution than move in with grown children. Butler and Lewis (1982) remind families and professionals not to fall prey to slogans like "keep them in their own homes" as they believe it sometimes may be inappropriate or even cruel.

Home Care—It Doesn't Always Work

For a number of years, we have been witnessing a shift in emphasis from institutional-based health care to home health care. Much of this trend is a result of attempts to curtail the rapidly rising cost of health care services. Proponents of the move argue that people respond better to care provided in a familiar surrounding, and that most people prefer their home to an institutional setting. However, I feel we must carefully evaluate this trend, especially as it relates to those most likely to be affected, namely the people with Alzheimer's disease and their families.

As an administrator of a home-health agency, I hear numerous stories of families attempting to care for their disoriented, dependent, and often combative member. Home care services supplement the role of the caretaker and provide needed guidance, as well as a respite from their daily demands. Unfortunately, the caretaker is often an aged spouse whose energies and resources are rapidly being compromised. Other family members are frequently not available to help to the extent needed. As the patient deteriorates, the need for more frequent home-care services becomes compounded with the problem of limited funding resources for the level of care needed.

For example, home-health care services available under Medicare and some private insurance carriers are limited to care that is medically necessary and rehabilitative in nature. The demented patient who has deteriorated to dependency in personal care rarely has needs that are covered by third-party insurers. Medicaid, on the other hand, will provide partial reimbursement for supportive care for income-eligible recipients. Frequently, these services are limited in extent and provide little help to the family facing round-the-clock care. Homemaker services can help the family with personal care, maintenance, and respite. However, we are now witnessing a far greater demand for services than what is available through the various funding sources. Similarly, adult day-care programs struggle with the problems of transportation and limited resources to provide for the needs of the aged adult. Families eventually face the choice of leaving their own employment, hiring full- or part-time help, or finding an affordable nursing home.

But will the families of the future Alzheimer's patient have the nursing home as an alternative to home care? As the move toward prospective payment systems continues, I see an emphasis on short-term, less costly care. Hospitals are expecting nursing homes to provide the rehabilitation needs of their acute-care patients. Medicaid requirements are beginning to mimic the short-term, post-hospital criteria used by Medicare and place further restrictions on the level of care reimbursed. I predict that nursing homes wil find the private paying patient and those with fewer care demands more desirable as they attempt to curb costs and live within a prospective payment system.

Already I see nursing homes place limits on the proportion of Medicaid patients they will serve. Beds are often only available to persons with sufficient resources to afford the full cost of care for a set time span. Some homes are refusing admission to patients who are severely demented and require extensive care. Local government-sponsored nursing homes, which have always been overburdened, are turning to management companies to become more cost-effective. No matter how one views the evolving scenario, the plight of the Alzheimer's patient is dismal.

I propose that the nation's health care providers and planners, as well as our legislators, re-evaluate the trend toward deinstitutionalization in relation to the needs of the severely demented individual. By providing disincentives to institutions to care for the long-term patient, we force the demented patient to receive less-than-adequate care. And although the required care is not medical in nature, it nevertheless requires the skill and expertise of experienced, quality-care personnel with patience and insight to make judgments based on non-verbal clues. I implore those with the power to change public policy and health care systems to evaluate the effect of the current trend and propose solutions that will not jeopardize the welfare of the Alzheimer patient and his family.

An editorial by Sylvia Schraff (1985). Reprinted by permission of the *Journal of Gerontological Nursing*.

Making the difficult decision between home or nursing home care should be done only after extensive assessment and collaboration among physicians, social workers, family members, and the elder. When home care is chosen, coordination of services to meet elder and family needs and continual reevaulation are essential if home care is to be successful.

Summary

Long-term care includes a wide variety of health and social services provided to elders in their homes, within the community, or in institutions. The need for long-term care is increasing drastically in our country with the current demographic shifts in the population; however, the availability of services has not kept pace with the need. Long-term care may be financed through federal and state funding sources as well as private funding sources. Although these multiple funding sources have increased accessibility to long-term care, strict reimbursement requirements and gaps in service are a major barrier to delivery of long-term care services.

Home-health care services include medical, dental and nursing services, rehabilitation services, homemaker/home-health aide services, monitoring services, adult day care, and nutrition services. However, families still bear the brunt of the emotional and physical strain of caring for a frail elder in the home.

Institutional services include skilled nursing facilities and intermediate care facilities. Women comprise the majority of nursing home residents and minorities are underrepresented in nursing home populations. Elders in nursing homes may receive inadequate care because of high prescription drug use, poor nutrition, little patient-physician interaction, encouragement of dependency, and the boredom and under-stimulation of an institutional environment. Nursing home advocates and a patient's bill of rights can help ensure that elders in nursing homes have their needs met.

Appropriate planning for long-term care includes a number of considerations: functional ability of the patient, personal financial resources, availability of a caretaker at home, accessibility of formal services, and the client and family's personal preferences.

Chapter 13

Activities

1. If you were preparing to enter a nursing home, what five personal items would you consider most important for your comfort and well-being? Contact a local nursing home and question them about types of personal effects permitted in their facility.

2. Tour a local nursing home. Inquire about the following: daily costs, admission requirements, personal items permitted, how roommates are matched, available interaction between resident and the community, activities offered within the home, and nutrition services. Observe the activity of the residents. Are services available for residents' families? Use a check list (a good one is People's Medical Society 1986) to gather added information. For a group project, compile your work, developing a directory of nursing homes for the public.

3. Compile a list of home care services for elders in your community. Check with the local Area Agency on Aging. What services are not available that are discussed in this chapter?

4. Would you prefer home or institutional care? Why? What health problems would convince you that your own institutionalization was necessary?

5. Using material from this chapter and other information about health needs of elders, design a topic outline for nurse's aide training in a nursing home. How might it differ from training home-health aides?

6. Given unlimited funds to build a skilled nursing home, what would it be like? Include physical environment, staffing, food service, rehabilitation, social and educational activities, admission procedures, patient's rights, services for families, mechanism of resident input on decision-making, and interaction with the community. Remember that most residents have moderate to severe disabilities.

7. You have just been hired as a nursing home administrator. List five policies or procedures you would want to implement to enhance the residents' quality of care. What arguments would you use to convince the Board of Directors of their cost-effectiveness or benefit to patients?

Bibliography

AARP News Bulletin. 1985. Nursing home costs would impoverish most in two years. October 26(9): 6.

Barhydt-Wezenaar, N. 1986. Home care and hospice. In Jonas, S., ed. *Health care delivery in the United States.* New York: Springer, 237–62.

Bennett, C. 1980. *Nursing home life: What it is and what it could be.* New York: Tiresias Press.

Brickfield, C. F. 1986–87. The Catch-22 of home care (editorial). *Modern Maturity* Dec–Jan: 15.

Butler, R. N., and M. I. Lewis. 1982. *Aging and mental health.* St. Louis, Mo.: C. V. Mosby.

Elwell, F. 1984. The effects of ownership on institutional services. *Gerontologist* 24 (1): 77–83.

Feller, B. A. 1983. Americans needing help to function at home. *NCHS Advance Data* No. 92, Sept. 14, 1983.

Goffman, E. 1961. *Asylums.* New York: Doubleday.

Goldstein, V., G. Regnery, and E. Wellen. 1981. Caretaker role fatigue. *Nurs Outlook* Jan.: 24–30.

Gubrium, J. 1975. *Living and dying at Murray Manor.* New York: St. Martin's Press.

Hing, E. 1987. Use of nursing homes by the elderly: Preliminary data from the 1985 National Nursing Home Survey. *NCHS Advance Data from Vital and Health Statistics* No. 135 May 14. Hyattsville, Md.: US Public Health Services.

Holmes, D., J. Teresi, and M. Holmes. 1981. Differences among blacks and whites in knowledge about and attitudes toward long-term care services. *Quarterly Contact* Natl. Center and Caucus on Black Aging. 4(4): 1, 8.

Hu, T., L. Huang, and W. S. Cartwright. 1986. Evaluation of the costs of caring for the senile demented elderly: A pilot study. *Gerontologist* 26(2): 158–63.

Kane, R. L., and R. A. Kane. 1980. Long-term care: Can our society meet the needs of its elderly? *Annu Rev Public Health* 1:227–53.

Kart, C. S., and B. Beckham. 1976. Black-white differentials in the institutionalization of the elderly. *Social Forces* 54:901–10.

Manton, K. G., and K. Liu. 1984. The future growth of the long-term care population: Projections based on the 1977 National Nursing Home Survey and the 1982 Long-term Care Survey. Quoted in Special Committee on Aging, U.S. Senate Information Paper, *America in transition: An aging society, 1984–1985 Edition*. Washington, D.C.: U.S. Govt. Printing Office.

Mendelson, M. A. 1974. *Tender loving greed*. New York: Random House.

Moss, F. E., and V. J. Halamandaris. 1977. *Too old, too sick, too bad: Nursing homes in America*. Germantown, Md.: Aspen Systems Corp.

Nocks, B. C., M. Learner, D. Blackman, et al. 1986. The effects of a community-based long-term care project on nursing home utilization. *Gerontologist* 26(2): 150–57.

Older Women's League. 1982. *Till death do us part: Caregiving wives of severely disabled husbands*. Grey Paper No. 7. Issues for Action. Older Women's League, 1325 G Street, NW, Washington, D.C. 20005.

People's Medical Society. 1986. *How to evaluate and select a nursing home*. PMS Health Action Series, 14 East Minor St., Emmaus, PA 18049 ($4.95).

Schraff, S. H. 1985. Home care—it doesn't always work. *J Gerontol Nurs* 11(2):5.

Sontag, S. 1978. *Illness as metaphor*. New York: Farrar, Straus and Giroux.

Stilwell, E. 1977. Editorial. *J Gerontol Nurs* 3:11.

Stone, R. 1986. Aging in the eighties, age 65 and over—use of community services. *NCHS Advance Data* No. 124. Sept. 30, 1985.

Strahan, G. 1987. Nursing home characteristics: Preliminary data from the 1985 National Nursing Home Survey. *NCHS Advance Data from Vital and Health Statistics*. No. 131, Mar. 27.

Sullivan, K. 1987. Spousal impoverishment reform high on OWL 1987 agenda. *The OWL Observer*, Older Women's League, January 1, February 1, 8.

Tobin, S., and M. Lieberman. 1976. *The last home for the aged*. San Francisco: Jossey-Bass.

U.S. Department Health and Human Services. 1981. Characteristics of nursing home residents, health status and care received: National Nursing Home Survey, United States, May–Dec., 1977. *Vital and Health Statistics,* Series 13 (51). Washington, D.C.: U.S. Govt. Printing Office.

U.S. House of Representatives, Select Committee on Aging 1987. Exploding the myths: Caregiving in America. Comm. Pub. No. 99–611. Washington, D.C.: U.S. Govt. Printing Office.

U.S. Senate, Special Committee on Aging. 1974. *Nursing home care in the U.S.: Failure in public policy*. Washington, D.C.: U.S. Govt. Printing Office.

Waldo, D., and H. Lazenby. 1984. Demographic characteristics and health care use and expenditures by the aged in the United States: 1977–1984. *Health Care Financ Rev* 6(1).

Ward, S. Y. 1983. Home health care. In Ernst, N. S., and H. R. Glazer-Waldman, eds. *The aging patient*. Chicago: Year Book Medical Publishers. 222–41.

Wetle, T. T., and D. A. Pearson. 1986. Long-term care. In Jonas, S., ed. *Health care delivery in the United States*. New York: Springer, 214–36.

Dying, Death, and Grief 14

We are all survivors of the deaths of others. We are all individuals who will someday die.

Richard Kalish (1985)

Introduction

A text on health and aging is not complete without a discussion of dying, death, and grief since death occurs more frequently among elders than other age groups. Although this seems elementary, it has not always been true. In 1900, those age sixty-five and older comprised only 17 percent of all deaths. Currently, 70 percent of deaths each year involve those age sixty-five and older (National Center for Health Statistics 1986). Reductions in infectious disease, death from childbirth, and infant mortality have contributed to this changing pattern. Not only are deaths more common among elders, but elders must confront the deaths of family and friends more often than younger groups.

Most professionals working directly with elders, especially those in the health and social services, will inevitably confront death, whether they work with people who die while in their service, or deal with others' grief. To be effective, they will also have to confront their own attitudes toward death and dying. This chapter will address issues commonly faced by the dying, the bereaved, and those working with them.

Death Defined

The moment of death used to be easy to determine: a person was pronounced dead when the heart stopped beating. Nowadays, ascertaining when a person is dead is more complex. Advances in medical technology now enable heartbeat and respiration to continue and, with intravenous tube feeding and waste removal, body organs may function without direction from the brain.

Today, death is most commonly defined as the cessation of higher brain function as evidenced by the lack of recorded waves on an EEG (electroencephalograph). Brain cells involved in higher thought and voluntary action are very sensitive and will die within about four minutes without oxygen. Therefore, if the heart or breathing stops, the person must be revived immediately or important brain function will be lost. If the heart and breathing are revived after four minutes, they may continue despite the loss of higher thought and voluntary motor function. However, if the brain centers have been deprived of oxygen for five minutes or more, the chance of return of all or even part of higher brain function is slight.

Even though the definition of death is clear, in reality, many decisions made about life and death matters are not. For instance, a person may not be technically dead because brain activity is present on an EEG, but if he has been in a coma for a long time, then what? Or if a person's higher brain functioning is almost nonexistent and machines are prolonging life, what should be done? The decision to remove the machines and pronounce someone dead is largely an ethical one that can be influenced by a number of variables, such as the patient's financial status, age, degree of former disability, prognosis, and family and physician attitudes. Efforts to save a patient whose heart stops will likely be more dramatic for a woman in her twenties than for an elder who is already partially paralyzed by a stroke. Some hospitals or physicians do not attempt radical life-saving measures on elder patients. There is less incentive to lengthen the life of an older person

It is important that those who are dying have a concerned person to depend upon.

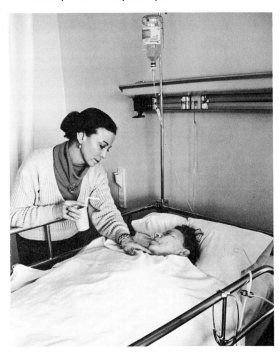

with a terminal illness because it is supposed that they will die soon anyway. On the other hand, many elders sustained by machines would otherwise have died without them.

Who Should Decide?

The advances of technology have created a number of ethical dilemmas. Most will agree that maintaining life at all costs is not necessarily better than death. Should life be artificially prolonged if there is a minute chance of recovery? Who should decide when a life is no longer of worth and death should be allowed? These are emotion-laden moral questions that laypersons, physicians, philosophers, theologians, and the court system are still debating. Although it is accepted that a conscious, mentally stable adult has the right to refuse any type of medical treatment, when the decision needs to be made the dying

Mr. Rosen's Long and Painful Death

by Daniel Foreman

As far as I am concerned, Mr. Rosen—a pseudonym for one of my patients—died weeks before I knew him. Yet medically he was still considered alive when I met him.

He was in the hospital's intensive-care unit for almost two weeks before he was transferred to my care on the general medicine floor.

After his heart attack, as the ambulance arrived to race him to the hospital, his poorly functioning heart failed to deliver precious oxygen-rich blood to his brain. Mr. Rosen received expert treatment, but while bodily function resumed elsewhere, it was permanently lost in his brain.

Irreversible brain death had occurred: blood-starved brain cells cannot be rejuvenated.

The patient I met was comatose. He was lying flat on his back, eyes dilated with a blank stare. Whirring machinery encircled him, fortress-like, fending off death.

Mr. Rosen's case is not unique. Dozens of patients each day enter the twilight between life and death. Sustained by technological gadgetry, they are infrequently "cured" and rarely regain consciousness. Machinery forestalls a death that otherwise would have already occurred.

As Mr. Rosen's doctor, what troubled me was that by keeping him breathing I was almost certainly increasing the family's suffering, contributing to the overburdened costs of the medical system and inflicting pain on my patient through endless blood tests, torturous suctioning of his breathing tube and catheters at every orifice.

Usually, resident physicians, grouped as more experienced doctors with first-year interns, begin the day visiting each patient, reviewing charts, clarifying orders and directing patient care. As Mr. Rosen's intern, however, I received little supervision. "Do what you want," I was told. "Call if there's a problem."

Providing medical care in the face of certain death saddens a doctor. Those with the choice often minimize their involvement.

So, nearly every morning I was the only doctor to visit Mr. Rosen. For the most part, he was to me simply a group of numbers. His past and his personality were irrelevant to his hospital care. I checked his blood count, his blood pressure, his potassium levels: These concrete parameters defined his existence.

With such dispassionate care, Mr. Rosen's death stretched into months. When his blood pressure dropped, he received intravenous fluids. When infections threatened to overwhelm his system, he was quickly treated with powerful antibiotics. The feeding tube pumped a continual ooze of nutrition. The respirator monitored, supplemented and, when necessary, replaced his breathing. Down the hall, his heart rhythm blipped on the nursing station monitor, confirming normal functioning.

The cost per day of such care is astounding. But even more expensive is the toll on family members, who visit daily while they struggle to be hopeful and optimistic. If one day Mr. Rosen twitched, his wife would ask if he was doing better. The next day he'd swell with fluid overload, and she'd ask if he was worse. But beyond day-to-day detail was the continuum of death.

The pain inflicted by this sort of persistence mounts exponentially. Wife and family cannot allow themselves to get beyond their sorrow and resume a happier life. Like quicksand, Mr. Rosen's lingering death drew them down. No one could leave for a much-needed vacation; relationships were put on hold, other commitments were neglected.

Anger often mounts as dying stretches into months. Emotional costs are compounded by the financial drain, and family resentment and guilt often intensify in an atmosphere of anger. How can one justify anger toward a loved one because he simply does not die?

Under the circumstances, imagine how particularly stressful are the issues surrounding "code status"—choosing the degree of aggressive care that should be used when the body next stops. In this age of medical-legal complexity, no doctor will make this decision for a patient's family. Those who do are frequently sued. The patient's family, like a consumer in a supermarket, is asked to select a package of care. But in the midst of guilt, anger and family dynamics, such choices are nightmares.

With an aging population, these complex issues are crucial. Their complexity is exacerbated by an economy that cannot afford the "luxury" of its own capabilities. For whom and for what do we extend the limbo preceding certain death? The family and the doctor are constrained by the difficult legal requirements and emotional ties. We all suffer passively as the patient lingers.

Sadly, though, I rarely have heard doctors discuss our dilemma. Rather, the subject, and even the patient, are avoided whenever possible. Highly trained technically, we often lack the emotional grounding to confront the pain of inevitable death. While medical care is implemented reflexively out of both legal and philosophical obligations, a sense of guilt and regret exists in many of us who prolong such a grim course.

Weeks after I was transferred away from Mr. Rosen, I heard he had died. His wife, I was told, had rushed to the hospital and had been inconsolable. Just as I had been emotionally distant while Mr. Rosen persisted, I was absent at his death.

person may not be in a position to decide. The rights of families or physicians to decide the extent of treatment a dying person should receive is not clear. Is one entitled to determine another's end of life? If yes, then who should decide? The issue is compounded by the fact that those with little chance for recovery hooked up to life-sustaining machinery use a tremendous amount of expensive hospital resources that could be employed to assist those with a better prognosis.

Euthanasia is the painless putting to death of one suffering from an incurable condition. Voluntary euthanasia occurs when the dying person wants to be allowed to die, while involuntary euthanasia is accomplished against the will of the dying person. *Passive* euthanasia is withdrawing or withholding treatment that would otherwise prolong life, allowing death to occur naturally. In contrast, active euthanasia occurs when someone takes an active step to deliberately end another's suffering or empty existence, such as giving an overdose of medication. *Active* euthanasia is considered murder in our country. The differences between active and passive euthanasia are not clear-cut. The case of pulling the plug after one is on life-support equipment is sometimes considered passive because it allows the death to progress naturally, but it is active in that it is an intentional, conscious act to end life (Foreman 1975).

Chapter 14

'Mercy Killer Gets Life'

A 75-year-old man who used a mercy killing defense was convicted of first-degree murder yesterday for shooting his ailing wife, and a judge sentenced him to life in prison.

Roswell Gilbert had testified that he shot his wife, Emily, 73, out of compassion because of her suffering from progressive senility and a bone disease.

Judge Thomas Coker Jr. immediately sentenced Gilbert to life in prison, with a 25-year minimum, mandatory term. Because the state waived the death penalty, Coker noted, Florida law allows no other punishment for first-degree murder.

"He's numb right now," said defense lawyer Harry Gulkin, adding that he will appeal.

Witnesses testified that Mrs. Gilbert had longed for and begged for death.

Gilbert sat stoically as his only child, Martha Morgan, burst into tears when the verdict was read after five hours of deliberation.

Mrs. Gilbert, 73, who was killed March 4 in their apartment, suffered from Alzheimer's disease and from osteoporosis, a painful bone disintegration.

Gilbert was indicted on a first-degree murder charge after he admitted shooting his wife.

Supporters of Gilbert said the conviction and sentence will aid their cause to legalize mercy killing.

Defense lawyer Joe Varon begged jurors in closing arguments yesterday to ignore laws and set legal precedent with an acquittal.

But prosecutor Kelly Hancock had urged jurors to ignore pleas for compassion. "Sympathy cannot play a role," he

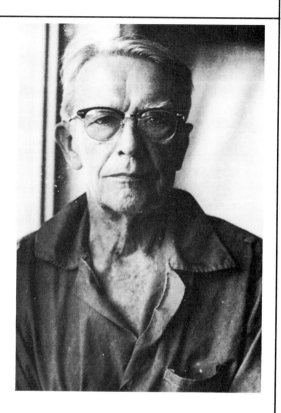

said in his closing arguments. "It was an act of convenience. He didn't solve her problems; he solved his."

Gilbert testified that his wife's senility and pain were increasing. Often confused, she sometimes referred to him as "the bastard" and was terrified that he would desert her.

On March 4, crying and in pain, she begged for death, he and two other witnesses testified.

"I know it's murder but so what? Some things are more important than law," testified the gaunt, silver-haired defendant. He had called police and turned himself in after the shooting.

The majority of Americans favor some type of euthanasia, believing one has the right to have death hastened in some cases (Kalish and Reynolds 1981). Although few physicians believe in active euthanasia, one report indicated that 87 percent approve of passive euthanasia and 80 percent have practiced it (Weddington 1981). Common ways that physicians hasten the death of their patients is ordering a TKO, meaning the nurses should endeavor "to keep open" the patient's intravenous feeding tube, but not supply enough nutrients to maintain life (*Los Angeles Times* 31 Oct. 1983). Another common euthanasia technique is called *snowing* in which the physician prescribes excessive doses of painkillers, even exceeding the lethal dose (Kluge 1975).

Should an individual be able to choose to end his or her own life if suffering from an incurable condition? Most states have now enacted legislation that honors the wishes of those who decide in advance that they do not want to be kept alive on machines when there is little or no hope of recovery. In some states, individuals who do not wish life-sustaining procedures can sign a legal document called a living will. The law requires the document to be signed and witnessed when a person is fully mentally capable. Without the document, the decision of how long a person should remain on life support is usually made by a physician and family members.

Allowing people to die can be humane or it can be an excuse to provide sub-optimal medical care. Some fear that legislation permitting euthanasia will be abused and the poor, elderly, and mentally ill will be killed against their will when medical intervention would help. Perhaps as a response to this fear, a group of physicians proposed a form requesting doctors to use super-human methods to maintain life (reported in *American Health* 1985). They assert that elders and the poor may desire such a form to prevent physicians from giving inadequate care or pulling the plug to save costs. An example of the form follows:

> I wish maximal medical care to be provided to me to prolong my life without regard to my physical or mental diagnosis, condition or prognosis and without regard to financial cost. . . . This declaration shall be honored by my family and physician(s) as the final expression of my legal right to preserve my life until the actual moment of my death.

Deciding to Die

A living will gives individuals more control over the circumstances of their death. However, the ultimate right to choose one's own death is suicide. The act of suicide may range from an irrational act done by a mentally unstable individual or a premeditated, rational decision to end physical or mental anguish. Suicide is a serious problem for all age groups, but elders commit disproportionately more suicides than other age groups. In 1980, those over sixty-five comprised 11.3 percent of the population, but accounted for 17 percent of all the suicides (National Center for Health Statistics, 1983). However, suicide rates are underestimated because many suicides are not reported as such—for example, drug overdoses, failure to take life-sustaining drugs, intentional starvation, and accidents.

White males over age seventy-five have the highest suicide rates of any population group. Elder males are more than five times more likely to commit suicide than females. While suicides among women peak in the forty-five to sixty-four age group, suicides among men continue to rise with each decade of life. In the sixty-five to seventy age group, male suicides outnumber those of females' five to one; by age eighty-five, the ratio is increased to ten to one (National Center for Health Statistics 1987).

Chapter 14

The Living Will

To My Family, My Physician, My Lawyer and All Others Whom It May Concern

Death is as much a reality as birth, growth, maturity and old age—it is the one certainty of life. If the time comes when I can no longer take part in decisions for my own future, let this statement stand as an expression of my wishes and directions, while I am still of sound mind.

If at such a time the situation should arise in which there is no reasonable expectation of my recovery from extreme physical or mental disability, I direct that I be allowed to die and not be kept alive by medications, artificial means or "heroic measures". I do, however, ask that medication be mercifully administered to me to alleviate suffering even though this may shorten my remaining life.

This statement is made after careful consideration and is in accordance with my strong convictions and beliefs. I want the wishes and directions here expressed carried out to the extent permitted by law. Insofar as they are not legally enforceable, I hope that those to whom this Will is addressed will regard themselves as morally bound by these provisions.

Signed _____

Date _____

Witness _____

Witness _____

Copies of this request have been given to _____

_____

_____

_____

To Make Best Use of Your Living Will

You may wish to add specific statements to the Living Will *in the space provided for that purpose above your signature.* Possible additional provisions are:

1. "Measures of artificial life-support in the face of impending death that I specifically refuse are:
   a) Electrical or mechanical resuscitation of my heart when it has stopped beating.
   b) Nasogastric tube feeding when I am paralyzed or unable to take nourishment by mouth.
   c) Mechanical respiration when I am no longer able to sustain my own breathing.
   d) _____"

2. "I would like to live out my last days at home rather than in a hospital if it does not jeopardize the chance of my recovery to a meaningful and sentient life or does not impose an undue burden on my family."

3. "If any of my tissues are sound and would be of value as transplants to other people, I freely give my permission for such donation."

The optional Durable Power of Attorney feature allows you to name someone else to serve as your proxy in case you are unable to communicate your wishes.

Should you choose to fill in this portion of the document, you must have your signature notarized.

If you choose more than one proxy for decision-making on your behalf, please give order of priority (1, 2, 3, etc.)

Space is provided at the bottom of the Living Will for notarization should you choose to have your Living Will witnessed by a Notary Public.

Remember . . .

- Sign and date your Living Will. Your two witnesses, who should not be blood relatives or beneficiaries of your property will, should also sign in the spaces provided.

- Discuss your Living Will with your doctors; if they agree with you, give them copies of your signed Living Will document for them to add to your medical file.

- Give copies of your signed Living Will to anyone who may be making decisions for you if you are unable to make them yourself.

- Look over your Living Will once a year, redate it and initial the new date to make it clear that your wishes have not changed.

Reprinted with permission of Concern for Dying, 250 West 57th Street, New York, N.Y. 10107; (212) 246–6962.

Maleness is the greatest risk factor for suicide, but other factors are significant. White elder males commit suicide at three times the rate of black elder males. Nonmarried persons of all ages are more likely to commit suicide, especially those who have recently lost their spouse or live alone. Elderly widowers are at high risk for suicide. Those who have experienced painful illness, retirement, loss of income and increased dependency are also at risk (McIntosh et al. 1981; Miller 1979).

Unlike younger groups, most elders who attempt suicide rarely make suicide attempts that fail (Kreitman 1977). Elders may be more successful at suicide because they have fewer social supports, use lethal weapons more often, and have poorer recuperative powers (McIntosh 1985). Further, they may be more determined to kill themselves and less likely to attempt suicide for attention or to hurt another person.

Most elders provide behavioral and verbal clues to suicide prior to the act. Miller (1978) noted that 60 percent of elders who committed suicide had given others verbal or behavioral clues. Robbins et al. (1977) reported that two-thirds of elder white men had previously commented on their suicidal intent. Previous suicide attempts, preoccupation with suicidal thought, agitation, or expression of hopelessness are important indicators. Elders who plan suicide may purchase a firearm, stockpile pills, make funeral arrangements, or give away valued possessions. Verbal clues may be direct, "I'm going to kill myself," or indirect, "I'm tired of life, what's the point of going on?" Crises—such as the diagnosis of serious illness, death of a spouse, retirement, or recent move—may increase risk of suicide. Family, friends, and professionals should be alert to prolonged depression or hints about suicide and should openly discuss the topic. Contrary to popular belief, talking about suicide will not set off those who are depressed, rather it may decrease their isolation.

It is common for elders to reach out to professionals prior to committing suicide. One study found that about three-fourths of elders who committed suicide had visited a physician within a month prior to suicide (Grollman 1971). Elders may visit physicians with vague somatic complaints that mask their anguish and helplessness. Unfortunately, few physicians are trained to recognize suicide symptoms. It is important that those who work with elders be aware of verbal, behavioral, and situational clues to suicide. Many suicides may be prevented by identifying high-risk elders and referring them to appropriate help (Osgood 1985). Unfortunately, formal suicide prevention and psychological services are not reaching most elders in need (McIntosh et al. 1981).

Suicides have a great impact on the survivors who often feel guilty for not having noticed the victim's trauma, or not intervening soon enough. Many survivors feel responsible for the victim's action. Further, because suicide is not a socially acceptable means of dying, survivors of a suicide may receive less social support from friends. For these reasons, those close to suicide victims may need counseling and support to allay their feelings of guilt, responsibility, depression, and self-blame.

Where Death Occurs

Institutions have taken over the physical and emotional care of the dying that was historically the role of the family. Currently, over 70 percent of the United States population will die in a hospital, followed by a smaller number in nursing and board and care homes (Veatch and Tai 1980). This trend is mainly due to a number of factors: the decrease in extended families in America, disengagement of family members from the dying, absence of family members in close proximity due to social mobility, and the medical technology available in hospitals to meet the

After 60 Years of Marriage, Couple Decides to Leave World Together

Julia Saunders, eighty-one, had her hair done. Her husband, Cecil, collected the mail one final time, paused to chat with a neighbor. Inside their mobile home, they carefully laid out a navy blazer and a powder-blue dress.

After lunch, the Saunderses drove to a rural corner of Lee County and parked. As cows grazed in the summer heat, the couple talked. Then Cecil Saunders shot his wife of sixty years in the heart and turned the gun on himself.

Near the clothes they had chosen to be buried in, the couple had left a note:

"Dear children, this we know will be a terrible shock and embarrassment. But as we see it, it is one solution to the problem of growing old. We greatly appreciate your willingness to try to take care of us.

After being married for 60 years, it only makes sense for us to leave this world together because we loved each other so much."

On the floorboard of the car, Cecil and Julia Saunders had placed typewritten funeral instructions and the telephone numbers of their son and daughter.

Then they consummated their suicide pact, becoming two of the more than four thousand elderly Americans authorities say will commit suicide this year.

"What struck all of us was how considerate, how thoughtful they were to all concerned about killing themselves," said Sheriff's Sgt. Richard Chard, who investigated the August 19 murder-suicide. "They didn't want to impose or be a bother to anyone. Not even in dying."

Julia's dimming eyesight, heart congestion and a stroke had driven Cecil to place his wife in a nursing home earlier this year. But she became hysterical over what she said was poor care there, and Cecil brought her home, said neighbors at the mobile home park where the couple had lived since 1974.

"You never saw him without her," said Vera Whitmore, sixty-seven. "If there ever was true love, they had it. I think they were just tired of living and couldn't wait for God to take them."

The Saunderses had hot dogs and beans for lunch, then drove their Caprice to pastureland 5½ miles from their mobile home, parking on the grassy shoulder.

As thunderstorms rumbled in the distance, they talked.

"I can picture in my mind them sitting there," Chard said. "Maybe they spoke about how things were when they were young. Then he leaned over and gave her a farewell kiss."

The bodies were found by workers from nearby Owl Creek Boat Works who called the police.

In Philadelphia, a police officer stood by as the Saunderses' son, Robert, fifty-seven, was told of his parents' death. His parents wanted no tears shed over their decision to die. The note they left for Robert and his sister, Evelyn, fifty-one, ended with a wish:

"Don't grieve because we had a very good life and saw our two children turn out to be such fine persons, Love Mother and Father."

Source: *Minneapolis Star and Tribune*, Oct. 4, 1983, p. 12A. Used by permission.

health needs of the dying (Fulton 1979). This transfer of responsibility has also altered the way the dying are cared for. Families are motivated to care for their dying largely because of emotional ties whereas institutions are motivated by economic gain. Because hospitals focus on control of physical problems, care is less personal and seldom meets the emotional or social needs of the patient. The advent of advanced medical technology and drugs have extended life, but they also prolong the dying interval. Prolonged life extension isolates the terminally ill, and places added strain upon the family.

A number of factors influence where death occurs. Health condition, amount of care required, availability of a willing caretaker, and sufficient community services are major factors that influence whether a death will occur in a hospital or at home. Those who live alone are more likely to go to an institution or hospital to die than those who live with family. Married men are more likely to die at home than married women since wives are more likely to care for dying spouses than husbands are. The cost of care is another factor influencing where an elder dies. Depending on the situation, hospital, nursing home, or home care may be the least expensive alternative. As mentioned earlier, Medicare will pay costs incurred at a hospital, but seldom reimburses the care provided by a home health aide. Personal preference also plays a role. Most elders prefer the familiar surroundings and personalized care at home, but some do not want to burden their families and prefer hospitalization (Kalish and Reynolds 1981).

Although most elders die in hospitals, some experts believe that they may not be the most appropriate place. Physicians generally subscribe to the view that death is pathological not natural and rank cure more important than care. This is not to say that they are uncaring, but that their work is oriented to saving lives and controlling death rather than alleviating symptoms and meeting the psychosocial needs of the dying. Further, the bureaucratic nature of hospital policies and procedures depersonalize the patient in favor of medical efficiency (Stephenson 1985).

Elders who are disabled and slowly dying, but whose death is not imminent or preventable with modern technology are often placed in nursing homes. When elders enter a nursing home, they, their families, and the nursing home staff recognize that they are coming there to live out their final days. However, nursing home personnel are generally not trained to deal with the special needs of the dying and may neglect dying individuals. Additionally, dying elders are often confused or comatose during the dying process, providing further impetus for inadequate care (Kalish 1985).

Home-care services can ease the burden of physical care for the family. However, a wide range of services at low cost is available in only a few communities (see Chapter 13). A relatively new service for the terminally ill and their families is hospice care. The first hospice inpatient facility was set up in London in 1967 as a reaction against the disease-centered hospital care of the dying. However, in the United States, hospice services are more often provided to the terminally ill in the home or in special wings of participating hospitals. Hospice programs use multidisciplined teams composed of clergy, physicians, social workers, and trained volunteers who offer medical services, personal care to the dying, emotional, and spiritual support for the dying, respite care, and grief counseling for bereaved family members.

Hospice care differs from conventional medical treatment in that patients are not admitted to the program unless the individual and physician believe further treatment and cure are no longer possible. Hospice attempts to keep dying patients at home as long as possible, with the understanding that if their condition worsens and they require hospitalization, the support services will continue.

Attitudes Toward Dying and Death

Elders are less likely to fear their own death than younger persons. They are more likely to be fearful of the process of dying than death itself. Common fears include fear of prolonged illness or disability, being a burden on others, separation or rejection from loved ones, being dependent, and being in pain (Kalish 1985). Because death is a common occurrence among elders, it is not unusual that elders fear death less and think about death more than younger age groups (Kalish and Reynolds 1981). Some elders may talk about funeral arrangements or disposition of belongings; others may reminisce, taking stock of their lives. Many elders cope with their impending death by preparing for it. Elders are more likely to have drafted a will, made funeral arrangements, paid for a cemetery plot, and arranged for someone to handle their affairs than younger people (Kalish and Reynolds 1981).

A number of studies indicate that attitudes toward dying and death are related to age. Until the age of seven or eight, children generally believe that death is not permanent. Gradually, children recognize the finality of death, but not for themselves. However, by age ten or so, the fact that they, too, will die is recognized (Nagy 1948).

Adolescents spend much time and energy struggling with their personal identity and immediate futures. During this time, it is difficult for them even to think about themselves as middle-aged. Death is recognized, but is not personally relevant (Kastenbaum 1969). However, many adolescents do think a lot about death and when questioned, many high school students admit to a fear of death (Koocher et al. 1976). Other reports show that the brighter the student, the higher the fear and the more frequent the thoughts about death (Maurer 1964).

Young adulthood is a period of height of energy and drive. Preparation for success in life is the principal focus. Thus, dealing with dying or death would mean to face rage, disappointment, frustration, and despair (Pattison 1977). Middle-aged individuals are more likely to think

Children recognize the finality of death, but do not spend much time considering their own death.

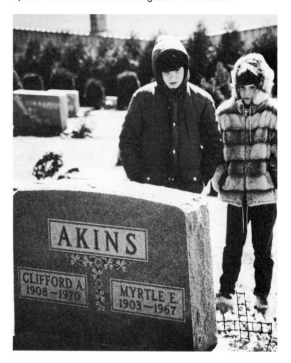

about personal death. One study indicates that middle-aged adults had a higher fear of death than adults younger or older than they (Riley 1970), but other studies do not support this finding (Kalish and Reynolds 1981). Middle-aged individuals are more likely to say "life is too short" and commonly reevaluate life goals—what has been accomplished and what remains to be done. Time no longer stretches out endlessly as it did in adolescence and young adulthood.

Studies consistently report that fear of death diminishes with advancing age (Kalish 1985). This reduction of the fear of death with advancing age may be due to a number of factors. Kalish (1985) asserts that death becomes more familiar with advancing age because older persons generally have more experience with the death of others than younger groups. In addition, the death of parents makes death more of a reality since parents generally die before their children. Further, the urgency of staying alive diminishes

---

Assess Your Attitudes Toward Your Death

Complete the following sentences, sharing your responses with your classmates. You may want to question people of other age groups to determine differences in attitudes.

Before I could die happily I feel I would have to . . .

My greatest fear about my own death is . . .

If I were to die today, my biggest regret would be . . .

I would like the following things around me when I die . . .

When I think of my own death, the saddest thing is . . .

Before I die, I would like to . . .

After I die, I want people to say . . .

When I die, I hope that . . .

I would like to have at my bedside when I die . . .

When I die, I will be glad to get away from . . .

When I die, I would like my funeral to be . . .

I want to die at age . . . because . . .

If I were to die tomorrow, my biggest accomplishment would be . . .

I would like to die at home if . . .

I want the cause of my death to be . . .

I would consider suicide when . . .

I want to be permitted to die when . . .

---

when individuals no longer have dependent children to care for. Finally, death is expected in the later years, so older persons are more prepared and resigned to it.

However, some studies show little differences in feelings about death based on age. Lowenthall et al. (1975) questioned a sample of individuals from adolescents to elders and reported surprisingly few differences between the life stages in their responses to death. Studies show that religious belief and education are stronger predictors of death attitudes than age (Kalish 1976; Lowenthall et al. 1975; Riley 1968). Other factors such as past experience with death and illness, cultural beliefs, and state of physical and mental health influence attitudes toward death.

Institutionalized elders are likely to welcome death as a release from continued disability and pain. Many have already experienced withdrawal from family and friends, lost much of their autonomy, and been separated from the pleasures in life that made it meaningful. Some who are not institutionalized, but who suffer from severe functional disability, depression, financial problems, loss of loved ones or rewarding activity, may also welcome death as a means to end the heavy demands of daily living.

Coping with Impending Death

When diagnosed as terminally ill, the social status of the sick person changes radically. Even though an individual was previously an important, contributing member of the community, s/he is now on the way out and therefore less valued. The sick individual may be ignored by many former acquaintances because of their discomfort with death. On the other hand, the sick person may no longer desire to interact with more than a handful of friends and family. As a result, the social sphere of the sick person becomes very small. Many former activities and broader interests disappear as the sick person becomes more focused on the tasks of dying and activities directly related to survival.

Stages of Dying

Based on her extensive work with the dying, Kübler-Ross (1969) proposed a process that dying individuals undergo in order to cope with their impending death. She described five distinct stages through which many terminally ill patients pass, each a defense mechanism against the fear of death. Kübler-Ross observed that the stages were not absolutes as both the time spent in each stage and the sequence varied among individuals and many stages overlapped. The five stages are as follows:

Denial: When first learning that they are terminally ill, many patients register shock and disbelief. They reject the diagnosis, thinking that the lab reports must be mistaken or that the physician made a wrong diagnosis. This stage is generally short unless the family continues to deny the illness.

Anger: The diagnosed terminally ill patient will bemoan, "why me?" The patient may become resentful that others are healthy while s/he must die. Individuals may express anger at their family, health professionals, themselves, or the anger may be unfocused. Irritability and complaining are common.

Bargaining: During this stage, death becomes a reality, but the individual attempts to postpone the time of death by bargaining. Most deals are struck with God, even if one has never talked with God before, and most are secret. During this period, the dying individual may seek out alternative treatments—such as faith healers, unusual drugs, or vitamin supplements—to postpone death.

Depression: When it becomes obvious that a bargain cannot be struck, depression occurs. Death is recognized as inevitable and the feelings of loss become overwhelming. Whereas before the individual may have been talkative, crying, agitated, or seeking sympathy, during this stage the individual often withdraws from visitors and mourns silently. Mourning for loss of capability and lost relationships allows an individual to prepare for death and to attempt to make sense of life and death.

Acceptance: Individuals at this stage are often devoid of emotion and disengaged from the outside world. Many limit contact to one or two people who are very close. The dying are often tired and weak, and days are spent in sleeping, resting, and reminiscing.

Kübler-Ross' work was revolutionary because it sensitized the public and professionals to the needs of the dying. However, her research has been criticized on a number of counts. For one, there are no clear, observable behavior patterns for each stage; differentiation among stages relied on her subjective interpretation of the patient's emotions or motivations. Critics question her findings because they believe her subjects' emotions were probably highly vulnerable to suggestion and manipulation. Additionally, some feelings reported may have been the result of drugs since this variable was not controlled in her study (Stephenson 1985). Finally, reviews of the literature have not confirmed her findings (Schultz and Alderman 1974). Hinton (1972) reported that depression and anxiety appeared in the last two months of life in one-half the patients he studied and both increased toward death.

Another problem with the Kübler-Ross model is that many health professionals erroneously interpret the stages as a prescription all must follow for a good death. In some instances, it leads to labeling patients and attempting to move them to different stages rather than helping them deal with their feelings and accepting their individuality (Fitchett 1980).

Other research has revealed that Kübler-Ross's stages of dying are not a natural, common way to deal with death and that there are many other emotions associated with the dying process. Many experts agree with Schneidman's description of the dying process: "Rather than the five definite stages discussed above, my experience has led me to posit a hive of affect, in which there is a constant coming and going. The emotional stages seem to include a constant interplay between disbelief and hope and, against these as background, a waxing and waning of anguish, terror, acquiescence and surrender, rage and envy, disinterest and ennui, pretense, taunting and daring and even yearning for death—all these in the context of bewilderment and pain" (1973, p. 7).

Since Kübler-Ross, many other researchers have attempted to more accurately characterize the dying process. In particular, Pattison (1977) defined three stages of the living-dying interval: acute, chronic, and terminal. In the acute phase, individuals face the knowledge of their imminent death and may react with anxiety, denial, or anger. In the chronic phases, individuals begin to confront their fears of dying such as loneliness, pain, and what will happen after death. The final or terminal phase signals the end of hope and the beginning of withdrawal from the outside world upon realization of the inevitability of death. The goal of treatment for the dying, according to Pattison, is to help them cope with the first phase, help them live through the second, and move them toward the third.

Both Kübler-Ross and Pattison infer that acceptance of death is a final, desirable stage. In fact, research has shown that those who accept that they have a serious condition, but believe they can postpone their death have higher survival rates (Holden 1978). Studies show that those who passively accept impending death have lower survival rates than those who express their anger and resentment at their dying, make demands on family, friends, and medical personnel, and ask for help when needed (Derogatis et al. 1979).

Kalish speaks for many when he expresses his views on his own dying process: "For some people and under some circumstances, acceptance of death is certainly the way to an appropriate death. For others, it is not. Perhaps anger, even fury, is the most appropriate way to die: what a mockery death is; how destructive it is; how absurd it is— there is nothing good about death, at least about *my* death and I have no intention of being peaceful or submissive or accepting!" (1985, pp. 135–136).

Rights of the Dying

Dying people are very vulnerable. The process of dying takes a lot of physical and psychic energy. Sedatives, painkillers, and some treatments can further reduce energy and cause disorientation and diminishing capabilities. As strength decreases, the dying are progressively less able to carry out daily activities. Because those who are dying are generally in a weakened state, family members and professionals are responsible to ensure their rights are not violated. The following section discusses some of these rights.

Right to Open Communication About Death

The majority of Americans of all ethnic backgrounds believe individuals have the right to know about their impending death and would want to be told if they were dying. Because individuals commonly deny that they are dying in the early stages, it is generally most sensitive to inform them first that their condition is serious and allow them to ask more questions as they are ready to hear it. Knowledge of impending death allows dying persons to complete certain tasks before dying and to close their life in accordance with personal wishes. Additionally, full awareness of impending death allows an individual to make responsible decisions, such as where to die and what treatments to allow.

Right to a Painless Death, to the Extent Possible

A common fear among elders is that their death will be painful. However, severe pain among the dying is not common and most patients can become pain-free with proper medication. It is generally held that painkillers, including strong, addictive morphine or opium, should be given freely to the dying who are in severe pain, if requested.

Right to the Presence of Concerned Others

Elders are more likely to die in lonely, isolated conditions than younger people. In fact, one of elders' greatest fears is abandonment at the time of death. A high proportion of elders may spend their dying interval without a concerned person to help make medical decisions or advocate adequate medical treatment. It is imperative that those who are dying alone be assigned a nurse or volunteer. The importance of a support person, especially during the final days, becomes apparent as the dying generally begin to lack interest in all visitors except one or two significant persons.

Right to as Much Control Over Environment as Possible

Because the dying so often experience loss of control over their environment and declining health, it is imperative that health professionals and family allow the dying person as much control as possible. Allowing patients some choice over meals, frequency of nursing interruptions, visiting hours, roommates, and medical treatments can greatly enhance their feelings of autonomy.

Technological advances have made the dying process more impersonal.

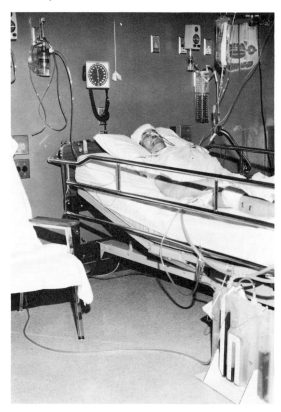

Right to Have All Treatments Fully Explained and to Refuse Treatment

The dying, like other patients, have the right to have all medical treatments fully explained including a description of the prognosis, methods of treatment, and potential risks, benefits, and side effects. Individuals have the right to refuse treatment for their illness and to seek out alternative treatments, even those not condoned by the medical profession. For instance, chemotherapy, a common cancer treatment, has a questionable success rate and is accompanied by many uncomfortable side effects, including hair loss and nausea. Because of this, many patients refuse the therapy, opting for a more comfortable, although perhaps shorter, life. As discussed earlier, patients have the right to refuse all heroic, artificial

Chapter 14

efforts to sustain life. On the other hand, it should not be assumed that all elders are ready to die and would refuse life-sustaining measures. Elders should have the right to all the technologically advanced equipment and treatments available to younger groups to prolong life.

Tasks of the Dying

Individuals who know they are dying often feel compelled to complete a number of tasks before they die. The importance of certain tasks and the time spent on each varies with the degree of disability, the nature of the illness, the time left to live, the personality of the individual and the environment, but will generally center around six themes (adapted from Kalish 1985 and Butler and Lewis 1982):

Completing Unfinished Business
Individuals vary in the types of activities they wish to complete before death. The unfinished business may include reuniting with a distant family member, completing a photo album, or sharing intimate feelings with their family. It is important to let the dying person decide what tasks to accomplish and the ways the family and the health worker can help.

Dealing with Medical Care Needs
The dying need to understand their diagnosis and prognosis, learn of alternative treatments and pain control methods, and decide on life-sustaining treatments. Further, they need to tell others what measures should be taken if their condition worsens to a point where they are no longer in control. They may complete a living will or direct a family member to make medical decisions. The dying individual also needs to be involved in the decision whether to die in a hospital, nursing home, or at home.

Allocating Time and Energy Resources
We all have thought of what we would do if we knew we had five or six months to live. The usual answers—such as traveling or accomplishing a creative feat—generally include tasks that require more mental and physical energy than most dying persons possess. How much time and energy a dying individual can allocate depends on the nature of the illness and its progression. As the disease progresses, individuals generally become weaker and must be selective about which tasks can be accomplished before death and which must be left behind. Additionally, dying persons must choose who to spend time with during their last days.

Arranging for Death
Another important task for the dying is to arrange what will happen after death. The dying person may need to make a will and distribute valued possessions to loved ones before death. Many make decisions on cremation or burial and donation of body organs. Some plan the details of their funeral. Others arrange for people to take care of finances and insurance policies and the care of pets after death.

Reviewing Their Life
The dying often spend time reminiscing about their life and its meaning. They contemplate what it means to die and their belief in an afterlife. Many individuals turn to religion or God during this time to give them hope or justification for their suffering.

Caring for the Dying

Most frail older people are cared for at home by a family member. When the task becomes overwhelming or the sick person needs specialized care, hospitalization usually occurs. Wherever the person is dying, the family is generally intensely involved, whether at home or in an institution. Caring for a terminally ill patient brings about profound changes in family roles and interactions. A parent, once the caregiver for his or her children, now must depend on them for physical care and emotional support. A husband may have to learn homemaking skills to care for an ailing wife. Caretakers must cope with feelings of loss and grief, while dealing with the physical, emotional, and financial needs of a dying loved one. Family members may become lonely or overwhelmed with responsibility, resent the dying individual, but feel very guilty for their feelings. For instance, the care of a very sick older person may require tremendous personal commitment and financial resources. At times, the caregiver may guiltily wish for the sick person to die. Although emotionally draining, caring for the dying can help the later grieving process.

Since one of the greatest fears of the dying is isolation or abandonment, perhaps the most crucial element of caring for the dying is to reduce this fear by being a trustworthy companion. Further, open communication with the terminally ill about their illness and treatment, day-to-day concerns, death fears or anxieties, and life reminiscences can reduce isolation and bolster their feelings of control. If the family member is institutionalized, the caretaker may also serve as patient advocate to ensure adequate care as well as encourage patient compliance with medical treatments. However, many find it difficult to associate with someone who is dying and do not visit or if they do, interact ineffectively. These feelings occur not only with the family and friends of the dying person, but also may be present in professionals assigned to work with terminally ill patients. Kalish (1985, pp. 266–268) discusses a number of reasons why people may have difficulty relating to dying persons (see below).

Caring as a Health Professional

Many who work in health and social services fields will necessarily deal with death and dying. However, many health professionals are inadequately prepared to deal with the physical or psychological needs of the dying or their own response to it, making their work frustrating and depressing (Dickenson and Pearson 1980–1981). Further, many people do not care to work with the dying but do so because of a lack of career alternatives.

Professionals, like the rest of the American population, do not like to be confronted with death. Physicians who see their role as restoring an individual to health and productivity may have special problems dealing with the dying. By viewing their role in this way, they face inevitable personal failure. Some may feel hesitant to waste their training on terminal patients. Additionally, it is often difficult for physicians and nurses to work with dying patients without intense feelings of failure and emotional conflict as they watch the patient deteriorate and die. On the other hand,

Difficulty in Relating to Dying Persons

Developing personal or professional relationships with the dying and the bereaved, are difficult for a number of reasons. In these types of relationships, individuals are confronted with several unique sources of stress that may lead them to withdraw the attempt. Some of these stressors relate primarily to the dying, others primarily to the bereaved, and some develop in both kinds of relationships.

First, the future of dying people is a particularly limited one; we are reluctant to invest a lot of our time and energy for individuals who will not be around to relate to or be productive in any fashion. Their social value becomes less. And many people desire to work only with individuals who have a potentially promising future. The dying are disengaging; others are disengaging from them. The impetus to care for and to care about them diminishes.

Second, dying people remind us that we will also not live forever. They remind us that we, like they, are transient, impermanent, subject to decay and death. Many of us don't like the reminder and don't want to work in a setting in which we are constantly reminded of our mortality.

Third, when we begin to think about our own mortality and transiency, we are also required thereby to consider the ephemeral quality of what we accomplish. The novel we write, the educational program we develop, the sales campaign we devise, the computer software we create, the fine wood cabinet that we design—none of these will last forever.

Fourth, death is loss, and we don't like to have to encounter a series of losses. It is bad enough that we must suffer the pain from the inevitable losses of people we love; we don't want to add to our pain by developing new relationships with people we know are going to die.

Fifth, the dying remind us that we cannot completely control our environment. A girl just entering her teens suffered a serious epileptic seizure. Although she was eventually stabilized on medication, so that she had no more seizures, the event was always fresh in her memory as an example of the suddenness with which

life can change, the absurdity of a condition within one's own body that comes unexpectedly, as if from nowhere, and has the potential of depriving life of some of its most basic satisfactions—even for depriving life of life, since a seizure at the wrong moment can lead to death. Each of us, at every moment, potentially has the seed of death within our body, and each of us, at every moment, confronts the potential of death from outside ourself. And we do not always have the power to control either the internal or external environment from which this potential emanates. Neither, of course, are we necessarily without power, but working with people who are dying is a constant reminder that change, absurdity, and chance are always in our lives. It is easier to ignore dying and death and to pretend to ourselves that we are really in charge of everything.

Sixth, dying people often look peculiar, talk strangely, have an unpleasant odor and are not able to offer some of the normal amenities of normal relationships. This is especially true during the later stages of some illnesses.

Seventh, people who are grieving, and, in fewer instances, dying often express a level of emotionality that we find difficult to handle. It is troublesome for me, whether functioning as your friend or as a professional who is trying to provide help and support, to be with you when you are so upset about events in your life and I am powerless to diminish your anguish to any appreciable extent. I then need to handle both your pain, which also pains me, and my powerlessness, which adds to my pain.

Health professionals need support from the administration and their peers to enhance their effectiveness in working with the dying.

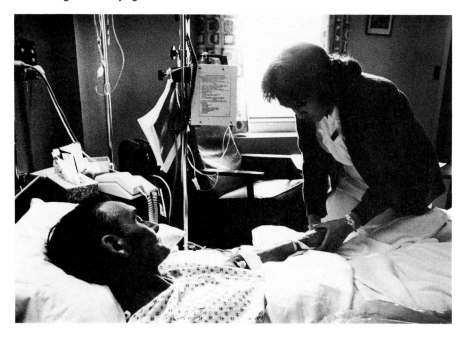

if emotional involvement is withheld from the dying, the professional may be less effective. Harper (1977) asks the critical question: how can professionals genuinely care about their patients by giving totally of themselves, yet totally preserving themselves?

Those who work closely with dying patients need to have deep compassion for the terminally ill and their family, while preserving a distance from the death that keeps them from falling into depression every time a patient dies. Harper (1977) has conceptualized a process that new professionals undergo as they learn to be progressively more comfortable in working with dying patients. She envisions the process to take from one to two years. The stages are described as follows:

Intellectualization
During their initial confrontation with death, those beginning to work with dying people are very intellectual regarding their tasks. There may be an abnormal desire for medical knowledge and the patient and disease are discussed in an intellectual, detached manner. This is generally a period of brisk activity. Tangible services to the dying and their family are provided, but no emotional involvement is displayed and conversations with the dying are impersonal. The professional is uncomfortable, but concerned. However she or he is unable to discuss death or dying with the patient. Although the worker knows intellectually that death will occur, this knowledge is emotionally unacceptable and may cause withdrawal from the patient and family.

Emotional Survival

This is a difficult period. The move from intellectualization to emotional survival occurs when the professional realizes that death and suffering are unavoidable. As professionals confront the death of their patients, they are forced to deal with the reality of their own death and mourn and grieve for it. They may also pity the patient as they feel guilt and frustration at the contrast between their own health and another's illness. They may try to fight back against death or illness, or question death. At times the professional is too emotional to face the patient.

Depression

This is the most crucial stage, often referred to as the "grow or go" stage. At this point professionals may either quit their job or learn to accept the reality of death. They begin to question their ability to help the dying and their families. Feelings of anger, hurt, depression, or grieving are commonly expressed. These emotions need to be acknowledged in order to accept death and accept their value in caring for the dying. On the other hand, if the depression or frustration is too great, the professional may begin to avoid interactions with the dying and may resign.

Emotional Arrival

In this stage of mitigation and accommodation, the professional experiences a sense of freedom from such debilitating emotions as identification with the patient's symptoms, preoccupation with own death, guilt feelings about personal health, and incapacitating depression. Although the professional is not necessarily free of pain, he or she is free from its debilitating effects. Sensitivity to the needs of the dying is sharpened, enabling a more appropriate emotional response.

Deep Compassion

During this stage of self-realization, professionals relate compassionately and sensitively to the dying while fully accepting their impending death. They learn to channel feelings of compassion into constructive and appropriate activities that assist the dying individual and the family. In this final stage, professionals have a full awareness and acceptance of their own death and so are able to help patients deal with their death compassionately. After reaching this stage, which takes one to two years, the caregiver has matured both professionally and personally.

For professionals to learn to effectively care for the dying, they need information on the psychological needs of the dying and the bereaved. Historically, medical schools have offered little death education. In 1980, only 13 percent of medical schools had a course on how to relate to dying patients and their families (Dickinson 1981). Dickinson and Pearson also reported that medical students who took a course in relating to dying patients were better able to deal with the terminally ill and their families than those who did not. Further, the report documented that skills necessary to work with the dying can be learned.

Health professionals also need to develop skills to assist the dying patient, the grieving family, and their own personal death. Not only is it important for schools of medicine, nursing, and social work to include curricula on working with the dying, but formal and informal discussions are necessary in the medical setting throughout professional practice.

Caring for the dying takes greater personal and time investment than working with any other patient population. However, this investment is seldom recognized. Often those who are serving dying patients are the lowest-paid paraprofessionals—nurses aides in hospitals or nursing homes. Nurse's aides are commonly overburdened with more sick people than can be effectively served, increasing their physical and emotional load on them.

No matter what the level of professional training, burnout (emotional and physical exhaustion) is common among those who work with the dying. Burnout is characterized by job dissatisfaction, cynicism, withdrawal from the dying and their families, and, in some cases, termination of employment. If professionals do not deal with the stress of working with the dying, they will not only reduce their effectiveness with the dying and their families, they will also damage the quality of their personal life. Those professionals who work alone, such as home health aides and visiting nurses, need special support.

Hospital or nursing home administrators can support those who work with dying patients by providing inservice training on the psychological, physiological, and social needs of the dying and how to communicate with the dying and their families. Institutions may also offer both formal and informal support to staff, allowing them to vent their personal problems in working with the dying. Supervisors can also help employees work through the complex emotions associated with work with the dying. Supervisors may serve as role models for new professionals who are learning to give good care without burnout. However, supervisors need to be aware that not all employees are qualified to work with the dying and some staff may need to be transferred. Further, supervisors need to recognize that even the most competent staff need a periodic time-out from working with the dying (Harper 1977).

Grief

Grief is a natural, even necessary response to the death of a loved one and is generally manifested as an acute sense of despair. The process of grieving is very complex, involving a whole host of physiological, psychological, and social reactions. The grief response is highly individual and dependent on personality, whether death was preventable or appropriate, and the intensity of the previous relationship. Additionally, the number of past losses experienced, the number of other love relationships, and the available social supports influence the extent of grief. For instance, a long dying period may be easier to cope with

than a sudden, unexpected death. Grieving may invoke multiple, contradictory emotions: despair, anger, detachment, sadness, denial, guilt, and depression.

The Grieving Process

Many experts have attempted to classify stages of grieving in much the same way stages of dying are categorized. The following section describes the three stages of grief identified by Stephenson (1985): reaction, disorganization and reorganization, and reorientation and recovery. However, it is important to keep in mind that these stages do not account for the wide range of healthy, individual responses to the loss of a loved one. Further, these stages may sometimes be interrupted—grief is put aside for a while, then is endured again when reminded (Rosenblatt 1983).

In general, during the *reaction stage,* individuals do not initially feel the full impact of their loss. They are commonly emotionally stunned, but their feelings are repressed as they do what needs to be done. Soon, however, those who grieve succumb to the urge to cry out in an effort to regain the lost object and internal tensions are released in a torrent of tears. Conflicting emotions are common: anger—at self, God, or the dead—may appear. Feelings of guilt about what one should have done for the deceased are often motivated by a desire to restore the lost loved person.

After a failed attempt to recover what was lost, disappointment and despair set in and a phase of *disorganization and reorganization* is entered. Normal activity patterns may seem useless or hurtful as grieving individuals realize the loss of part of themselves with the death of a loved one. For instance, an elder widow who spent the last year caring for her sick husband may not know what to do with herself since her time and energy had previously been focused on his needs. Individuals may obsessively review the past, be unable to sustain normal activity, or feel they are losing their mind. The phases of profound disorganization are interspersed with periods of clarity as the individual succeeds at new activities and behaviors. The internal reorganization is necessary for the individual to find meaning in life and to initiate a new lifestyle.

Finally, individuals enter a stage of *reorientation and recovery*. Rather than feelings of profound despair when the loved one is remembered, the individual becomes able to reminisce with only a touch of sadness. The bereaved begin to make sense of the loss and incorporate new activities and meanings in their lives. Successful resolution of grief is accomplished when the individual can reintegrate into the external world. As the bereaved regain control and sense of personal worth in the absence of the other, they move forward into new activities and relationships with only fleeting periods of depression or sadness.

Although the stages of dying end, the grieving process may continue indefinitely, its intensity decreasing with passing years. The time it takes to adapt to the loss of a loved one varies widely among individuals. It is lengthened by an avoidance of situations or thoughts that cause pain because of their associations with the deceased. If individuals continue to refrain from doing things that bring back memories of the deceased or resist breaking down, it may take longer to get over the loss.

Some degree of physiological disturbance is common among the bereaved. Worden (1982) describes common symptoms: hollow feeling in the stomach, tightness in the chest and throat, breathlessness, muscle weakness, and lack of energy. Further, after a loved one dies, the survivor is more likely to become ill or die than others their age who have not survived a recent loss. A number of studies chronicle the deterioration of health status, especially among widowers. Survivors commonly experience insomnia, changes in appetite and weight, increased consumption of alcohol and other drugs, and increased physician visits and hospital admissions (Rowland 1977). A review of the literature (Stroebe and Stroebe 1983) concluded that widowers suffer more than widows both psychologically and physiologically.

I Miss My Husband

The pain is as sharp and deep as the day he died. People think because I can speak of him calmly, sometimes with a smile, that I am over it. You don't love that much and live that close and get over it. Ever. Sometimes I hurt so much I want to run to someone, be held fast, have my head stroked. But he is the one I would have run to His arms would have held me, his hands stroked my head. Now there is no one. No comfort. Only pain . . .

Men exhibit significantly higher mortality and morbidity rates shortly following the death of their spouse. Studies also show that elder widowers have higher rates of alcoholism, suicide, and depression than their married counterparts. Although the effect is not as great, women exhibit a higher illness and mortality rate two to three years after the death of their spouse.

Some individuals cannot cope with the loss of a loved one and instead exhibit a number of inappropriate grief reactions. Individuals who have difficulty accepting their own death or those mourning a suicide, homicide, sudden death, unconfirmed death, or death where the mourner felt partially responsible are more likely to have difficulty coping with the death of another (Simpson 1979). Grief reactions may vary. Some individuals act as if nothing out of the ordinary has happened. Others may deny that the death occurred and continue interacting with the dead. Individuals may become so severely depressed and overcome with feelings of guilt or worthlessness that they may be suicidal. Others may manifest physical symptoms similar to those of the dying person or become seriously ill. This may result from personal neglect, stress, or grief. Some individuals retreat into social isolation or numb their pain with alcohol or other drugs.

Maladaptive coping strategies must be transformed into normal reactions before the individual can accept the death and go on living. Psychotherapy can help those who have repressed their grieving to deal more healthfully with their emotions. Volkan (1975) developed a re-grief therapy to help individuals understand the reasons they have not finished grieving and assist them in completing the grieving process.

Assisting the Bereaved

Methods to assist the bereaved to cope with the death of a loved one are highly variable and depend on the situation and personality of both the helper and bereaved. It is not uncommon for those approaching a newly bereaved person to be unsure how to act. Even though visits to the bereaved may be uncomfortable, friends should not avoid the bereaved or avoid discussion of the loss because of not knowing what to say. Visits and sympathy during the grieving process can be tremendously helpful in reducing social isolation and helping the bereaved express their grief.

Some physicians prescribe drugs to help individuals deal with grief, but this practice has recently been criticized. Mild sedation closely following the death can relieve exhaustion and severe insomnia. However, the negative effects of sedatives may outweigh their usefulness. Tranquilizers and sedatives prevent the griever from experiencing the pain that ultimately must be faced. The bereaved may be drugged during the funeral and miss this experience to grieve at a time when social support is available.

A number of resources are available for the bereaved, but these vary significantly among communities. Psychotherapy can help the bereaved release emotions, reminisce, or orient themselves to the future. Group therapy may be

"What is to come we know not. But we know that what has been was good." William Henley.

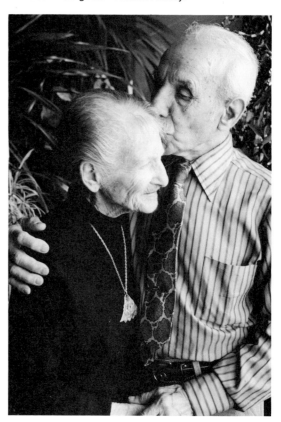

especially appropriate for widows and widowers, enabling them to deal with their grief and problems of living alone while facilitating social interaction. Perhaps the most inexpensive, accessible programs for the bereaved that offer both social and psychological support are widowhood programs. Some utilize volunteers, themselves widowed, who contact a recently bereaved person (from obituaries or funeral home referral) to provide psychological support. Other programs utilize social gatherings or discussion groups of widows or widowers headed by a professional or trained layperson.

Summary

It is important to learn about dying, death, and grief when studying aging and health because death occurs more frequently among those age sixty-five and older than any other age group. Further, elders are more likely to confront the deaths of friends and loved ones than younger persons. Death is defined as the lack of brain waves on an EEG. Modern technology allows the prolongation of life, but many ethical questions about euthanasia and the right to die accompany it. Suicide is an extension of the right to die and an important issue among elders. More elders, especially white males, take their own lives than any other age group.

The dying can choose to die in a hospital, at home, or in a nursing facility. The dying have certain rights such as the right to full knowledge of their condition and treatment, and the presence of supportive others. Further, dying individuals have certain tasks to complete such as finishing projects, planning funeral arrangements, and deciding on medical treatment protocol.

Caring for the dying is physically and emotionally draining and family and professional caretakers must cope with their own feelings while meeting the needs of the dying. Professional caretakers pass through certain stages in learning to work with the dying. Grief reactions are inevitable following the death of a loved one. Support groups and professional assistance is available for those who need help in the grieving process.

Activities

1. Would you be more likely to sign a living will or the alternative asking for heroic efforts? Give reasons for your choice. Would you be willing to sign the document now? Discuss this issue with your family and friends. Find out statutes related to living wills and the right of families and the dying to refuse treatment in your state.

2. Make a will stipulating what should be done with your personal possessions in the event that you die and how your funeral should proceed. Discuss this with your family and close friends.

3. Question your parents and friends to determine who has made a will. Do you find it true that elders are more likely than younger persons to have plans for their death?

4. If you were given six months to live and knew your health would be failing considerably toward the end, what tasks would you wish to complete? What significant others would you like near you? Would you prefer to die in a hospital or at home? Why?

5. What services or programs in your community help bereaved elders (churches, senior organizations, funeral homes, hospitals). How are they publicized? What is the cost?

6. Design an administrative policy for a hospital or nursing home on care for the dying. Outline goals, policies, and procedures to meet the social, psychological, and medical needs of the dying and their families.

7. Visit either a local nursing home or hospital and question staff on their policies regarding the dying. Is there a special section for the terminally ill? Are the patients told they are dying? Are there professionals or volunteers available who are trained to work specifically with the dying? How do other residents react to the death of an elder? What is their policy on living wills?

8. Are there any circumstances in which suicide would be a solution for you? Discuss these with the rest of the class.

Bibliography

American Health. 1985. Hands off that plug! June, 91.

Butler, R. N., and M. I. Lewis. 1982. *Aging and mental health.* St. Louis: Mosby.

Dickinson, G. E., and A. A. Pearson. 1980–81. Death education and physicians' attitudes toward the dying patient. *Omega* 11:167–74.

Derogatis, L., M. Abeloff, and N. Melisaratos. 1979. Psychological coping mechanisms and survival time in metastatic breast cancer. *JAMA* 242 (4):1504–08.

Fitchett, G. 1980. It's time to bury the stage theory of death and dying. *Oncology Nurse Exch* 2(3).

Foreman, P. 1975. The physician's criminal liability for the practice of euthanasia. *Baylor Law Rev* 27:54–61.

Fulton, R. 1979. Anticipatory grief, stress and the surrogate griever. In J. Tache, H. Selye, and S. Day, eds. *Cancer, stress and death.* New York: Plenum.

Grollman, E. 1971. *Suicide: Prevention, intervention and postvention.* Boston: Beacon Press.

Harper, B. C. 1977. *Death: The coping mechanism of the health professional.* Greenville, S. C.: Southeastern University Press.

Hinton, J. M. 1972. *Dying.* Baltimore: Penguin Books.

Holden, C. 1978. Cancers and the mind: How are they connected? *Science* 200:1363–69.

Kalish, R. A. 1976. Death and dying in a social context. In R. Birnstock and E. Shanas, eds. *Handbook of aging and social sciences.* New York: Van Nostrand-Reinhold.

Kalish, R. A. 1985. *Death, grief and caring relationships.* Monterey, Calif.: Brooks/Cole.

Kalish, R. A., and D. K. Reynolds. 1981. *Death and ethnicity: a psychocultural study.* Farmingdale, N.Y.: Baywood.

Kastenbaum, R. J. 1969. Death and bereavement in later life. In A. H. Kutscher, ed. *Death and bereavement.* Springfield, Ill.: Chas. C. Thomas.

Kluge, E. H. 1975. *The practice of death.* New Haven: Yale Univ. Press.

Koocher, G. P., J. E. O'Malley, D. Foster, and T. Gogan. 1976. Death anxiety in normal children and adolescents. *Psychiatr Clin North Am* 9:220–29.

Kreitman, N. 1977. *Parasuicide.* New York: John Wiley and Sons.

Kübler-Ross, E. 1969. *On death and dying.* New York: Macmillan.

Los Angeles Times. 1983. Life support court edict leaves physicians cautious. 31 Oct.

Lowenthall, M., M. Thurnher, D. Chiriboza, et al. 1975. *Four stages of life.* San Francisco: Jossey Bass.

Maurer, A. 1964. Adolescents' attitudes toward death. *J. Genet Psychol* 105:75–90.

McIntosh, J. L. 1985. Suicide among the elderly: levels and trends. *Am J Orthopsychiat* 55(2): 288–93.

McIntosh, J. L., R. W. Hubbard, and J. F. Santos. 1981. Suicide among the elderly: A review of issues with case studies. *J Geriatr Soc Work* 4(1):63–74.

Miller, M. 1978. Geriatric suicide: The Arizona study. *Gerontologist* 18:488–95.

Miller, M. 1979. *Suicide after sixty.* New York: Springer.

Nagy, M. 1948. The child's theories concerning death. *J Genet Psychol* 73:3–27.

National Center for Health Statistics. 1983. Advance report of final mortality statistics, 1980. *Monthly Vital Statistics Report,* 32 (4, Suppl).

National Center for Health Statistics. 1987. Health statistics on older persons, United States, 1986. *Vital and Health Statistics,* Analytical and Epidemiological Studies, Series 3, No. 25. Hyattsville, Md.: Public Health Service.

National Center for Health Statistics. 1986. Births, marriages, divorces and deaths for April, 1986. *NCHS Monthly Vital Statistics Report.* 35(4).

Osgood, N. J. 1985. *Suicide in the elderly.* Rockville, Md.: Aspen Systems.

Pattison, E. M. 1977. *The experience of dying.* Englewood Cliffs, N.J.: Prentice-Hall.

Riley, J. W. 1968. Attitudes toward aging. In M. W. Riley et al., eds. *Aging and society (Vol 1): An inventory of research findings.* New York: Russell Sage Foundation.

Riley, J. W. 1970. What people think about death. In O. C. Brian et al., eds. *The dying patient*. New York: Russell Sage Foundation.

Robbins, L. N., P. A. West, and G. E. Murphey. 1977. The high rate of suicide in older white men: A study testing ten hypotheses. *Soc Psychiatry* 12:1–20.

Rosenblatt, P. C. 1983. *Bitter, bitter tears*. Minneapolis: Univ. of Minnesota Press.

Rowland, K. F. 1977. Environmental events predicting death for the elderly. *Psychol Bull* 84:349–72.

Schultz, R., and D. Alderman. 1974. Clinical research and the stages of dying. *Omega* 15(2):137–43.

Schneidman, E. 1973. *Deaths of man*. New York: Quadrangle/New York Times. 7.

Simpson, M. A. 1979. *The facts of death*. Englewood Cliffs, N.J.: Prentice-Hall.

Stephenson, J. S. 1985. *Death, grief and mourning*. New York: The Free Press.

Stroebe, M. S., and W. Stroebe. 1983. Who suffers more? Sex differences in health risks of the widowed. *Psychol Bull* 93:279–301.

Veatch, R. M., and E. Tai. 1980. Talking about death: Patterns of lay and professional change. *Ann Am Acad Polit and Soc Sci* 447(1):29–45.

Volkan, V. 1975. Re-grief therapy. In B. Schoenberg et al. eds. *Bereavement: Its psychosocial aspects*. New York: Columbia University Press.

Weddington, W. W. 1981. Euthanasia. *JAMA* 246(17):1949–50.

Worden, J. W. 1982. *Grief counseling and grief therapy*. New York: Springer.

Subject Index

t

Tardive dyskinesia, 118, 175, 248
Target heart rate, 274–75
Taste, 88–89
Team approach to care, 330, 332, 367–68
Telephone reassurance, 353
Temperature (*See* Body temperature)
Temperature receptors, 89–90
Testosterone, 44, 62, 95, 127, 297, 300, 305–6
Tetracycline, 61
Theories of biologic aging, 30–36
Thermoreceptors, 89
Thiamine, 228–9
Thymosin, 41, 91
Thymus, 41, 67, 68
Thyroid, 67, 125 (*See also* Myxedema)
Title XX (Social Security Act), 349, 352
Tooth loss, 72, 139
Tophi, 122

Tranquilizers, 175, 269
Transient ischemic attacks, 109, 206
Transinstitutionalization, 214
Transitions in later life, 195
Transurethral resection, 126, 304–5
Tricyclic antidepressants, 176
Triglycerides, 226, 263
Tuberculosis, 42

u

Uric acid, 122
Urinary incontinence, 128–29
Urinary system, 72–74
    age-associated changes, 73
    disorders of, 95, 128–29
Urinary tract infections, 140–41

v

Vaccination, 138, 139
Vaginismus, 297
Varicose veins, 67

Vegetarian diet, 250–51
Vertebral fractures, 124
Vertigo, 89
Veteran's Administration, 325, 349
Vision, 80–83
    accident susceptibility and, 144
    age-associated changes, 80–83
    diseases and disorders, 116–18 (*See also* each type)
Vital capacity, 70
Vitamin A, 228, 243, 244
Vitamin B, 228, 230, 243, 247, 251
Vitamin C, 40, 138, 230, 233, 243, 244, 246, 247
Vitamin D, 60, 230–31, 251
Vitamin E, 40, 231
Vitamin K, 231
Vitamins, 228–31
Vitamin supplementation, 234–35

w

Waste product accumulation theory, 33
Water, 51, 228
Weight reduction, 119, 125, 245, 250, 262–63, 268
Weight Watchers, 250
White coat syndrome, 105
Widowed, 290, 361, 395
Widowers' syndrome, 306
Widowhood Programs, 396
Wrinkling, 60, 61

x

X-Rays, 333, 334–35

z

Zinc, 138, 234, 243, 245, 247

Author Index

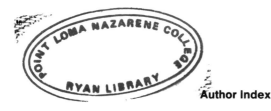
Author Index